THE
SOURCE

Unlock your natural energy, revitalize your health and change your life

Dr Woodson Merrell & Kathy Merrell

This edition first published 2010 by Rodale
an imprint of Pan Macmillan, a division of Macmillan Publishers Limited
Pan Macmillan, 20 New Wharf Road, London N1 9RR
Basingstoke and Oxford
Associated companies throughout the world
www.panmacmillan.com

First published 2008 by Random House Canada

ISBN 978-1-9057-4458-9

1 3 5 7 9 8 6 4 2

A CIP catalogue record for this book is available from the British Library.

Printed and bound in Great Britain by CPI Mackays, Chatham ME5 8TD

This book is intended as a reference volume only, not as a medical manual. The information given
here is designed to help you make informed decisions about your health. It is not intended as a
substitute for any treatment that you may have been prescribed by your doctor. If you suspect you
have a medical problem, we urge you to seek competent medical help.
Mention of specific companies, organizations or authorities in this book does not imply endorsement
of the publisher, nor does mention of specific companies, organizations or authorities in the book
imply that they endorse the book.
Addresses, websites and telephone numbers given in this book were correct at the
time of going to press.

Visit www.panmacmillan.com to read more about all our books and to buy them. You will also find
features, author interviews and news of any author events, and you can sign up for e-newsletters so
that you're always first to hear about our new releases.

We inspire and enable people to improve their lives and the world around them

CONTENTS

Introduction 5

Part I
Transforming Energy: Six Ways to Reclaim Your Vitality 19
1. Power Mind, Boundless Energy 20
2. Power Food, Your High Performance Fuel 58
3. Power Detox, Remove Toxins, Increase Vitality 95
4. Power Exercise, the Energy Factory 140
5. Power Rest, How to Recharge Your Battery 172
6. Power of Connection: Cultivate Spirit, Access Positive Energy 202

Part II
21 Days to Optimal Energy: Power Up, Cleanse, Maximize 229

Part III
Menus and Recipes 295

Recipe Index 346
Acknowledgments 347
Index 348

A Note on Using The Source

This book is divided into three parts: The why, the how, and the food. The 'why' of the book in Part I will provide powerful motivation for many of you who will be committed to taking on the 21-Day Plan after understanding the latest information on how your body makes energy and stays healthy. But for those of you who want to cut to the chase and skip the explanation of Part I, you may go straight to the 'how' – the Plan in Part II on page 207. The Plan puts the six fundamentals of Part I into action, providing a daily guide for powering up your energy and retooling your health. But promise that as you work through the plan over the next three weeks you go will back to Part I and read the background and science underlying *The Source*. Here you'll pick up on a wealth of useful information on how to increase your energy, and after reading the compelling evidence you will realize (as I have) that this is not a fad – this is the medicine of the future.

Introduction

CASE STUDY
OPENING UP

JUNE came to me late on a Friday afternoon over twenty years ago at the beginning of my private medical practice. She brought with her a dossier of tests, scans and results from procedures she'd undergone for four years in a quest to regain her wellness and youthful energy, on top of which she'd placed a cover sheet summarizing a chronology of her health events. Yet while she clearly wasn't well, the tests all showed that she wasn't ill, though she obviously felt awful and had no energy. At the bottom of her chronology page she had written, 'My goal is to regain my energy, recover my health, and not to have to worry all the time about if I can or can't make plans or feel well enough to live my life fully.' My heart went out to her.

June's problems were sporadic, but frequent enough to keep her from feeling well much of the time. She'd had a series of colds that deteriorated into chronic sinus congestion. After numerous visits to ear, nose and throat specialists, she'd had surgery for nasal polyps, which gave her some relief, but she continued to suffer from sinus infections every few months. She subsequently developed intermittent digestive problems with bloating and cramping, and trouble sleeping. For the past year she said she'd felt constantly exhausted. Too tired to exercise, June was overeating just to keep herself going.

Trying to make sense of all of the pieces of her puzzling fatigue, I looked for an overarching illness that could explain what had brought her to me with a sense of urgency about wanting better health, and in particular more energy. But I, like the many doctors she had seen before me, couldn't find anything specifically wrong with her. I took almost every moment of that one-hour first visit to elicit the details of her medical history, but, looking back, I now see that one of the most important moments was when I asked her what had occurred in her life when the troubles began. Initially, she said everything was fine – successful marriage, two children, thriving real estate career – but it turned out she was not leading the charmed life she tried to present to the world. She became quite emotional as she related to me that she'd grown in a different direction from her husband, was relatively estranged from her mother who'd recently died from breast cancer, and harboured guilt about not spending enough time with her children.

As our time ran out I realized with frustration that I didn't have much to add in terms of conventional diagnoses. Wanting to say something positive, I told her that over the weekend she needed to think about how to reduce the stress in her life. I asked her to return for a follow-up on Monday to go over the few tests I could think of that had not been done – and I hoped I'd have a diagnostic brainstorm in the interim.

What happened when she came back three days later set my practice on a new course. And ultimately this new direction for treating patients evolved into the programme at the heart of this book. On Monday, June walked into my office, dramatically more buoyant. She thanked me profusely for my time on Friday, and said she had not felt this good in years. I tried not to let my jaw drop – by medical school standards I'd done virtually nothing. She said that being able to open up about the stressors in her life was the best medicine she had had in four years. She felt as if an energy switch had flipped on inside her. She had felt so much better after admitting that she had these stresses that on Sunday she'd even gone out for a light jog. Having named some of the energy-draining situations in her life, she was now determined to face them and take charge of her life again.

I worked with June to overhaul her diet, to help her stick with a regular exercise programme, to reduce her stress, and to evaluate her home and office for potential environmental triggers of sinus infections. I also recommended that she use a few nutritional supplements. After two months, the sinus problems and bowel complaints disappeared, her sleep improved markedly, and June had more energy than ever before. Reflecting on the healing experience she'd been through, June told me that the most important part of her journey was that this new energy helped her feel connected again – to her family, to herself (with a better lifestyle) and to the world around her.

SINCE THEN, I have been constantly seeking ways to harness people's innate healing energy so that they can return to wellness. I have worked with thousands of people who, like June, came to me after visiting many other doctors, often finding little improvement. Many of them have had one health problem lead to another until they find themselves with a host of chronic issues that drain their energy and keep them from living life to the fullest. Many people who come to me are not sick, but they're working on getting there; for example, with recurring colds or headaches, nagging fatigue, digestive problems and unremitting stress that weaken them and make them susceptible to more serious illness. Many others are just pushing themselves way too hard, hoping not to get sick, but undermining their health in ways that will inevitably catch up with them. Sound familiar?

I did finally find the common thread that tied together all of June's varied problems – and most other people's chronic complaints. That common link is energy. My patients were losing vital, health-giving energy in at first little and then increasingly big ways. They weren't really sick, but they weren't well either. They needed to stop leaking energy and shore up their bodies, minds and spirits.

Creating Healing Energy

In order to develop a true healing programme to treat this widespread energy deficiency, I needed methods that worked quickly as well as methods that kept working long-term. There was no single medicine or magic pill – and to this day there is no single medicine or magic pill – that could cure any deficiency of vital healing energy. So I looked into the latest medical and scientific studies on energy to find out more about what energy is and why my patients didn't have enough of it. If I could figure out where energy comes from – the source – if I could figure out how we make energy and how we lose it, maybe I could help my patients get and create more of it and increase their capacity to heal and achieve their optimum potential. I immersed myself in the sciences of metabolism (how the body extracts energy from food) and cellular respiration (how cells make energy) and psycho-neuro-immunology (how the body communicates its needs across systems, for example, from the nervous system to the immune system). I examined the growing research into the effects of our emotions and psychological states on our health, and also investigated the latest science on the effects of environmental toxins on various systems in the body.

I uncovered a lot of connections between physical energy and mental energy that had not been part of my Western medical school curriculum at Columbia University College of Doctors and Surgeons, or my internship and residency at New York City's Roosevelt Hospital. It became clear that people needed to urgently identify their underlying energy problems in order to improve their health.

I also delved into other cultures' ancient methods for creating energy. I learned profound, beautiful ways that indigenous cultures view health – in all of which energy is at the core of their philosophy and practice. I sat at the feet of some great masters of Tibetan, Native American, Ayurvedic (Indian) and traditional Chinese medicine. Their systems see body, mind and spirit as a whole, a single energy system. Their treatments, including meditation, herbs, acupuncture and tai chi, have simple physical components but deep overall effects – especially on energy. I have found them to be surprisingly compatible with a modern Western medical practice and our daily lifestyle.

'The lifestyle changes you need to make are simple: they focus on balancing and regenerating energy.'

Besides these ancient traditions,

I also trained in newer complementary approaches such as homoeopathy, functional medicine (the nutrition science that studies food's effect on cell function and energy) and manipulative body work. And I kept going deeper into my study of energy until I arrived at the convergence of quantum physics and spirituality – two fields that actually share many views of the interconnected nature of energy and reality. Quantum physics has shown that matter at its most fundamental level operates as a web of interconnected energy fields in constant communication with each other.

Ultimately, I pulled everything I learned in my quest into a practical programme for creating healing energy and optimal health for my patients. For the last twenty years I have worked with many extraordinary people and helped them win back their health and regain a youthful, vital energy. Now, I want you to have that same experience – to feel as good as you can, and even better than you ever have. I want you to have *The Source* of health and energy. *The Source* presents the long-lasting six-step programme that I developed for my patients to increase their energy, as well as a complete 21-Day Plan for revitalization.

My goal for every patient – and now for you as you embark on the healing journey of *The Source* – is to help you transform from being an energy consumer to being an energy producer. You can live a fully sustainable life – without stimulants or cravings or prescription drugs or feelings of total burn-out. I will show you how.

I've seen from my own practice – and from reading decades of other doctors' and researchers' concerns in the medical literature – that more people than ever before need the help that *The Source* provides. We are suffering from an epidemic of fatigue in the West. While fatigue is not classified as a disease, it is debilitating and makes you more vulnerable to developing a disease. In the UK, 40 per cent of people admit to feeling extreme fatigue at work, and 44 per cent claim to feel constantly run-down. A Sleep Council study found that more than half of us feel so tired at work that we'd rather go home, and one in eight of us feels this way three or four times a week. What's more, a survey commissioned by Legal & General found that 42 per cent of the 5,000 people asked said that lack of sleep was their biggest health concern, followed by 34 per cent worrying about low-level, general fatigue. The cost of stress and fatigue to the UK economy is estimated to be more than £15 billion, and US research shows that fatigue triples the chance that workers will lose productivity. According to Action for ME, an estimated 240,000 Britons have been diagnosed with the most severe form of fatigue – chronic fatigue syndrome, or 'ME'. ME (myalgic encephalomyelitis) is not well understood, but it is believed to be an immune system disorder – when the body doesn't have the energy to heal itself – with possible viral origins. The accepted practice of running on empty in our 24-hour consumer society is a major health and economic issue. Pundits have quipped that it's taboo to say you're tired, but I think it's time to alter the national dialogue and begin to solve this pervasive problem and bring back our greatest natural resource – human energy.

The most common solutions to the perplexing dilemma of energy loss are counterproductive self-treatments – whether that means drinking more coffee, consuming caffeine-packed energy drinks like Red Bull, taking a sleeping tablet, or in the US (and increasingly in the UK), taking the new drug to increase alertness (Provigil). In the US, this drug racked up $800 million in sales in its first year on the market. But these things don't address the sources of your energy drains and they don't rejuvenate your inner source of natural energy.

Loss of energy is one of the top five complaints to doctors, but that's only the tip of the iceberg. It's been estimated that 66 per cent of people who visit their doctors while experiencing debilitating exhaustion never even mention the problem! This is primarily because of a widespread belief (mostly accurate) that doctors don't have a treatment for being tired. The truth is that only 3 per cent of people with fatigue are found to have anything wrong with them when they are tested for the many things that can cause fatigue, such as a hypothyroid condition, anaemia, heart disease, nutritional deficiencies, infectious diseases, immune deficiencies or autoimmune diseases. Interestingly enough, a survey of GPs in the UK found that one in three patients complains of being tired all the time (TATT), although this is not their primary reason for seeing a doctor. It's important to note that doctors are trained to stay within the precepts of Western medicine, using pharmaceuticals and surgery as their main tools. As a result, questions and recommendations about factors in their patients' lifestyles that should be a cornerstone of healthcare are often neglected. So many doctors have a difficult time helping their deeply tired patients – who often don't have an underlying medical disorder.

An Integrated Approach to Health

With *The Source* I offer a fresh, unique perspective on the possibility of energy creation that unifies Western medical science with Eastern mind-body and energy practices. As a doctor of internal medicine with a busy private practice, as well as an educator and researcher at both Columbia University College of Physicians and Surgeons and Albert Einstein College of Medicine, I have helped lead the development of a new medical discipline: integrative medicine. This new approach to health and healing, which emphasizes a partnership between doctor and patient, utilizes the best of indigenous, complementary/alternative and conventional approaches, which we individualize to each person's needs. Integrative doctors look at the whole patient, not just the disease, and we consider the emotional, spiritual, dietary, environmental and lifestyle influences that can affect health and healing. I would never tell a patient just to cope with exhaustion, because, to me, living each day with full vital energy is the essence of being well. I'm not a disease mechanic. My job description, and the goal of this book, is to promote your well-being. Energy is at the core of our quest for optimum health.

Lifestyle Changes

Many of the most common illnesses – such as hypertension (high blood pressure), coronary disease, diabetes and high cholesterol, as well as functional problems such as headaches, irritable bowel and arthritis – originate in your lifestyle. Patients beginning to slip into diseases primarily created by lifestyle mismanagement often come to me after they've seen a conventional doctor who's addressed the developing problem with medication and, sometimes, general advice on how to lead a healthier life. My patients and I have usually been able to prevent or reverse these problems with exactly the programme I put forth here in the 21-Day Plan. The lifestyle changes you need to make are really quite simple: they focus on balancing and regenerating energy. I get such great satisfaction when a person who thought he was sentenced to a lifetime of disease-management medications (such as statins for high cholesterol or steroid inhalers for asthma) makes transformative lifestyle changes that allow him to taper off, and eventually stop, the medication merry-go-round.

Over the years I have found that many people have a difficult time believing in the connection between energy, health and lifestyle – until they begin to understand that their mind, body, heart and spirit are part of an interconnected web, rather than a collection of parts. Every thought, every emotion, every heartbeat has the potential to resonate throughout the body due to the nearly instantaneous communication between cells that constantly takes place. Complex as these interconnections are, the process of making energy in the body has been very clearly demonstrated.

The Science of Personal Energy

From a strictly medical point of view, energy is a measurable biological commodity. Scientists working in biomolecular medicine have created a much clearer picture of how this common energy that powers life works and how the body creates energy. They have also made new discoveries about why the body begins to experience fatigue and slide into poor health. Working independently in myriad disciplines from neuroscience to exercise physiology to nutrition and mind-body medicine, researchers have begun to delineate the sources of energy in your body and identify new ways to tap them. In

The Source I will show you how to apply the results of these findings to create more abundant energy and achieve more vibrant health.

Your body stays near 37°C/98.6°F throughout your life, which could be for the better part of a century, by making its own thermal energy day in and day out. Scientists have identified the carriers of the energy your body creates; they are present in every cell of the body – everywhere from your skeleton to your brain – as tiny rechargeable battery-like packets of available energy called adenosine triphosphate (ATP). The act of making these molecules of energy, also known as energy metabolism, depends on some very primitive DNA called mitochondrial DNA. Mitochondria are like tiny factories – thousands of them are within each and every cell (with DNA as the plant supervisor) – and they work ceaselessly to transfer the potential energy from food, air and water into active human energy. With a complex cycle of chemical transformations that requires many essential vitamins and other nutrients, mitochondria are able to extract about 40 per cent of the energy available in food and turn it into ATP, the universal currency of energy in your body that can be used anywhere to do any kind of work, from fuelling your heartbeat, to providing the chemical energy to process thoughts, mustering the biological energy to attack a flu virus, or supplying the power to create a human life if you are pregnant.

The energy system in your body is highly dynamic, it constantly recycles energy, and it's exquisitely sensitive to change. Your activity level, your environment, the food you eat, the water you drink, your stress levels, your emotional state, the amount of sleep you've had – are all factors that can affect your energy-generating system. What makes the body's energy supply so susceptible to shifts in the biological machine is the fact that the energy packets of ATP cannot be stored. ATP is constantly made on demand, used up and quickly recycled, which makes the energy your body works so hard to manufacture quite fleeting – though almost infinitely replaceable if you properly care for and maintain your body.

The amount of energy your body is required to make every day is absolutely astonishing. At any given moment you've got about

90 grams (3 ounces) of energy (ATP) in your body – just enough to power ten seconds of intense exercise, or an all-out sprint to catch a train. And then your body starts all over again constantly remaking ATP thousands of times a minute. Even a sedentary person recycles an amount of ATP each day equal to about 75 per cent of his total body weight (an 82kg/180lb man would recycle almost 62kg/135lb of ATP just sitting on the couch with the remote control). A person running a marathon can recycle twice as much energy as a sedentary person – that would be a whopping 122kg/270lb of pure energy molecules processed by that same 82kg/180lb guy while running a marathon. Considering the hefty energy requirements for keeping a body going, it is no wonder that people develop problems and inadequacies with their energy-generating system.

Energy metabolism – which is how biologists describe the body's energy-making activities – plays an important role in health and ageing. The healthy functioning of mitochondria is a key component in longevity, according to a wide range of research – from a leading gerontologist in the UK to neuroscientists at UCLA in the US. Using this latest research, and my decades of experience with patients, *The Source* can improve your body's ability to extract and transform energy from your environment.

The message of energy philosophy behind *The Source* – that your body is designed to be an energy *creator*, not an energy *consumer* – is easily translated to daily living by following the 21-Day Plan. Exhaustion does not have to be the inevitable by-product of coping with continual stressful demands. I will teach you how to build your energy through all your waking hours. Your mental acuity and creativity will increase day by day, as will your health. As you work with the 21-Day Plan – with its numerous methods for relaxation, exercise, eating for energy, emotional balance, sleep, spiritual development and detoxification – you will find that all of your physical and mental systems function more efficiently and work together to support your energy needs. You will be at ease with your body; you will become more resilient; and you will feel an ever-expanding capacity for engaging in all activities with a full sense of vital energy and total well-being.

Specifically, *The Source* will show you:

- A new perspective on illness and health that stimulates and incorporates your inherent healing energy;
- The six essentials of energy creation: Power Mind (stress management), Power Food (diet), Power Exercise, Power Detox, Power Rest and Power of Connection (spirituality);
- The latest scientific breakthroughs on how the body generates energy and ways you can maximize your body's energy-making mechanisms;
- How to think about, conserve and create energy the way Eastern cultures do, with simple ways to practise energizing meditation and yogic breathing;
- Complementary/alternative approaches to curing fatigue and improving health, such as acupuncture, herbs and body work;
- A 21-day, step-by-step plan – complete with recipes – for increasing energy.

The book is organized into three parts: Part One, 'Transforming Energy, Six Ways to Reclaim Your Vitality'; Part Two, '21 Days to Optimal Energy'; and Part Three, 'Menus and Recipes'. Each part stands alone as a practical guide to energy creation. But taken together, all of the parts will magnify and deepen your understanding of how to increase energy and create a uniquely personal, healthy lifestyle.

Check for Illness First

Before I place anyone on the 21-Day Plan I always screen for illnesses that could be causing fatigue. My most important job is to make sure every person I see is as healthy as possible – especially that he or she has no underlying, undiagnosed medical problems that could be causing fatigue. I expect you're picking up this book because you've already sought medical answers to your fatigue without success. But don't abandon your regular check-ups. And as part of this general health care, it's important to have regular, periodic, screening tests, such as a colonoscopy by age sixty and a mammogram by age fifty

– or sooner, depending on personal or family risk factors. There are numerous routine tests that just have to be done, even if you think you're perfectly healthy. Your GP knows about them and can refer you. The 21-Day Plan presumes that you have been medically evaluated for existing conditions.

If you do have an existing medical condition, you can still embark on this plan along with your medical treatment, after clearing it with your own doctor. Almost everyone can follow this programme, except that you cannot take the juice cleanse on Day 10 if you have diabetes or are pregnant. People with heart disease and women who are pregnant should not take the saunas. And you should not take supplements without consulting your doctor, especially if you have any serious medical conditions or are on medication.

The following represent the most important categories of health concerns to have evaluated as part of a regular check-up, especially if you are experiencing ill health and fatigue:

Allergies • Anaemia • Arthritis • Asthma • Bowel Dysfunction • Cardiac Conditions • Chronic Infection • Diabetes • Headaches • Hormone Imbalance • Hypothyroid • Immune System Dysfunction • Liver Disease • Medication Side Effects • Nutrient Deficiencies • Poor Vision • Tooth or Gum Disease

The Power Up! Quiz

To determine your energy profile rate your honest answers on the following scale:

0 never **1** rarely **2** sometimes **3** most of the time **4** always

		Circle Your Score				
1	I wake up with good energy.	0	1	2	3	4
2	My energy is as good as it has ever been.	0	1	2	3	4
3	I look forward to each new day.	0	1	2	3	4
4.	I have a feeling of joy in my life.	0	1	2	3	4
5.	I am able to focus and finish tasks easily.	0	1	2	3	4
6.	I have a good memory.	0	1	2	3	4
7.	Exercise gives me energy.	0	1	2	3	4
8.	My physical stamina is good.	0	1	2	3	4
9.	I don't feel a need to rest during the day.	0	1	2	3	4
10.	I drink less than 2 cups of coffee a day.	0	1	2	3	4
11.	I drink a litre of water each day.	0	1	2	3	4
12.	I do not need stimulants.	0	1	2	3	4
13.	I get plenty of vitamins.	0	1	2	3	4
14.	I feel alert after meals.	0	1	2	3	4
15.	I'm not cranky.	0	1	2	3	4
16.	I consciously manage my stress.	0	1	2	3	4
17.	I am rarely ill.	0	1	2	3	4
18.	My moods are stable.	0	1	2	3	4

19.	My sex drive is good.	0	1	2	3	4
20.	I feel younger than my age.	0	1	2	3	4
21.	I am a vibrant member of my community.	0	1	2	3	4

TOTAL

YOUR ENERGY PROFILE

Less than 30: *Neophyte.* You never have enough fuel. You need to make the commitment to learn how to manage and create energy.

30–40: *Novice.* Although you are aware of your deficiencies, you are an energy novice who wants and needs to develop new habits that both conserve and generate energy.

41–51: *Initiate.* You are an energy initiate. You respect your energy needs and use about as much fuel as you spend. Your energy levels are at risk of plummeting during times of stress.

52–62: *Adept.* Impressive! You are very good at balancing your energy, but must learn to generate more juice.

63 or more: *Grand Master.* Congratulations! You are ready to explore energy generation on an advanced level, and are already using energy to keep yourself healthy.

Part one

Transforming Energy

Six ways to reclaim your vitality

Chapter 1

Power Mind, Boundless Energy

CASE STUDY
UNABLE TO SWITCH OFF

JACK was in his mid-forties and had a family history of heart disease. A new patient, he arrived stressed and in a state of absolute depletion, complaining that he'd been forcing himself to get out of bed every day like a robot. This represented a dramatic downshift from his characteristic world-beating attitude, which had fostered his career as a top executive for a major corporation. He admitted to being deeply concerned about his health due to constant exhaustion, headaches, recurring colds and the feeling of not wanting to get up in the morning. He said, 'Maybe I've got a blocked artery, or a brain tumour! God knows what I've done to myself.'

He was halfway through a multi-year contract that would make him eligible for a big pay-out, and he was planning to work right through that contract. Unfortunately for him, his company had developed catastrophic problems almost the day he arrived and he had been in a state of constant crisis management, working seven days a week.

I took all of the samples necessary for thorough testing and conducted a complete physical exam, which confirmed my initial impressions that Jack was basically healthy – by conventional physical standards. But in my opinion he was working on getting sick through a lifestyle that was completely out of balance with inordinate stress that he was managing poorly. He needed a break from the constant stress that was bathing his body in adrenalin, cortisol and other stress hormones that damage cells over time.

My initial comments about relaxation got nowhere. Like many people I see, Jack felt he was not a person who could relax. He said he couldn't sit for ten minutes and do nothing – his downtime consisted of a high-intensity workout at 6.30 in the morning. He knew he was under high stress, but so was everyone else, and he simply had to turn the company around and not whine about it. Meditation was out of the question – it made him feel anxious and nervous and defeated.

I decided to introduce him to the powers of relaxation by giving him acupuncture. Acupuncture, used in China for thousands of years to promote relaxation, has been a mainstay of my stress-management practice for decades. I had him lie down on an exam table with a pillow under his head, dimmed the lights, and gave him acupuncture on some primary stress points.

I returned to the room fifteen minutes later and removed the needles. He sat up with tears in his eyes. He said that he understood by the relaxation he felt during acupuncture how stressed he had been for the last two years. He asked if he could use my phone and called his office to tell his staff he'd be back in two weeks. He left that day for a truly life-saving holiday.

Three weeks later, Jack saw me again, ready to take control of his health and learn some relaxation exercises (he still won't call it meditation!). Then he got through the gruelling last two years on his contract, which he largely credits to his morning relaxation exercise (focussing on his breathing for at least five minutes before getting out of bed) and breathing techniques that he uses throughout the day.

JACK'S CASE of stress-induced fatigue is extreme; not many people would attempt to work four years without a break! What is not unusual about Jack's situation, though, is that Jack (like so many people who come to see me) had no idea that stress – and his failure to address it – was causing his exhaustion and lethargy. The majority of people I see in my practice wildly underestimate the amount of stress in their lives.

The Effects of Stress

When you experience stress, the energy that your body needs increases, often significantly. In the short term, most of us have the capacity and reserves to meet these energy needs, but over time – with chronic exposure to stress – the body may not be able to keep up. Initially Jack was energized by the challenges of his new job; he was almost addicted to the adrenalin rush, but as happens with so many people, he couldn't sustain life on overdrive. He was depleted, felt exhausted and, while he hadn't yet become sick, he was working on getting there.

Jack did not recognize that stress was the most pervasive detrimental influence on his health and energy. Nor did he know that managing it is possible and that the tools for managing it are very simple. Many people – including doctors – don't know this, either.

I spend the majority of my time as a doctor pulling people back from the brink of illness, and most often the first step is to put into place a programme of stress management that engages the power of the mind to reduce stress and the collateral damage caused by stress. By 'mind' I do not mean a series of thought processes in an isolated region of the brain that orders the body to do something. By 'mind' I mean your thoughts and emotions and your body working together as one entity. This was a novel concept thirty years ago, but has been established as a scientific fact – albeit an underappreciated one. Every cell in your body has a mindful intelli-

'Stress – and more important how you perceive it – is the single most pervasive factor that determines the state of your energy.'

gence that receives input, analyses it, and sends out messenger molecules through the nervous system and the blood stream to communicate with the rest of the complex, weblike matrix of your body. The intelligence of

'Thoughts effect physical changes, and physical changes cause a reciprocal change in thought.'

every cell in the body makes relaxation exercises such as meditation and breathwork so effective in combatting stress. Using the power of your mind to stop the stress that undermines your health is essential to your well-being and to maintaining your energy.

Stress – or as I like to think of it, the mind that's running on overdrive – is now considered to be a leading factor in numerous illnesses: notably obesity, cardiovascular disease, gastrointestinal disorders and chronic pain. By some estimates, up to 80 per cent of all illnesses are stress induced. Research shows that for some heart patients, mental stress is as dangerous as smoking cigarettes. Stress has been associated with slower, more complicated post-operative recovery, dysregulation of the immune system, and decreased blood flow to the heart muscle.

Not all stress is bad – athletes and concert pianists will tell you that a touch of anxiety enhances their performance. The type of stress that causes damage manifests as a chronic sense of pressure that is beyond one's control. Energy-draining stress can arise from anything that disrupts your balance: unrealistic deadlines at work, moving to a new home, marital disharmony or a new marriage, a change of job, financial difficulties – or all of the above. Your nagging concerns, your worries, your efforts to adapt to a new situation (whether welcome change or not) will take a toll on your energy.

We all try to compartmentalize our stress, but recent discoveries in neuroscience have shown that it is impossible to separate the workings of your mind and emotions from the mechanical functioning of your body. When you transform the pattern of your thoughts and emotions away from anxiety, fear, frustration and anger towards tranquillity, calm and hopefully a greater sense of joy, you also transform your energy. It is possible to harness the power of your mind

– especially via the use of the mind-body techniques detailed in the second half of this chapter – to achieve just such a transformation.

If you're wondering why your doctor hasn't mentioned any of this, consider that most medical scientists still work under the old paradigm that drugs and antibiotics and other magic bullets are the best way to cure disease and kill bacterial and other 'invaders' that make you ill. So scientists have for the most part used this radical new information about the body's global response to stress to search for more pharmaceuticals – antidepressants, anti-anxiety drugs and sleeping pills. Yet thousands of articles have proven that simple, non-drug, mind-body exercises can reduce stress, anxiety and depression and improve sleep. And after decades of experience, I have seen first hand that shock-and-awe medicines – while they can be useful in the short term and when dealing with advanced, severe problems – are often unnecessary. Simple, consistent, energy-promoting relaxation exercises and a realistic coping plan can counteract the deleterious effects of stress. You do not need the latest prescription medication to feel better.

Stress is not the only cause of energy depletion; you'll learn about other lifestyle factors in every chapter of this book. While most people know that a diet of cream cakes is bad for you, few realize a constant emotional diet of stress is equally bad.

With this book, I am here to help you just as I help my patients. With the information in Power Mind – and more incrementally with the 21-Day Plan – you can begin to transform the jagged stress in your life into a boundless stream of energy.

'By shifting from being at the mercy of your stress to being in control of your stress you can effect a dramatic increase in energy, and as a result you will be less likely to become ill.'

The Mind-Body Connection

I went to medical school in part because I wanted to understand the scientific reasons that meditation, yoga and other Eastern philosophies and health practices – all of which have energy as their core concept – effect changes in the body. The essence of the healing process in Asian medicine is tapping into vital energy or the life force called Qi (Chi) – for which there is no correlation in Western medicine. For example, in China acupuncture is understood to work by placing needles at specially designated points that access stagnant Qi (thought to cause illness or pain) and get it moving again. Such powerful practices had captured my imagination as a curious undergrad in the 1960s, but my Western mind craved a scientific explanation. When I entered the Columbia University College of Physicians and Surgeons in 1972, however, I quickly found there was little science available to explain them. Now, thirty years later, the story is very different. Scientists (spurred on by ever more powerful tools such as functional MRIs for watching molecules in action) have made tremendous headway in unravelling the mysteries of the mind-body connection. The massive volume of information has even spawned a scientific discipline called psycho-neuro-immunology (PNI), whose scientists try to understand the complex interplay between emotions and illness.

Mind-body research has brought about the equivalent of a Copernican revolution in physiology. The ideological wall that separates mind from body – constructed by scientific rationalists beginning in the seventeenth century with Descartes – has come crashing down. Whereas Copernicus figured out that the earth was not at the centre of the universe, neuroscientists – working on the level of molecular activity much smaller than a single cell – have figured out that the brain is not running the show from your head. Rather, intelligent molecules distributed throughout your body are constantly sending and receiving information that directs nearly instantaneous changes in cells widely dispersed throughout our bodies. To be sure, much of the information comes from the brain via highly developed nervous system structures, but input from the brain is not the only information your body has to act on. Your immune system, your heart, your gut and your endocrine (hormone) system all operate intelligently – independently and interdependently – through messenger molecules called neuropeptides. You think and feel with every centimetre of your body!

You are what pioneering neuroscientist Candace Pert calls a 'bodymind', a complex web of informational, electromagnetic and chemical messengers constantly processing and responding to the environment, to thoughts, to emotions and to physical processes. Pert dubbed these messengers 'molecules of emotion', because so many neuropeptides (such as the feel-good hormones serotonin and endorphins) are associated with emotional states. These products of our intelligence operate on a global level throughout the body telling the DNA inside our cells what to do. For example, when you are stressed and start feeling depressed, not only is the serotonin in your brain reduced, but the intestinal cells, the cells lining your blood vessels, the platelets in your blood vessels are all reacting with their own serotonin production. On the other hand, laughter has been shown to help prevent blood-vessel complications in diabetes and improve the balance of immune antibodies throughout the body – especially for people with allergies and rheumatoid arthritis. In a wonderful study from Japan, breastfeeding mothers who laughed while watching the Charlie Chaplin movie *Modern Times* had higher levels of the beneficial hormone melatonin in their breast milk, which reduced their babies' previously diagnosed allergic skin reactions to latex and dust! The mind's intelligence (and sense of humour) is transmitted by a complex network of nerve fibres and chemical messengers that are located everywhere in your body – not just in the 2kg/5lb above your neck.

'Simple, non-drug, mind-body exercises can reduce stress, anxiety and depression and improve sleep.'

The body's ability to adjust to its own milieu is nearly instantaneous. The very content of your thoughts, and the corresponding neuropeptide activity generated by them, can change the rate at which

'Your immune system, your heart, your gut and your
endocrine system all operate intelligently – independently
and interdependently – through messenger molecules called
neuropeptides. You think and feel with every centimetre of
your body!'

your body uses energy from moment to moment. In landmark studies of transcendental meditators conducted at Harvard by Dr Herbert Benson, a founding father of the mind-body medicine movement, overall energy consumption dropped by as much as 17 per
cent with the simple act of meditation. 'They were burning less body
fuel by thinking differently,' says Benson. If you come away with
nothing else from this chapter, I want you to remember that your
thoughts are part and parcel of your body. If you are at all engaged
in transforming your health and energy, you must also be engaged in
transforming the content of your thoughts and emotions.

Stress: the Gateway to Poor Health

When my patients try to shrug off their stress as unavoidable, I try
to make them see that stress is like a gateway drug to more serious
stuff. Stress leads to other, more damaging states – such as depression and anxiety (it is estimated that 20 per cent of the nation has
undiagnosed anxiety, and for half of them, anxiety interferes with
normal life). Unmanaged stress sets up a vicious cycle that becomes
self-perpetuating – for example, people develop recurring headaches
or irritable bowel syndrome from chronic stress; or they turn to un-
productive emotional outlets – like heavy drinking or smoking –
that displace the original stress but cause all sorts of other problems,
not the least of which is significant loss of energy. Your mind has the
power to make changes that will reduce stress, save energy and avoid
negative emotional states that sap even more energy once they are
set in place. My patient Jack was about to reach this tipping point

into the more serious stuff. His cellular batteries, the mitochondrial DNA inside each cell responsible for making energy, were beginning to get worn down from all the stress. Research now even shows that stress can reduce the number of cells in a primary memory centre of your brain and shrink a segment of your cells' DNA, called a telomere, a protective cap on the end of each chromosome that determines your biological age! If it all boils down to shortening your life, will you begin to do some of the relaxation exercises that reduce stress? I hope so. First, let's go on a little tour of the body, so you can understand how the Power Up! stress-reduction programme works.

The Anatomy of Stress

The body has three main mechanisms geared specifically towards handling stress: the autonomic nervous system (ANS); the hypothalamic-pituitary-adrenal (HPA) axis; and the neuropeptide web. Familiarity with these systems will help you understand the latest research that shows how relaxation exercises turn down the volume on your stress-response mechanisms.

Autonomic Nervous System (ANS): Your Fight-or-Flight Mode

The body's massive nerve fibre network, the autonomic (automatic) nervous system is responsible for continual, subconscious functioning of all vital organ systems – heart, lungs and intestines, to name a few. Recognized as being responsive to stress as early as the nineteenth century, the ANS speeds up vital systems and provides a burst of energy in response to stress – preparing you to run from the proverbial sabre-toothed tiger or modern mugger. It accomplishes this through two mirror-image operating modes: sympathetic, also known as the fight-or-flight mechanism, which releases adrenalin to speed up metabolic processes in response to a perceived threat; and parasympathetic, which releases the neurotransmitter acetylcholine (via the body's longest and largest nerve, the vagus) to slow down and reverse the frenetic activity caused by the sympathetic response.

> ### *Your Body's Response to Stress*
> *When you have stressful thoughts, your entire body goes into stress-response mode by initiating physiological processes that consume energy and can damage cells, leading to fatigue and, ultimately, to disease. When you have positive thoughts you stimulate positive changes in the brain that improve cell functioning throughout the body, including down-regulating inflammatory processes that cause chronic pain and negatively affect the immune system.*

Sympathetic activation halts digestion (considered non-essential when preparing to fight or flee) and accelerates blood pressure, heart and respiration rates, causing the body to expend considerably more energy during stress. Scientists now also believe that the sympathetic system is involved in helping the body decide when to store food as fat, and when to use it for energy. The parasympathetic response (which can be deliberately activated with relaxation exercises such as a single yoga session) seeks to calm down the physiological processes that have been put into hyperdrive by stress.

Hypothalamic-Pituitary-Adrenal Axis (HPA Axis): Your Stress-Hormone Highway

First identified as a stress-response mechanism in the 1950s, the HPA axis is a network of glands that deliver information through hormones in the bloodstream, originating in the body's master gland, the hypothalamus (located in the lower part of the brain) and ending in the adrenals, two walnut-sized endocrine glands sitting on top of the kidneys. This basic survival mechanism, responsible even for shocking a newborn's body into drawing its first breath, causes the adrenals to bathe the body in adrenalin and cortisol, the principal regulatory hormones sent out in response to stress and in preparation for injury. Cortisol reduces inflammation, which is important because reducing inflammation is part of the initial healing process. However, repeated elevation of cortisol levels is destructive: in its efforts to reduce inflammation cortisol also suppresses the immune system, and when chronically elevated cortisol raises blood pressure, increases blood sugar by blocking the effect of insulin, dampens memory, and causes the body to store visceral fat, the worst kind. All of these cortisol-driven processes in response to stress require significant energy expenditure. Studies have shown that relaxation exercises result in lower cortisol and adrenalin production in response to stress.

Neuropeptide Web (NPW): Your Biochemical Internet

First identified in the 1980s, this body-wide network of hormone-like chemical messengers, the neuropeptides, and their receptors gave a revolutionary new understanding of the mind-body connection, and helped explain how the body can respond so quickly to perceived stress. The neuropeptide web makes it possible for your psychological and physical states to have a back-and-forth exchange. Scientists were astounded to find that molecules that were associated with emotions (and thought to be limited to the brain) – such as endorphins, serotonin and dopamine – could actually be manufactured and received in cells throughout the body. In fact, the cells lining the intestine produce more serotonin than the brain. The most celebrated neuropeptide, serotonin is responsible for maintaining mood, and provides the basis of action for the SSRI family of antidepressants such as Prozac. The cells lining the blood vessels also synthesize their own serotonin to help control blood pressure (a basis for the new triptan drugs for migraines). Likewise, substances previously only associated with the immune system (inflammation and immune response control molecules such as tumour necrosis factor and interleukins) are now known to be made in abundance in the emotional centres of the brain. And the immune cells (white blood cells) produce 'brain' neuropeptides such as the pituitary's ACTH (which causes the release of cortisone), as well as endorphins, thyroid-stimulating hormone and growth hormones. Discov-

THE STRESS HORMONE SUPERHIGHWAY

Stress – both from external sources and from stressful thoughts – sets off a cascade of hormones including adrenalin and cortisol, which cause your heart to beat faster, your breathing rate to increase, your digestion to slow, and a number of other physiological responses that cause wear and tear on your body over time.

ery of this neuropeptide web means that the stress response is far-reaching, with implications for every cell and organ system in the body. Through the neuropeptide web, the body responds to stress (both physical and psychological) with alterations in billions of cells' DNA leading to thousands of new chemical reactions in each cell that require tremendous energy production – all in the blink of an eye. By the same token, the body's response to a loving thought is equally dramatic, and infinitely more beneficial.

Relaxation Is Proven to Combat Stress

The effects of these three stress-response mechanisms have been subject to much research over the past decade, especially in mind-body science. The research so far has teased out the particularly dramatic effects that stress has on immunity, heart health and the functioning of the digestive tract. By mapping the pathways of the autonomic nervous system, the HPA axis and the neuropeptide web, scientists have begun to provide an explanation for the mechanism behind the link between stress and many different disease processes. Research has also established a firm connection between relaxation exercises and buffering of the three stress-response mechanisms.

Some of the most dramatic and compelling research on the control of stress has been done with the relaxation response, beginning with Herbert Benson's pioneering work beginning in the 1970s. Thousands of studies since then have shown that very simple techniques (meditation, guided imagery and yoga among others) evoke a measurable decrease in the activity of the stress-response mechanisms and improve health and energy. The relaxation response works throughout your body: it activates the calming parasympathetic response system of the autonomic nervous system, reduces output of stress hormones from the HPA axis and alters neuropeptide balance in the neuropeptide web – for example, increasing endorphins and serotonin.

The work on stress and heart rate variability over the last couple of decades parallels equally dramatic work on the effects of stress on many other organ systems. For example, researchers have found that stress (even something as purely cognitive as telling a lie) inhibits gastric activity after eating, which can cause indigestion. Scientists have proved that the sympathetic pathway of the autonomic nervous system acts as the inhibitor of digestion. By the same token, voluminous research shows that the relaxation response elicited by yoga, guided imagery and meditation reduces the sympathetic activity of the autonomic nervous system, offering a no-risk method for improving digestion. In addition to relaxation exercises, certain supplements (herbs, vitamins, minerals and others) that I will describe later in this chapter can also help tame stress. As someone who has exhaustively studied the literature and put it to practical use for decades, I can tell you with great certainty that the same pattern crops up over and over again: stress activates mechanisms that, over time, cause low energy and poor health, and stress management is a simple way to reverse this damaging cycle.

We've all had the experience of stress making us ill. Now

Heart Rate Variability

A specific example of how stress effects your physical functioning is found in studies looking at heart rate variability. Like the brain, the heart has its own measurable energy field. I was amazed when I first learned that the heart's energy is 5,000 times greater in strength than the energy produced by the next most electromagnetically active organ, the brain. The electromagnetic impulses of the heart can be measured up to 3 metres away, and it's thought that others may sense your heart's energy by picking up on its energy field! Researchers have been able to take advantage of the heart's formidable power output by recording changes in its rate, called heart rate variability (HRV). This measure of the duration between successive heartbeats allows scientists to put together a detailed picture of the heart's response to stress.

One hallmark of an individual who handles stress well is greater heart rate variability – a sign of the heart's sensitivity to changing demands. Greater variability shows the heart is able to quickly return to a slower, resting state rather than constantly being in a fixed autonomic nervous system overstimulation mode (through chronic exposure to adrenalin and other stress-induced hormones and neuropeptides). Unfortunately, millions of people are walking around with hearts that have been under too much stress – their heart rate variability is frequently out of whack, even in their sleep. This significantly increases the work of the heart – and such increased energy expenditure has been shown to result in heart disease as well as general fatigue.

science has explained that this happens through the intelligence of our cells reacting to even just a stressful thought with biological changes all the way down to the smallest particles of DNA and the cell's energy-generation mechanisms. Today we are only beginning to understand the subtleties of mind-body medicine, but you must accept the fact that the daily experience of life and its challenges directly affects your health and energy. Stress is a known risk factor for illness and the greatest potential drain on energy. Actively working to transform your stress (the 21-Day Plan is a good jump start) is the single most powerful way to take back your vital energy and feel ten years younger.

Good Stress vs Bad Stress

Several years ago a patient brought me a pillow embroidered with this bit of wordplay: 'Stressed spelled backwards is desserts'. I keep the pillow in my reception room in the hope that people will reflect on it as they wait to see me because it encapsulates one of the most important elements of stress management (not to eat more dessert!). It is often your perception and handling of an event, and not the nature of the stressor, that determines its effect on you.

I mentioned earlier that for athletes and concert musicians, stress can lead to constructive outcomes – the adrenalin rush that releases a burst of energy before a match or performance can improve their playing. However, research has found that this is only true when a person has prepared thoroughly for a task. The more control you perceive yourself to have over a stressful situation, the less damaging the stress will be. (For athletes and musicians control comes through practice and the resulting confidence.) In a fascinating study conducted at Yale University in the US, adult men who were given no

The Relaxation Response

The opposite of the stress response, the relaxation response is a group of beneficial physiological changes that occur when a person achieves a state of psychological relaxation. It is most easily achieved by practising any mind-body relaxation technique that focuses attention repeatedly on a sound, word, thought, phrase, visual image or even a muscular activity that allows you to disregard other thoughts.

control over a laboratory-induced stress session for 20 minutes experienced a reduction in the activity of their natural killer cells (the first line of immune defence) that suppressed their immune systems for as long as 72 hours later. Those who were given control over the stress had no reduction in natural killer cell activity; their immune systems remained strong. In another study, painful stress after surgery was shown both to suppress immune function and to promote metastasis of cancer cells, but the proper use of pain medications to relieve the painful stress was shown to reduce those negative effects. The lesson is that health and immunity are not about stress per se, but about how you perceive and manage it.

Your Stress Tipping Point

Nowhere is the perception of stress better illustrated than in the latest research on the link between Type A personalities and heart attack risk. For many years scientists thought that all Type A personalities – hurried, high-achieving, risk-taking people – had a greater chance of developing heart disease than non-Type A personalities simply because Type As invite more stress into their lives. However, it turns out there are healthy Type As and unhealthy Type As – the difference is in their emotional coping style and how they perceive the stressors in their lives. A higher risk of heart attack exists only for Type A personalities in combination with a hostile coping style (characterized by anger and frustration in response to stress). Type A people with positive attitudes and optimistic coping styles live longer and have no greater risk of heart disease than the general population. The veil of emotions through which you perceive your stress to a large degree determines the toll it will take on health and energy.

Let's revisit Jack, whose case history introduced this chapter. He was

'Ensuring that you don't reach your tipping point and gaining the perception of being in control are the keys to a good stress-management plan.'

definitely a Type A person, but he'd undergone a change in coping style, from feeling hopeful to feeling frustrated. This is a problem that people often develop when stress becomes chronic and fatigue sets in. Jack had in fact developed the two most damaging forms of stress. His was constant (remember he wouldn't take a holiday) and it had begun to feel beyond his control (he felt he was at the mercy of the misfortunes of the company he was running). In the medical world psychologists have come up with rather intimidating terms for these problems: allostatic load – I call this the tipping point – which is the amount of stress you can take before it makes you ill; and locus (or perception) of control, which is the amount of control you perceive you have over a given stress versus perceiving the stress as imposed upon you. Making sure you don't reach your tipping point, and gaining the perception of being in control are the keys to a good stress management plan.

Incredibly, I have found that it is in the most difficult periods of people's lives that they tend most often to underestimate the amount of stress they have, and therefore do nothing to cope with the additional burden. Jack's lack of self-awareness and absence of coping mechanisms put him on the brink of chronic fatigue and illness. At his first treatment with me, I was able to induce physical changes (slowing his metabolism with acupuncture by activating the parasympathetic nervous system, releasing mood-enhancing neuropeptides such as endorphins and serotonin) that altered his physical awareness and his mental outlook and put some distance between Jack and his stress. Jack got a glimpse of what he could achieve by shifting his chemistry from stress-driven back to its natural balance, something he would later learn to do daily with relaxation exercises.

TAP INTO THE SOURCE

1. Two Ways to Turn Bad Stress Into Good Stress
• **Move Your Tipping Point:** The point beyond which cumulative exposure to stress causes fatigue and illness is a moving target. For each person,

the tipping point is different and it can vary from day to day. There are many stories about people who survive catastrophic emotional or physical situations and tragedies and go on to lead healthy lives. On the flip side we all know people who collapse at seemingly trifling stress (the delivery man never showed up). The point is that you simply cannot allow stress to accumulate, no matter which kind of stress affects you. You've got to come up with ways to offload your stress. You probably can't take a holiday every other week, but you can constantly downshift your stress response with relaxation exercises. Over time, relaxation exercises can move your tipping point, increasing your limit of tolerance so that stressful situations don't bother you as much, and allow you to maintain your energy for other challenges.

• Create the Perception of Control: The thought (even if it seems initially like an illusion) that you can exercise personal choice in a stressful situation has been found to be the single greatest predictor of effective stress management – regardless of whether or not you actually have control! Taking conscious steps to control your stress, even if it's something as simple as taking calming breaths just before a major meeting, is an important part of the transformation towards a more energetic life.

2. What's Your Coping Style?

Often the biggest obstacle to developing a stress-management plan is your accustomed coping style. Making an assessment of your coping style can begin to help you improve it. The first step is to think about how you typically cope. In my experience, people generally fall into one of five basic coping categories:

• **Helplessness:** You are overwhelmed, incapable of reacting.
• **Denial:** You don't recognize the presence of stress; eventually it catches up with you.
• **Stoic acceptance:** You may recognize stress, but repress it rather than attempt to deal with it.

- **Fighting spirit:** You are not afraid to engage the stressors, often head-on, but sometimes this can lead to exhaustion.
- **Resilience:** You look for links between thoughts, feelings and reactions, and come up with a reasonable coping strategy.

Regardless of your accustomed coping style, I want you to move towards resilience. The ability to detach from your stress, to place it in perspective, and to come up with a plan for coping is the healthiest approach. When you are resilient you make the decisions; your emotions don't run the show. You are able to come up with a plan because you are not denying or repressing the need for one (in a recent study, suppressing emotions was associated with heart disease, especially for women). And for the most part you are able to let go of the stress. Daniel Goleman, psychologist and author of the bestselling book *Emotional Intelligence*, has succinctly defined the desired attitude as self-awareness. 'Self-awareness is not an attention that gets carried away by emotions, overreacting and amplifying what is perceived. Rather, it is a neutral mode that maintains self-reflectiveness even amidst turbulent emotions ... It is the difference between, for example, being murderously enraged at someone and having the self-reflexive thought, "This is anger I'm feeling."' Many people might think this sort of detachment requires decades of psychotherapy, but, at the risk of sounding like a broken record, practising relaxation exercises – like those detailed in the second half of this chapter – helps to cultivate just such a healthy perspective. For example, by practising a brief breathing exercise in the 21-Day Plan, you can stop the cascade of stress responses triggered by an experience, and thereby provide a little distance for reflection.

'It is often your perception and handling of an event, and not the nature of the stressor, that determines its effect on you.'

Back in the 1950s my mother constantly reminded my brothers and me of the message of a popular New York minister and author, Dr Norman Vincent Peale, who promoted the idea of the power of positive thinking. At the time we were too young (and certainly not introspective enough) to realize the importance of his message. He was even perhaps a bit ahead of his time (one of the first in a long line of self-help gurus), yet he was saying things that humankind has known for millennia: the key to a healthy life is in using the power of positive thinking. It is not what confronts you but rather the attitude you bring to a situation – and the tools you have for managing your attitude – that matters most. Now, as a doctor, I have seen first hand what my mother and Dr Peale knew decades ago: thoughts have the power to transform lives. Your thoughts are the best medicine you have for dramatically improving your health. Your mind is the best tool you have for dramatically increasing your energy supply.

3. A Guide to the Best Relaxation Exercises

Practising just one of the recommended relaxation techniques – whether it's meditation, breath work, yoga or tai chi – will bring positive energy into your life. Some of the techniques in this guide – such as breath breaks – simply trigger the relaxation response, while others, like acupuncture, have broader applications. It really doesn't matter which technique you choose; numerous published studies have shown that all relaxation techniques – which promote an altered state of relaxed concentration or focused reverie – have beneficial effects, including a decrease in energy consumption. The laboratories of Herbert Benson's Mind/Body Medical Institute at Harvard University in the US have demonstrated the healing influence that relaxation techniques can exert over numerous medical conditions such as high blood pressure, irregular heartbeat, chronic pain, insomnia, impotence, the side effects of cancer therapy, surgical recovery and fatigue. Mind-body relaxation techniques are a means of releasing tension in the mind and halting the destructive march of the biochemical processes set in motion by that tension. The release of mental anxiety (which affects your entire physiology) in turn allows healing energy to flow.

The top stress-management techniques described here – all

elicit the relaxation response – have been used with great success by thousands of my patients. Many of these techniques were developed by other cultures over many years – in some cases thousands of years ago. Most of these techniques have been subject to rigorous testing by Western scientists over the past thirty years. There is something for everyone here, whether you dislike sitting still or can't stand to hear the word meditation. You can do this for yourself, and in fact you probably already know how. The best general description I've ever heard of the type of relaxation exercise that down-regulates the stress response comes from Belleruth Naparstek, a gifted psychotherapist and author of *Staying Well with Guided Imagery!* Belleruth likens the altered state of relaxation achieved through these exercises to what you do when you get into a crowded lift.

When we are in a crowded lift, and strangers are uncomfortably close to us, our defence is to stare straight ahead, concentrating on an imaginary spot on the lift door or on the floor indicator above the door, blocking out our perceptions of the people breathing down our necks.

This is a perfect example of turning down the volume on a stressful situation. You don't have to be a monk sitting on a mountaintop to be able to evoke an altered state, where all distractions cease. Many experts have found ways to achieve the goal of relaxation, the point at which your body's systems are operating with the least amount of effort. The best way to find what works for you is through trial and error.

Have fun! Relaxation is a therapeutic intervention you can't overdo.

Establishing Breath Breaks

The supply of oxygen to your cells is a major determinant in how much energy you make. By simply increasing the oxygen supply in your blood with deep breathing exercises, you will be able to make more energy and elicit the relaxation response, which simultaneously allows your body to utilize less energy. Breathing involves chemical, mechanical and cerebral control mechanisms at many levels of the nervous system, all of which are put into overdrive when you experience stress. Compared with other vital functions such as heartbeat, breath rate is by far the easiest to influence voluntarily. While breath work can be exceedingly powerful, especially when performed at an advanced level (such as kundalini yogic breathing or Holotropic breath work), I consider it to be an entry-level relaxation exercise – it can be easier for the novice than meditation. You focus attention on your breath (the sound and sensation of the air moving in and out of your body) so you don't have to find a mantra or phrase to repeat. The goal is to take deeper, slower breaths, which allows a general deceleration of the metabolism and stress-response systems, along with a corresponding conservation of energy and improved alertness.

Patients have told me that this exercise transformed their lives by automatically reducing their stress. The key to this profound breathing technique is to take abdominal breaths, which means that the abdomen, rather than the chest, expands as you inhale. (By involving the diaphragm, you draw oxygen deeper into the lung cells and recruit muscles and neurotransmitters that significantly enhance the effects.) It's best to sit up straight with shoulders back to expand your lung capacity. As you become more aware of your posture

---

Your *Power Up! Breath Break**

1. Inhale slowly to the count of four – with abdomen expanding, chest relaxed, listening to your breath.
2. Pause for one count.
3. Exhale slowly and completely to the count of six – with abdomen deflating, shoulders relaxed and engaged, listening to your breath.
4. Pause for one count.
5. Repeat four times.

* Sit up straight for this exercise, shoulders back.

through these exercises, you'll notice that you spend much of the day with shoulders slumped forward taking shallow chest breaths that promote anxiety.

You can take breath breaks any time – in the office, in the car, in a conference room or on a plane. By following these basic instructions you will unfailingly experience a softening of your upper body's usual tension, and a slower, more relaxed breathing pattern – even after you finish the exercise. Studies of this technique show that it results in slower pulse, lower blood pressure, relaxed intestinal muscles, lower cortisol and blood carbon dioxide levels. The nervous system alone utilizes about 20 per cent of the oxygen you take in, so by reducing the nervous system activity you preserve energy. I recommend using this technique as often as you can – preferably every hour or two. Whenever you pass a mirror or window where you can see your reflection, check your posture and practise your breath work. If you do only one thing to increase your energy, this breath break would be my choice.

The 'M' Word: Meditation

Many people are wary of meditation because of its association with sacred, esoteric, Buddhist or Hindu religious practices. Some also worry that practising meditation is somehow at odds with their own religious beliefs. But from my perspective meditation can be used with any religious practice. It is simply a tool for using the power of the mind, a very simple way to rest the mind – to let go of normal, everyday thought processes, especially the hundreds of worried, fearful, jealous, angry or frustrated thoughts that tend to crowd into our consciousness, even when – sometimes especially when – we don't want them to. By allowing you to take a step back from the constant workings of the mind, meditation helps you gain greater insight into your thought processes and greater control of your emotions. It is the ultimate healing tool because it works subconsciously, on an energetic level where healing – and illness – take root. Practically speaking, meditation is a wonderful exercise for building a more re-

Take Two Oms and Call Me in the Morning

Many beneficial physical changes occur with meditation. Numerous published studies have demonstrated the positive effects: lower cortisol production in response to stress; less sympathetic (accelerating) and greater parasympathetic (calming) activity in the nervous system; improved heart rate responsiveness; reduced oxygen consumption; increased positive neurotransmitters, serotonin and endorphins; increased (relaxing) alpha brainwaves; increased immune responsiveness; and reduced pro-inflammatory molecules (cytokines). Meditation balances physiological processes – halting stress in its tracks, reducing energetic needs and allowing energy to regenerate.

silient coping style, for cultivating self-awareness, and for quieting self-destructive tendencies. In short, it's just what the doctor ordered as part of an effective stressmanagement programme.

Meditation at its most basic level, as it is used for stress management, is nothing more than slow breathing with a mantra – a neutral or positive word, phrase or prayer repeated over and over again, such as Om, Peace, Now or Calm. The rhythmic repetition of the mantra is an effective way to slow your breathing (by activating the calming parasympathetic nervous system) and to take your mind off anxious thoughts, thereby further dampening your stress response. There are a number of different meditation techniques, but the two most commonly practised are single-pointed meditation – the afore-

'Rather than spending your energy ruminating on the past or worrying about the future, you will find through meditation that your body has boundless energy for being in the here and now.'

mentioned slow breathing, focusing on a mantra – and mindfulness meditation, which is basically slow breathing with the intention of keeping your mind in the present moment in an emotionally positive way. For example, when washing your hands, you consciously think of the beauty and usefulness of your hands and of the water running over them (not the dozens of things you haven't got to yet today). Meditation is quite simply a change in thought patterns for the better. It is a direct way of replacing energy-draining negative thought patterns with energy-generating positive thought patterns.

Since the late 1960s when The Beatles introduced transcendental meditation to the public, researchers have been studying the mechanisms and effects of meditation. One juicy research tidbit came recently from the University of California where researchers were able to demonstrate a 50 per cent reduction in lab-induced pain (as measured in the brain during an MRI) after people practised meditation for five months. And another study from the University of Massachusetts Department of Medicine showed that psoriasis patients who practised a brief mindfulness meditation during light therapy (the standard treatment) had significantly faster healing than people who didn't meditate during treatment. One of the most astonishing recent studies came from the University of Calgary in Canada, where investigators were able to determine that meditation caused beneficial changes in the mix of T-cells (immune cells that fight cancer) in breast and prostate cancer patients. Every year new studies are published that attest to the power of meditation to effect beneficial changes throughout your body.

Prepare to Meditate

The nuts and bolts of how you meditate are relatively simple. It is best to sit with an erect spine in a comfortable position – if you lie down you might fall asleep. (It is not necessary to sit with legs crossed, though this is a good position for aligning your spinal cord from head to hips.) Choose a single point of focus: a neutral word such as the Sanskrit 'Om', 'Peace', the sound of your breath – the exact mantra is less important than finding one that helps you let go of your thoughts. Especially in the beginning it is best to meditate in a darkened room in order to reduce stimulation and allow thoughts – and awareness of the outside environment – to recede more easily. When you become aware that you are engaged in conscious thoughts, notice them, release them and return to the single point of focus. These are the basic instructions.

In the 21-Day Plan I ask you to do this for two minutes when you wake up each morning, at a time when your stress hormones are nearly doubling from their resting rate. This is a good practice for every morning, whether you're on the plan or not.

With practice, you will be ready to move on to the next level of meditation, allowing the focal point to dissolve and entering a deeply peaceful state. This is the sweet spot of meditation. Once you are able to let go of the mantra without conscious thoughts crowding in, you've reached a profoundly calm place – it's been described

A Happy Mantra

One of my favourite mantras comes from Thich Nhat Hanh, the luminous Vietnamese monk who has published more than forty books explaining Buddhism to the West. He offers a wonderful point of focus for beginners with these two sentences: 'Breathing in, I feel calm. Breathing out, I smile.' You can simply say or think 'calm' when you inhale, and 'smile' when you exhale. Many people have told me this practice refreshes them even in the midst of total stress.

Another example of a mindfulness exercise that can be practised whenever you wash your hands throughout the day:

'Water flows over these hands.
May I use them skilfully to preserve our precious planet.'

FROM *THE ENERGY OF PRAYER* BY THICH NHAT HANH

as nothingness or emptiness, but I think of it as being completely in the present. The negative thoughts of past and future worries that constantly swirl in your subconscious have quieted. Rather than escaping from those thoughts, which is what happens when you watch television, for example, meditation allows you to release negative thoughts. It's not just the effect of the 15 minutes you are meditating – the nervous system is reset to a less reactive state for many hours afterwards. With practice, meditation permanently cultivates a more tranquil and positive mental attitude, which makes for a more effective coping style.

Mindfulness meditation differs from single-pointed meditation in that it has an object – your body, your feelings, your mind, the objects of your mind. It may seem a little Kumbaya, but the idea is to radiate love toward the object. Mindfulness requires full attention. The idea is to keep your focus in the present moment, not letting in other distracting thoughts. It is the opposite of multitasking.

The beauty of a meditation exercise is you can repeat the same one over and over again, and receive ever-deepening benefits of enhanced tranquillity and greater energy each time. The only limitation will be your own desire to get it right. There is no 'right way'. The process of meditation is what provides the benefits. There is no goal because the point is to be in the present moment. Rather than spending your energy ruminating on the past or worrying about the future, you will find through meditation that your body has boundless energy for being in the here and now.

Biofeedback

Biofeedback is what I call meditation for engineers. It is a decades-old, well-documented stress-reduction method that employs an electronic device to guide you through a relaxation technique. Usually the device provides an audio or visual cue to slow the breathing to less than ten breaths per minute, a therapeutic zone shown in studies to reduce sympathetic activity, blood pressure and stress. Biofeedback devices (from companies such as Presage, StressSweeper and

Wild Divine) employ sensors – commonly attached to the fingertips – that record the biological markers of relaxation such as electrical skin resistance, and provide feedback (such as a change in tone of the audio cue heard through a headset) to signal the progress of your relaxation response. Studies have shown the ability to see how well you're doing significantly enhances any relaxation exercise's effectiveness, and the device itself provides a focus that keeps your mind from wandering to stressful thoughts.

Video games have opened up a new realm of possibility for biofeedback. One of my favourite new products is a series of software programmes from The Wild Divine Project (www.wilddivine.com), which uses phenomenal healers such as Deepak Chopra, Dean Ornish and Andrew Weil as interactive guides to the meditation session. The Wild Divine finger monitors plug into a USB port, and the software provides visually fanciful meditative imagery on the computer screen. In one segment you have to coax a rabbit out from behind a hedge simply through relaxation (my thirteen-year-old daughter is much better at this than I am!). The most extraordinary aspect of biofeedback is to be able to see how quickly you can improve your relaxation skills with a little practice.

Guided Imagery

Guided imagery is basically meditation with imagination. Many people find that it is easier to manage stressful thoughts with the distraction of specific imagery. The image can be preprogrammed and provided by audio recording, a book, computer software or a therapist; or it can be a spontaneous image springing from your own imagination. The image has to be detailed enough so that it occupies sufficient cognitive space to stop you from reengaging with thoughts, worries and concerns – so that it halts the cascade of stress responses. Often people start with a programmed image and then elaborate on that image with their imaginations.

Guided imagery can be extremely powerful, and has been found in recent studies to be especially effective in pain management and in helping insomniacs fall asleep faster by managing unwanted presleep worries. At the University of Washington Human Interface Technology Lab, cognitive psychologist Hunter Hoffman and his colleagues have been alleviating pain with a software programme called Snow World. When a burn patient's bandages are changed it can feel like the experience of being burned all over again, so during wound care, patients wearing virtual reality goggles are immersed in an arctic landscape populated by smiling snowmen zipping about igloos and glaciers. Patients report a dramatic drop in pain, primarily, researchers believe, due to the complete shift of attention from the activity of wound care to the virtual world. It's also very likely that the snowy images help 'put out the fire' in the viewer's minds.

For stress management, an image has to be relaxing, which var-

Mountain Stream Meditation

You are sitting on the bank of a clear, cold mountain stream;
You are surrounded by tall trees in an ancient forest;
You feel the gentle pressure of the soft forest floor underneath you;
You inhale deeply, taking in the crisp mountain air;
You become aware of the sound of birds in the trees above;
You watch beams of sunlight filter through the trees;
You see patches of deep-blue sky overhead;
You begin to focus on the site of the running water before you;
You watch the inches-deep water flow over rocks in the stream;
You notice pebbles moving along the streambed;
There is nothing else but you and the stream;
There is nothing else but you and the water;
You are one with this place;
You breathe in the rhythms of the stream;
You are the stream.

ies tremendously from person to person. If someone had a terrible experience on the beach, then the ocean would not be a good image. For others, the ocean can be profoundly calming. First choose the general image, then fill in the details. Opposite is one exercise that uses a mountain stream to create a relaxing world. The exercise will be more powerful if you evoke the place by listening to a recording of the sounds of the forest while you meditate.

4. Stress-Busting Body Work
Acupuncture

I have been using acupuncture in my practice for over twenty years, and consider it to be one of my most powerful tools for reversing the effects of chronic stress, as well as for treating a multitude of stress-related conditions such as headaches, irritable bowel, asthma and chronic back pain. In my experience, having acupuncture is a bit like having your car serviced – everything just works better. The Chinese say that acupuncture raises and rebalances Qi (or vital energy). Western medical research has demonstrated that it works through the nervous system, reducing inflammation, changing neurotransmitters, and turning down the stress responses of all the body's systems. Many of my patients such as Jack report feeling energized and able to take further action to reduce their stress after just one session, which is about as close a definition to increasing vital energy as I can imagine.

Acupuncture is administered by inserting ultra-thin needles (six acupuncture needles can fit inside one hypodermic) at specific points depending on what the session is meant to address. The needles are so thin that most people don't notice them when they are going in. (General stress points are located in the shoulders, neck, hands and lower legs.) Treatments always require more than one needle placement because the idea is to provide balance – where one point is stimulated, an equal and opposite point must also be stimulated.

As you receive the treatment, you usually either lie down or sit in a comfortable, supported position – usually in a darkened or softly lit room to enhance the relaxation. The needles' superfine points glide into the top layer of skin almost imperceptibly, creating a slight pinch. Many people report a sensation of invigoration – something like a shiver (what the Chinese call the De Qi sensation) – when the needles are inserted, followed by a sense of relaxation. A single session can last from 10 to 30 minutes. Dramatic effects can be achieved with one treatment, but a series of treatments produces more lasting results.

Many people ask me how I know where to put the needles, and the answer to that question always leads back to China, where I first studied acupuncture in the late 1980s when the government was beginning to foster more scientific dialogue between East and West. The general position for all acupuncture points is in the

How Does Acupuncture Work?

Hundreds of studies have been published since the late 1970s demonstrating that acupuncture buffers all three stress-response mechanisms. While acupuncture works by releasing tension at the point where the needles are inserted (locally it increases blood flow and decreases muscle strain), it also works at a distance from where the needles are inserted, generating beneficial changes in neurotransmitters. Similar to the relaxation response, but often more immediately powerful, acupuncture lowers sympathetic and raises parasympathetic activity in the autonomic nervous system and balances hormone levels in the hypothalamic-pituitary axis that governs the nervous systems' response to stress. Numerous studies have established that acupuncture can produce a dramatic shift in the neuropeptides' governing mood, for example, sharply raising the level of feel-good endorphins. In short, acupuncture can significantly reduce stress, and its calming effects can last for days afterwards.

muscular trigger point (the mid-point of a muscle, where nerve fibres and tension are most concentrated). The Chinese amassed a huge body of evidence through trial and error beginning 2,000 years ago that established the acupuncture points most effective for eliciting global benefits. An experienced acupuncturist knows when he's hit the right spot by the feeling of De Qi. (Novices often learn to identify points with electronic sensors that measure changes in electrical resistance on the skin.) Historically, acupuncture in China has been used as part of a larger holistic system of traditional medicine that includes dietary changes, herbs, massage and other techniques, but in the last century acupuncture has been recognized both in China and in the West as effective when used by itself.

For the extreme needle-phobic there are other options for accessing acupuncture points. Laser acupuncture, magneto-acupuncture (employing magnets) and acupressure (using the hands to target points) are all alternatives to needling, in descending order of effectiveness. Laser and magnet therapy require a licenced acupuncturist. Acupressure (or shiatsu) is a massage technique that can be deeply effective, and sometimes even difficult to endure as the tender trigger points are pressed and released.

Yoga

It is near impossible to go anywhere these days without seeing someone with a yoga mat in a bag over her shoulder, and considering the benefits it's hard to argue against the craze. One of the world's oldest forms of exercise and mind-body techniques (continuously practised in India for over 3,000 years) yoga is the mind-body movement therapy most extensively studied by Western science – with numerous controlled studies comparing yoga to other restful non-yoga interventions, sham yoga or no intervention. The many schools and styles of yoga include general stretching, breathing and relaxation (hatha); strenuous energizing breath work (kundalini); deeply meditative and restorative (pranayama, Kripalu); therapeutic, oriented towards working with medical conditions (Iyengar); and intensely aerobic (power, urban, Ashtanga or Jivamukti yoga). Much of the benefit of yoga stems from moving and stretching the body in profound, often unaccustomed ways – often while doing yoga you will find yourself in a position you haven't assumed since childhood – and the breath work and mental focus required. The challenging postures and deep breathing (known as prana) accomplished through yogic techniques developed over thousands of years and constantly updated by the many gifted yogis practising in the West today offer a vast resource of healing potential.

In numerous clinical trials yoga appears to have widespread beneficial effects on fitness, stress reduction and energy levels. A single yoga session can involve the entire nervous system and thousands of muscles, many of which are accessory groups that haven't been activated in years. The most powerful aspect of yoga is actually the breath work, which requires relaxed chest muscles and conscious control of the diaphragm in order to draw the air deeper. The overall effect is to energize corners of the body you forgot even existed, while calming the mind. By coordinating the rhythm of the breath with movement (for example, timing moments of exertion with exhalation) studies suggest the practice of yoga improves regulation of the autonomic nervous system. This vagal stimulation is thought to trigger a series of parasympathetic (calming) responses that buffer the effects of chronic stress. Amazingly, it doesn't take much yoga at all to achieve measurable results.

The very real therapeutic effects of yoga perhaps explain its popularity. Once you learn the basic postures, you can practise yoga in a very small space in a relatively short time – at home, in the office, or on the road. If I had only one type of bodywork to recommend it would be yoga. It's a terrific way to reduce the perception of stress in your life, focus your attention on something that is good for you, and energize the forgotten recesses of your mind and body.

For more on yoga refer to Chapter 4.

1. *Cat*

2. *Staff*

3. *Downward-facing dog*

4. *Cobra*

5. *Warrior 1*

6. *Mountain with bound arms*

Six Gentle, Energy-Generating Yoga Postures

Here are some of my favourite energy-generating yoga postures. Getting into one of these postures requires specific steps. You should consult an instructor or an instruction video, and follow all of the preparatory steps required to complete the posture before attempting to try any of these.

The Power of Yoga

Studies of yoga suggest the following beneficial effects*

After One 30-to-60-Minute Session	After Three to Eight Sessions	After Thirty Sessions
Lowers heart rate	Reduces cortisol (the master stress hormone)	Reduces depression
Lowers blood pressure	Reduces blood pressure response to stress	Reduces anxiety
Reduces fatigue	Activates anti-inflammatory pathways	Accelerates cardiovascular recovery time from stress
Reduces hostility	Increases heart rate responsiveness	Improves glucose tolerance
Induces digestion	Raises endorphin and serotonin levels (feel-good hormones)	Decreases visceral fat
Dilates arterioles	Reduces the biochemical stress response	Reduces risk factors for arteriosclerosis, hypertension, and cardiovascular disease

* Compilation of numerous studies.

Tai Chi

Tai chi is an ancient Chinese martial art that developed as an off-shoot of Qi gong, a major branch of traditional Chinese medicine. tai chi combines controlled breathing with precise physical movements designed to build Qi (pronounced chee), or vital energy. Like yoga, there are multiple styles of tai chi (chen, yang, old wu, wu and sun are just a few) all of which combine deep, diaphragmatic breathing with specific postures. Tai chi is a fluid practice; it entails performing a series of continuous movements that resemble a graceful slow-motion dance. Once restricted to highly secretive teaching within Taoist monasteries, tai chi classes are now more widely available. In my experience, patience is the only mandatory requirement for learning tai chi – not only because it is a slow-motion practice, but also because the postures are incredibly precise and require excellent muscle control.

Studies from several countries (of both healthy and chronically ill adults) suggest tai chi has similar effects on stress reduction as yoga – including lower blood pressure, reduced stress response and enhanced heart function. In a fascinating study from the Cousins Center for Psychoneuroimmunology of the University of California at Los Angeles Neuropsychiatric Institute, practising tai chi for fifteen weeks improved older adults' immune response to a shingles vaccine. Advanced practitioners claim to be able to manipulate energy (for example, releasing blocked energy) and nothing in my experience causes me to think this cannot be done. Several investigations offer evidence that tai chi reduces perceived stress and enhances stress-related coping, which is most likely a result of the focused attention required. In studies of elderly people, tai chi dramatically improved alertness, balance and coordination. Quite simply, tai chi is a profound movement exercise that sharpens your mind, improves muscle tone and control, and is very likely to get your juices – and energy   flowing.

5. Supplements to Aid the Nervous System
If you are under a doctor's care for a medical condition, check with your doctor before taking any new supplements.

Nutriceuticals (nutritional supplements)

L-theanine: L-theanine is an amino acid, a natural nutrient comprising protein that is now sold in capsule form. L-theanine is one of my favourite calming aids: I liken it to a natural valium, but without the drowsiness. It is found in abundance in green tea (average 2 per cent) – one reason that the stimulants in green tea (theophylline, caffeine) provide a calming rather than a jagged lift. Studies have shown it reduces sympathetic nervous system activity – lowering heart rate and improving heart rate variability. It has also been shown to support the immune system, even increasing the efficacy of some anti-cancer drugs. Much of L-theanine's calming and protective effect on the brain comes from its ability to block glutamate receptors – brain cell components that excite our nervous system, and that need to be dampened for relaxation. Theanine has been shown to aid in raising beneficial brain neurotransmitters, including GABA, serotonin and dopamine. (Precautions are minimal.)

SAMe (S-adenosyl-methionine): SAMe is a very important nutrient for mood support. It is an active form of the amino acid methionine – the body converts the methionine in our food to SAMe. In this more active form, acting as methyl donor, SAMe has been shown to do three things, and do them well for many people: (1) help reduce arthritic symptoms (acting as an anti-inflammatory), (2) help the liver detoxify, and (3) improve depression. SAMe provides the substrates the brain needs to make more mood-enhancing neurotransmitters, especially serotonin. (Precautions include needing medical guidance first if using SSRIs, and Parkinson's medications, and it can be overstimulating for some.)

5-HTP (5-hydroxy-tryptophan): 5-HTP is another amino acid derivative. Its base, tryptophan, is also effective as a calming and antidepressant aid (serotonin is made from tryptophan) – but was removed from the market in the 1980s when a contaminated batch from Japan caused debilitating lung problems. Since then the more active form 5-HTP has safely been on the market, and used successfully to help induce a state of relaxation and improve mood. (Patients – especially those on SSRI antidepressants, anti-seizure medications, and with Parkinson's and Down's syndrome – must consult their doctor before using.)

Magnesium: Magnesium is the second most common mineral in the body after calcium, and is extraordinarily important in many critical biological processes. It has been shown to help relax muscles, reduce vascular spasm in migraines and heart attacks, bronchial spasm in asthma, intestinal spasm in constipation, and blood vessel tension in hypertension. It also helps block the excitatory NMDA receptors in the brain, which is part of the explanation for its ability to calm some people. (Due to its huge range of physiological effects, and difficulty in measuring accurately in the blood, magnesium supplements should be used only with professional guidance.)

Botanicals (Herbs)

Chamomile *(Chamomaelum nobile* {Roman chamomile} or *Matricaria recutita/chamomilla* {German/English chamomile}): Certainly the best known of the relaxing herbs, chamomile has been used for centuries for its ability to calm the mind and body. It helps with stomach upset as well as emotional upset. Because of its pleasant taste, it is most commonly used as a tea or tincture. (Precautions pertain to its causing relaxation – with care in the daytime – and since it is in the ragweed family, people with these allergies should use with caution.)

Lemon balm *(Melissa officinalis)*: This is another good-tasting herb that can be used as a relaxing tea. It has many active ingredients and, beside relaxation of the nervous system, has been shown to reduce stomach agitation (dyspepsia) and oral herpes. One interesting study showed reduced agitation in Alzheimer's patients. (Sedation is the main precaution.) Other calming herbs, such as valerian and passion flower, are better used as sleep inductors and are discussed in Chapter 5.

Lavender oil *(Lavandula officinalis/angustifolia)*: Lavender oil has been used for centuries as a calming or sleep aid (depending on amount employed). Plus it smells beautiful. Lavender is administered by placing a couple of drops in an essential oil diffuser, or by diluting it with a neutral oil (such as almond oil) and rubbing into the skin – its active ingredients can be absorbed through the skin. (Don't take lavender oil internally, and be aware that its use can make you drowsy.)

Homoeopathy: I was raised with homoeopathy and use it daily in my practice for stress management, digestive disorders, upper respiratory allergic and asthmatic problems, and musculo-skeletal injuries to name a few. It is a medical discipline, first developed by a German doctor in the nineteenth century, that utilizes dilute amounts of natural substances to stimulate the body's healing processes – in a manner likened to that of vaccines. A core concept in homoeopathy is the restoration of a person's vital energy   leading to balance and amelioration of physical and psychological problems. Homoeopathy is not intended to be primary treatment for serious or life-threatening diseases – it is too gentle for that. But for more limited physical problems and for emotional issues it can be very beneficial. It is best used on the advice of a homoeopathic practitioner who will take an extensive history. While reduction of stress and balancing of mood as both cause and effect in illness is a central part of homoeopathic practice, there is no such thing as a homoeopathic valium or valerian – each person's remedy is established by the totality of his or her unique characteristics and symptoms.

Chapter 2

Power Food, Your High Performance Fuel

CASE STUDY
YOU ARE WHAT YOU EAT

KATE, a working mum in her late thirties, came to me complaining of all-day fatigue which, despite her hectic life, surprised her because she felt she had a healthy lifestyle and had recently lost a few kilograms with a lower calorie diet. After quizzing her extensively on her new eating habits I discovered that she was consuming a diet high in wheat, and with too many refined carbohydrates. This resulted in late morning cravings for sugar, as well as for other foods that in susceptible people can drain rather than support energy. She also had been consuming caffeinated beverages that were contributing to a late afternoon crash.

The first step was to eliminate suspected food allergens – energy-draining foods. For the coming month she would have to avoid a number of the most common food sensitizers (wheat, eggs, nuts, red meat, dairy, caffeine and alcohol), after which she would add them back one at a time every three days. This is the most accurate way to tell what foods your body reacts poorly to – better than any blood or skin test.

Right away Kate felt a difference when she eliminated wheat. She realized that she literally crashed after eating pasta! I recommended substituting nutritious 'Old World' whole grains such as spelt and kamut. We added nutrient-dense foods (such as morning energy shakes) and energy-enhancing non-caffeinated beverages throughout the day. Much to her surprise her energy zoomed back. Whenever she started back on wheat or caffeine, she felt a near-immediate decrease in energy.

FOOD MEANS DIFFERENT things to different people. For foodies it's an art form to be celebrated and almost worshipped; for chronically overweight people it's a public enemy and sometimes secret lover; for the office-bound it's the hassle to get something, anything, delivered quickly; for many food represents the drudgery of daily preparation and for others it represents the sustenance of home. But for all people eating serves only one true purpose, and that is to provide fuel to support all of the body's processes. The most fundamental of these processes, necessary for any other cellular action to take place, is the creation of energy within the cell. Underlying life is energy: from energy all else flows. With the 21-Day Plan, I'm going to reconnect you with the power of the energy in your food.

Over the last half-century, as major food corporations have been liberating us from the labour of cooking from scratch, we've grown increasingly distant from the process of nourishing ourselves. We don't have to grow our food (an activity that imparts a tremendous appreciation for its energy and life force), we often don't have to cook it, and sometimes we don't even have to touch it with our hands, so clever is the packaging. It's no coincidence that, as food has become more convenient and is increasingly cultivated at greater distances from the majority of the population, we have as a people grown fatter and increasingly fatigued.

'With this book I'm hoping you will see the wonder in the process that takes the potential chemical energy available in nature and transforms it into high-energy bio-molecules of life used to power every system in your body.'

Food and Energy

Once a morsel hits your palate it begins the conversion into vital energy – this is one aspect of the food supply chain that hasn't changed a bit over the millions of years that people have been eating. But not all food holds the same potential to be transformed into energy. In the 21-Day Plan you will learn how to eat for more energy and health.

From a biochemical perspective your body is a massive nano-technology manufacturing facility. Every day, food provides the raw materials your DNA uses to operate, maintain, repair and, in many cases, replace parts. Most people think you only need DNA in order to inherit traits from your parents in the womb, but that couldn't be further from the truth. DNA is the seat of intelligence in every cell that directs all processes within the cell on an ongoing basis – whether it's a pancreas cell producing insulin or a stomach cell aiding digestion. One of its critical functions is to make sure the cell survives by monitoring the cell's environment and regenerating itself. As part of that process your DNA is programmed to replace almost every cell in your body every six months throughout your life. DNA provides the blueprint, but the integrity of the construction of this continually recycled you depends largely on what you eat. Energy, manufactured in each cell by special DNA located inside a tiny structure called mitochondria, drives this process of biofabrication, and the quality of your energy stems from the quality of your food.

When you eat processed foods full of synthetic preservatives, colourings, and flavourings, your body spends a great deal of energy separating out the artificial ingredients from whatever nutrients it can find.

'When you eat whole plant foods your genes have the key to unlock the energy of the sun that is stored in leaves and stems, roots, seeds and flowers.'

The importance of eating whole plant foods has become increasingly clear with cutting-edge research from the field of functional medicine, a new scientific discipline founded by brilliant nutritional biochemist Dr Jeffrey Bland, which explains at a molecular level how food – along with all aspects of lifestyle and environment – contributes to health and energy. Functional medicine offers a revolutionary new way of looking at food: the nutrients in food are molecular messengers that guide each cell's DNA. It turns out that whole plant foods carry incredibly sophisticated, health-promoting signals for your genetic blueprint. For example, the incorporation of fish or flax oil into your diet reduces the tendency for cell damage in chronic inflammatory conditions such as heart disease and arthritis. In this way food can be your best preventive medicine, helping you to avoid genetic predispositions to disease. By making food choices that deliver more pro-energy molecular messages and fewer energy-draining molecular signals you can reprogramme your body to maximize energy and I will show you how.

Energy-Boosting Foods

Much of what I have learned treating patients over the years has to do with first eliminating foods that muck up the body's ability to heal itself and create energy. Like Kate, many people spend their days eating energy-draining foods. My role has been to rein in those impulses by teaching how and why some foods drain energy and others enhance energy. One way to remove energy drains is to detect food allergies and sensitivities that are symptoms of runaway inflammation set in motion by the immune system. Another way is to reduce or eliminate artificial stimulants. You should also avoid certain foods like burnt red meat, fried foods and refined sugar; the consumption of these can lead to the creation of harmful chemical by-products called free radicals, which damage DNA and cause premature ageing of cells. As you cut out foods with a negative effect on energy you will also begin to add foods with beneficial effects, which form the heart of the 21-Day Plan.

The medical establishment has been slow to leverage the importance of food to people's health and well-being, but there have been some very helpful advances in public policy. I am a great fan of food labels, which have become increasingly detailed as the chemistry of prepared foods has become more complex. It's crucial to know what you are eating and to make choices that will promote energy and health rather than fatigue and accelerated ageing. With this chapter you will have what it takes to understand what you are buying and eating and to reclaim the energy that nature has to offer.

It's fashionable today to talk about food in terms of evolution and to note that our metabolism – which was fixed several hundred thousand years ago – and our instinct to eat when food is abundant haven't changed along with our lifestyle. Our ancestors were active hunter-gatherers, but we've become sedentary web surfers in a society overflowing with sugar-dense, fat-heavy, chemical-laden foods. Yet there are also many more clean and healthy foods available than at any time in recent history. Another aspect of evolution that I think is even more important is the increase in the average lifespan. When there was a high probability of being killed by a sabre-toothed tiger or smallpox or bubonic plague before the age of 40, it hardly mattered if you were suffering damage from free radicals or toxins that degrade health over the long term. But if you want to live to a ripe old age (the average in the UK is now 75 for men and 79.9 for women) cumulative damage matters. As you age (which is just another word for sustained damage to DNA), your cells get more and more depleted – think of wrinkles, but on the inside – and your body becomes less efficient at making energy, which is the basis for all functions. By consuming wholesome foods that cause minimal damage and promote maximum repair of cells, however, you can stave off the ageing process, dramatically increase your energy and begin to reverse many common health problems. With this book, you will learn how to eat for the new longevity.

Don't feel bad if you discover that your diet requires a great deal of revamping. You're in good company. Many senior medical school students don't know the first thing about food and nutrition, and I know many doctors who still don't understand it well. Advances in biochemistry and genetics are happening so quickly that it's an effort to keep up with learning about the role food plays in creating energy and health. The best advice I can give is to keep your diet simple and make changes thoughtfully so they will be lasting changes. Altering your diet is not something you can do overnight. If I could I would turn back the clock on our collective dining lives – to an era when processed and packaged foods were not so readily available and every high street wasn't replete with a coffee emporium selling scones and caramel lattes. Since I can't, my goal is to help you embark on a thrilling journey back to nature – to connect you with the energy of the sun stored in plants, available to us as fruits and vegetables – and to bring life and vital energy to the daily process of nourishing your body.

Making Energy

All of the cells in your body that are making energy every microsecond use the same fuel for their molecular fires – food and oxygen delivered by the bloodstream. While sugar is the primary food ingredient combined with oxygen to make energy, there are dozens of other substances (called co-factors) essential for energy creation, all of which your body has to acquire from what you eat. When your body digests food, it breaks down every mouthful into glucose (a simple sugar) and dozens of other nutrients (vitamins, minerals, fatty acids and amino acids) that it absorbs and sends into the blood supply. To oversimplify the process: the bloodstream delivers sugar, nutrients, water and oxygen to each cell, and your cells' internal energy factories (the mitochondria) then use the nutrients to combine the sugar with oxygen and create energy. A heart attack caused by a clogged artery is basically a shutdown in the fuel supply to the heart. Without the regular delivery of nutrients and oxygen the heart can't make energy, and goes into arrest – quickly dying if the fuel line isn't restored.

Every single one of the trillions of cells in your body can unlock the energy inherent in food and transform it into a sort of universal energetic currency called adenosine triphospate (ATP), available for any purpose. A precise molecule of energy, ATP is made in the mitochondria of each cell. Even more amazingly, each cell has the ability to determine how much energy it needs at any given moment. At the core of the process of energy creation is a tiny structure within the cell called the mitochondrion – this is the body's energy factory. Each cell contains multiple mitochondria, depending on the cell's function. An energy-guzzling heart muscle cell can contain up to 100,000 mitochondria (comprising two-thirds of the heart's volume), whereas a short-lived sperm cell contains about ten mitochondria – with all due respect to the sperm, that's like the difference between a high-performance car battery and a triple-A. But the number of mitochondria (most cells contain about 3,000) is only one reason cells can make different amounts of energy.

The mitochondrion also has its own intelligence, that is, it contains its own DNA (inherited strictly from your mother) separate from the main DNA in the cell's nucleus. That mitochondrial DNA, when it's functioning properly, is immensely adaptable – capable of jump-starting its energy production rate on demand via a complex system of cell surface receptors, inner cell enzymes, and transport proteins – all of which regulate the amount of fuel entering the cell and the amount delivered to its energy factory. This dance between regulatory mechanisms within the cell makes your body capable of incredibly intelligent energy creation. For example, it allows your body to produce and consume much more energy when running a marathon than it will when you're sitting for a long car ride.

Once ATP has been made from sugar and oxygen in the cell's mitochondrial forge, it is released into the system as pure energy,

The Energy 'One-a-Days'

Here are some of the most important vitamins and minerals required for making energy: Vitamins B1 (thiamine), B2 (riboflavin), B3 (niacin) and B6 (pantothenic acid); biotin; iron; calcium; magnesium; vitamin C, zinc and copper.

leaving behind a sort of shadow molecule that goes back into the cell and waits to be once again transformed into ATP, like a microscopic rechargeable battery. On average an ATP molecule of energy (of which your cells create billions every moment) gets recycled a thousand times per day. The process also generates heat, water and toxic by-products called free radicals, but it results in the ultimate prize – that intangible animating substance we call energy. The ability to generate energy in each cell evolved over aeons (molecular paleontologists have dated the origin of mitochondria back 1.6 billion years); our prowess for creating energy is what makes it possible to sustain the improbable complexity of the human body.

Your Body's Energy Factory

This miraculously complicated metabolic transformation from food and oxygen into energy is called the Krebs cycle. Trying to fully understand it has made medical students quake in their boots for generations, but increasingly the Krebs cycle (and the nutrient spectrum required to complete it) has become the focus of nutritional science, and a rich area of research for preventive medicine. The upshot of what scientists have learned about the Krebs over the past decade is that having a supply of nutrients sufficient for completing the cycle ceaselessly every day – and for keeping the mitochondria clear of damaging free radicals – is crucial to optimal health and energy.

In an ideal world – where people eat a nutrient-dense, unpolluted diet and live stress-free, active lives – the mitochondria are efficient energy-generating machines capable of capturing 40 per cent of the energy stored in food. Unfortunately, we don't live in an ideal world, and don't feed our systems the fuel needed to keep those millions of machines in good working order. All of the essential substances for making energy (see opposite) must enter the body via food – or in the form of supplements. I was shocked to find out a few years back that most people lack a full supply of the nutritional building blocks of energy when a definitive study from the Harvard School of Public Health determined that the majority of the adult

Maximize Your Energy

In addition to often missing key nutrients for energy generation, your body's energy-making mechanisms are constantly under assault from environmental pollution (see Chapter 3) and three damaging internal processes – oxidation, inflammation and glycation (see the 'The Three Enemies of Energy', below).

The mitochondria are routinely gummed-up, weakened and sometimes even killed by these damaging processes, all of which are exacerbated (and some even created) by poor eating habits. The good news is you can eat foods that maximize your body's energy-generating capacity and minimize destructive processes in the cell discussed in detail later on. In the 21-Day Plan you learn how to do this by following the simple, delicious menus and recipes every day.

population is deficient in vitamins and minerals. These deficiencies are considered to be subtle – you may not have beri-beri (a shortage of B vitamins), for example, but your body is struggling to keep up with the nutritional demands of making energy. Without sufficient nutrients, your cells have to beg borrow and steal from wherever they can (tissues, organs, neighbouring cells), setting up a process of depletion that can lead to fatigue and ultimately disease.

The Energy in Food

In conventional science the 'energy' in food refers to the calories (the lion's share of which comes from sugars and fats). The traditional scientific world view has come to realize that consuming too many calorie-dense foods is at the heart of many of our most common medical ailments – obesity, diabetes, heart disease, even cancer are significantly linked to overeating calorie-dense foods. But the new science – based on our recently acquired understanding of the biological processes that take place inside a single cell – conceives of the energy in food as all of the constituents that contribute to the creation of energy: the calorie-carrying macronutrients (carbohydrates, proteins and fats), along with the essential micronutrients including amino acids, vitamins, minerals, enzymes and a host of other compounds that protect your DNA.

Chronic overconsumption of macronutrient-dense sugars and meats and chronic underconsumption of micronutrient-dense plants is a problem of epidemic proportion. I am always shocked by the fact that counting the potatoes in chips and tomatoes in ketchup makes those two plants the most widely consumed vegetables in both the US and the UK. Since one of ketchup's main ingredients is sugar and chips have more calories from the saturated fat in which they're cooked than in their potato base, this represents an extremely unhealthy state of affairs.

Empty, sugar-rich calories can give you a quick boost, but they ultimately do more harm than good. Your cells require a simple sugar molecule as the basic ingredient for making energy. A sugar (or glucose) molecule's usefulness as an energy source, however, depends on several elements: how quickly that sugar gets absorbed, and whether or not it comes with a posse of nutrients that help convert the sugar into energy and clear the cell of free radicals created by the conversion process. Eating sugar alone, say, in a doughnut, without essential nutrients forces the cell to use up some of its stores of micronutrients to convert the sugar into energy, and that sets off a process of depletion.

Your cells also require protein to provide amino acids used for many critical cell functions like building muscle, hormones and

'The best sugar source for energy comes from complex carbohydrates (whole grains, brown rice, beans, lentils) that contain multiple energy-building and damage-controlling nutrients as well as fibre to slow the absorption of sugar to a steady stream.'

neurotransmitters, as well as providing a back-up energy source. The problem is that the proteins most commonly consumed in the West come loaded with unhealthy fats. Red meat, while it does carry many energy co-factors like iron, zinc, folic acid and the B vitamins, also delivers highly damaging saturated fats. The fats you need for optimum health are monounsaturated and omega-3 unsaturated fats (present in oily fish, nuts and olive oil, for example). These fats are key components in maintaining the integrity of your cells, and their constituent fatty acids can be used as fuel in an emergency. A switch from refined to complex carbohydrates and from animal fats to fats from plants and fish will go a long way in improving your energy and endurance.

Food pyramids foster the misperception that all foods fall into one of three distinct macronutrient categories – carbohydrates, proteins or fats. This has led to the demonization of foods like carrots and eggs, which contain essential nutrients beyond the starches and

Calories Are Kindling

The calories in food provide the combustible material for creating energy. Different foods have different energy potential based on their calorie content. Nutritionists calculate calorie content based on the heat liberated when a specific food is entirely burned up (in a device called a bomb calorimeter). Foods high in fat are the most calorie dense (over two times that of proteins and carbohydrates). A typical adult female who expends 2,100 kCal of food energy each day would have to consume 420 celery stalks, 105 carrots and 26 eggs, yet only 350g of peanuts or two average-sized pepperoni pizzas to meet her daily energy needs. Filling up on vegetables and consuming moderate quantities of protein and carbohydrates along with small amounts of healthy fats is the best way to keep your fire burning all day long.

fats that give them a bad reputation. The reality is that foods cross boundaries; many foods contain a mix of macronutrients and micronutrients. I am a strong proponent of eating broadly within a spectrum that contains a balance of macronutrients (ideally 40 per cent complex carbs, 30 per cent lean protein, 30 per cent healthy fats) packed with multiple micronutrients (see the Power Foods chart, page 86) including antioxidants, anti-inflammatories, vitamins, minerals and enzymes – all of which are essential for making and maintaining a vital energy supply.

At the risk of alienating dyed-in-the-wool devotees of meat-rich, the Western diet, it's best to eat lean, plant-based foods. The typical meat-sweet diet (one that is heavy in saturated fat and carbohydrates) is deficient in so many nutrients that it causes premature ageing of nuclear and mitochondrial DNA (that means it makes you look and feel older and more tired than you should, and predisposes you to many debilitating health problems). Taking a multivitamin will help you extract more energy from food by providing energy's manufacturing co-factors, specially if your diet is heavy on meat and sugar, but if you really want to achieve optimal energy and feel ten years younger, you'll want to eat primarily nutrient-dense, unprocessed, plant-based foods. The 21-Day Plan will take you through the baby steps you need to take to make this transition, and it will get you completely immersed in the nutrient-dense, energy-rich, plant-based diet. The 21-Day Plan involves interacting with produce (as I like to call it). Everyone who has done it reports a renewed sense of connection to the planet – and to the energy of the sun – by simply beginning to eat more glorious plants!

Talk to Your DNA

On a basic level, food is nothing more than a collection of genetic signalling molecules. When you eat a lot of sugar you signal your DNA to produce insulin. Tucking into a slab of Wagyu beef loaded with saturated fat can signal your DNA to create inflammatory molecules that among other mischief oxidize cholesterol, causing it to

> ### So-called Energy
> 'Energy' seems to be the food industry's code word for drinks
> and snack bars packed with caffeine and sugar, which provide
> an immediate rush often followed by a crash. These so-called
> 'energy' foods are actually energy substitutes: they mimic the
> effects of energy, but deplete your energy supply. If you use
> them as short-term fixes, make sure you also replenish essential
> nutrients and get real rest. For making energy, catnaps beat
> caffeine, hands down.

stick to the inside of your blood vessels. Eating fish signals your DNA
to create anti-inflammatory molecules to prevent this harmful oxidation of fats. Every time you eat, you ingest substances that interact
with your DNA, causing changes at the molecular level. If you want
to tell your DNA to create more energy, you have to send the right
signals.

Caffeine, probably the most widely used 'energy' food, does
not tell your DNA to make more energy, but rather tells your DNA
to activate your nervous system. This may improve your sense of
mental alertness, but the process of stimulating your nervous system
actually *expends* energy. By contrast, aerobic exercise utilizes energy
and burns calories, but it also causes the body to *create* more cellular energy factories. A jolt of caffeine consumes energy that in turn
produces a rogue's gallery of damaging by-products. As a result, your
DNA is told to clean up, which requires still more energy that could
in fact be used for other purposes, like staying alert.

The way to coax your body into making more energy available for every task is to eat foods rich in the raw materials of energy
manufacture, which signal your DNA to make energy. Sugar is the
necessary foundation for creating an energy molecule (your body
can make energy without sugar, but not at all efficiently), but the
type of sugar you eat is absolutely critical. When you eat a complex

carbohydrate, say a bowl of whole grain muesli, you get starch that's converted into sugar, but you also get fibre to control the delivery of sugar and make you feel full, and the germ (the nutrient-dense seed at the heart of a stalk of grain) that contains hundreds of different phytochemicals – including the energy essentials zinc, copper, B-complex vitamins and vitamin E. Complex carbohydrates such as whole grains or beans allow the body to generate energy efficiently and mop up free radicals, sending pro-energy metabolic signals to your DNA. Better yet, eat your muesli with almonds (that provide monounsaturated fats and amino acids, important energy co-factors) and a handful of blueberries (with antioxidants to sweep away toxic by-products.) That's the sort of snack that tells your DNA to manufacture clean energy.

Enemies of Energy: Inflammation, Oxidation and Glycation

There are three processes within the cell that unnecessarily consume large amounts of energy, produce premature ageing and cause widespread damage: *oxidation, inflammation* and *glycation*. All of these processes are affected by what you eat. Inflammation and oxidation are part of natural cell life, but when they happen in excess – from eating a typical Western diet, for example – they lead to cell damage and fatigue. The third cell-damaging process, glycation, is solely a result of sugar excess. Glycation is never a normal process, but it is becoming more prevalent in our society where highly concentrated sugar increasingly in the form of high fructose corn syrup (and glucose syrup) is pervasive. You'll find it in bread, ketchup, baked beans, salad dressings and breakfast cereal to name a few sources. Minimizing these three processes is crucial to having high energy and good health.

I am asking you, as I do many of my patients, to eliminate the worst offenders that cause these processes. I realize it's asking a lot; many inflammatory foods – such as sweets, meats and cheese – taste delicious. (Keep in mind that everyone's vulnerabilities are different; part of this programme is identifying which foods affect your body most.) But it's extremely important to protect cells from these three damaging processes, especially the cells in our most vital organs.

So here's the deal: I want you to read the case against these processes and decide for yourself. You be the jury and send down a verdict on the offenders. The sentence I recommend: banish the offending foods (see Trouble Foods to Avoid, below), and hold wild dinner parties with the many protective foods mentioned in this section and detailed in the Power Foods chart.

Inflammation

Inflammation is a powerful and wildly diverse immune response. Think of inflammation as your body's military defence network. It's a life-sustaining process by which the immune system identifies, attacks and repairs damage from potentially injurious substances – without it we'd have no effective immunity. Like all defence systems, inflammation's usefulness depends on its ability to recognize a substance as foreign, or not 'self' – its target can be bacteria, a virus, a toxin, food or even one's own tissue in the case of autoimmune disease. It can be seen in a broad range of anatomical events: from the redness, swelling and heat that accompanies a sunburn to the bloating, pain and diarrhoea of inflammatory bowel disease; from the formation of plaque in your arteries to the hives, swelling and trouble breathing initiated by a peanut allergy.

The retaliatory assault begins with a warning signal – that can be sent by just a single cell to far-flung locations in the body – carrying the message that defences have been breached, and a potentially destructive process is underway. The immune system's first line of inflammatory defence, led by white blood cells, sends out multiple chemical messengers that mobilize the body's resources both locally and systemically to remove the bad guys. The most important of these immune messenger molecules are cytokines. Cytokines signal cells throughout the body to spring into

'Increasingly, chronic inflammation is being suggested as the common link between *all* chronic illnesses.'

How Fats Affect Inflammation

When digested, fats are transformed into substances that can either create or quell inflammation. On the good side of the divide are foods that contain omega-3 fatty acids that are transformed into anti-inflammatory substances. On the bad side of the divide are foods (such as red meat) that contain omega 6 fatty acids, which are transformed into pro-inflammatory substances. Eating more omega-3s can reduce damaging inflammation in your body.

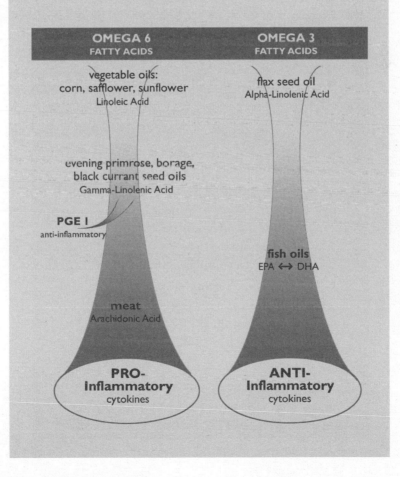

OMEGA 6
FATTY ACIDS

OMEGA 3
FATTY ACIDS

vegetable oils:
corn, safflower, sunflower
Linoleic Acid

flax seed oil
Alpha-Linolenic Acid

evening primrose, borage,
black currant seed oils
Gamma-Linolenic Acid

PGE I
anti-inflammatory

fish oils
EPA ↔ DHA

meat
Arachidonic Acid

PRO-
Inflammatory
cytokines

ANTI-
Inflammatory
cytokines

action and send in reinforcements. In response, the immune system sends out a full defensive assault team: natural killer cells are the samurai warriors that engulf invaders; tumour necrosis factor is the flame thrower that disintegrates molecules; platelets are field docs ordered to stop bleeding; fibrin throws a sticky mesh over the area to hold it together. All the while neighbouring cells release more cytokines to continue the inflammatory reaction. When the battle is won, to calm the warriors the body has a group of anti-inflammatory substances – manufactured by cells and absorbed from foods – that turn the process off.

Chronic Inflammation

Chronic inflammation occurs when the inflammatory machinery doesn't get turned off. This is the abnormal process central to such common illnesses as coronary artery disease, diabetes, arthritis, Crohn's disease and ulcerative colitis, obesity, Alzheimer's, Parkinson's and chronic fatigue.

And there are likely to be more. For example, cancer researchers are only beginning to unravel the incredibly complex behaviours of the immune system's inflammatory molecules, which are thought to be able to either halt a tumour in its tracks or encourage its growth.

Lifestyle can magnify the inflammatory response – poor eating habits, high stress levels and exposure to toxins (like tobacco smoke, air pollution and heavy metals) can throw off the body's ability to maintain the balance between promoting and quelling inflammation,

Are You Chronically Inflamed?
The symptoms: muscle stiffness, joint aches, asthma, allergies, irritable bowel, slow wound healing, gum disease, premature ageing, morning fatigue, longer or more frequent hangovers from moderate drinking, intense jetlag, recurring colds and sinus infections.

> ### *Power Foods that Fight Inflammation*
> *Salmon, trout, almonds, walnuts, pulses, cruciferous vegetables,*
> *dark leafy greens, tea, grape skin, citrus fruits, olive oil, turmeric,*
> *ginger, garlic and rosemary.*

thereby creating a chronic state. Food is a crucial factor in the inflammatory equation. Eating is the most constant and unremitting activity that can introduce pro-inflammatory 'foreign' substances into the body, and can also introduce substances that calm inflammation.

We now know that certain fats universally create inflammation and others quell inflammation. There are two main classes of bad fats. The first includes saturated fat in meats, poultry, eggs, dairy and some fish (shellfish, squid and octopus all have cholesterol) and polyunsaturated fats in corn and safflower oil, all of which can be converted to arachidonic acid, a toxic substance the body uses to make pro-inflammatory cytokines. The other category of bad fats is man-made transfats in margarine and baked goods, which directly cause inflammation. There are two categories of good fats as well: monosaturated (from olive and grapeseed oils); and omega-3 oils from flax, fish, nuts and seeds. These essential fatty acids (EFAs) are used by the body to make anti-inflammatory cytokines. Simply by switching from eating unhealthy fats to healthy fats you can dramatically reduce inflammation. Foods that contain good fats promote the creation of anti-inflammatory cytokines and allow your DNA to operate in an optimal environment, thereby using energy more efficiently. Which kind of fats would you rather have circulating in your system?

An Anti-inflammatory Diet
In addition to the mix of fats, the types of carbohydrate you eat also affect the level of inflammation in your body. Studies show that eating high glycaemic index (GI), refined carbohydrates that are quickly

absorbed into the bloodstream (such as white wheat flour breads and pastas, potatoes and white rice) causes an increase in inflammatory molecules. Conversely, when you eat low GI carbs (such as whole grains, beans and pulses) there is a marked decrease in circulating inflammatory molecules.

Food allergies are another common source of inflammation. Most people are not surprised to learn that classic food allergies (which cause an immediate, acute reaction) produce inflammation. But most people don't know about the prevalence of more subtle, delayed food allergies and sensitivities, which operate along slightly different inflammatory and immune pathways than immediate allergies. (For more on allergies see 'Hidden Allergies', page 82.)

While I want you to eat fewer foods that cause inflammation, I also want you to eat more foods that calm it. As scientists have been elucidating the complex immune process of inflammation they have also learned a lot about what stops it. Cruciferous vegetables, beans and pulses, nuts and seeds, olive oil, herbs and spices, and fatty fish all contain dozens of anti-inflammatory compounds – including bioflavonoids, polyphenols, catechins and anthocyanins. These compounds, which the human body cannot make, were developed by plants and fish to fight off their own inflammation and diseases, but can be used by our bodies to switch off the destructive activities of inflammatory molecules without weakening the immune response. Many of these compounds – for example, the flavonoids in turmeric – directly reduce the activity of the cell's internal DNA messenger that can force the cell into inflammation hyperdrive. Food changes the messages getting to your DNA. By eating foods that fight inflammation you free up your body's energy supply to be used for more productive pursuits and reduce the risk of developing one of the many diseases – including cancer, heart disease and diabetes – that are now associated with inflammation.

The body is perfectly capable of managing the inflammatory process with a proper, anti-inflammatory diet and healthy lifestyle – especially in the early stages of inflammation. Your daily sustenance should be low in inflammatory foods and high in foods that provide anti-inflammatory substances along with the substrates (primarily essential fatty acids) for manufacturing the body's own internal anti-inflammatory brigade. Hence the adage: *Food is your best medicine.*

Oxidation

This particular enemy arises from the love-hate relationship most life forms have with oxygen. Your ability to create energy efficiently – and support life – depends on oxygen. But while oxygen gives life to your cells, it also can be corrosive, with the ability to damage or oxidize cells (think of rust and tarnish). The very act of energy creation invites oxygen into the inner, most vulnerable part of the cell creating a number of highly destructive substances called free radicals as a natural by-product of energy creation. You are constantly ingesting, absorbing and creating free radicals, not only from your own metabolism, but also from certain toxic foods, air and water pollution, and sun exposure – they're everywhere!

These free radicals (most of which are known by the rather Jurassic title of 'reactive oxygen species') can easily damage your all-important DNA and harm other delicate cell structures, including membranes that hold the cell together and enzymes that constantly break down debris. The body has a number of compounds designed to very efficiently eliminate free radicals. These are home-grown antioxidants continually produced by the cells. Problems arise, however, when the free radical bad guys outnumber your internal antioxidant good guys. This is when your body looks to nature to send in reinforcements in the form of foods that provide additional antioxidants. Vitamins E, C, and the carotenes are prime examples, but there are hundreds of other compounds found in abundance in fruits (especially berries and citrus), vegetables (especially leafy greens and cruciferi like broccoli and cauliflower), fruit and green tea.

'By eating a diet full of colourful plants (a so-called 'rainbow diet') you will reduce oxidative stress and are very likely to reduce your chance of getting cancer and many other diseases.'

TAP INTO THE SOURCE

Reducing Oxidation

My mantra for dealing with oxidation is: reduce exposure; increase protection. It's critically important to reduce the cumulative burden of free radicals. Here's how:

- If you smoke, please stop – free radicals are only the tip of the toxic iceberg that is a cigarette.
- Avoid free radical-promoting foods (charred meats, refined sugar, transfats and fried foods).
- Another good fix is to exercise more and moderately (overly intense aerobic activity generates free radicals), and work out as far away as you possibly can from car exhaust and other pollution.
- Avoid overimbibing alcohol to the point of getting a hangover, which is basically an overdose of toxins and free radicals.
- Drink adequate amounts of water (minimum six glasses a day), which will support your body's ability to excrete the neutralized free radicals and other toxins.
- By practising relaxation exercises you can reduce the nervous system's enormous energy needs, and thereby reduce the free radicals that result from constant energy manufacture.
- You can make a dramatic impact on your body's ability to protect cells from free radical damage by simply eating more foods with antioxidants.

You will find a more complete listing of antioxidant foods in the Power Foods chart, but here is my short list of antioxidant foods to start eating now: blueberries, cranberries, green tea, broccoli, dark chocolate, carrots, spinach, kale, cantaloupe, sweet potato, tomatoes and citrus fruit. Colour is of the utmost importance because plant pigments are antioxidants.

In their wonderful book *Healing Foods*, naturopaths Michael Murray and Joseph Pizzorno write, 'Some experts have said – and we agree – that cancer is a result of a "maladaption" over time to a reduced level of intake of fruits and vegetables.' While this may be an oversimplification I believe there's a great deal of truth in it. At the very least, when you become a devotee of produce you will protect your mitochondria from oxidation, and as a result you will protect your energy supply.

Glycation

OK, here we go with the sugar bashing. You've heard it before, but it's an important part of the energy story. When the body has too much circulating sugar – which is almost always a result of eating too many rapidly absorbed sugars from overly refined carbohydrates – the resulting excess glucose molecules will eventually start sticking to proteins, in a process called glycation. Glycation transforms the molecular structure of cells, damaging their function and making them die an early death. I call this 'sugar ageing'; it happens every time your blood sugar spikes.

People often have a 'that's-not-me' attitude toward the concept of sugar ageing. This is partly due to a common misconception about how the body receives sugar. A food does not have to be made with table sugar (called sucrose) in order to deliver sugar to the cells. For example, white rice is rapidly converted into sugar even though it doesn't contain sucrose. Nutritional scientists have given us two ways to determine whether or not a food will cause a spike in blood sugar – glycaemic index and glycaemic load. Glycaemic index (GI) is a measure of how quickly sugar is absorbed from a food; glycaemic load (GL) is a measure of the amount of sugar a food actually delivers to the cells. Glycaemic *load* is the more relevant number. Eating low glycaemic *load* foods is the most critically important way to reduce glycation.

One hidden trove of sugars is the veritable mountain of new low-fat foods, which are routinely given

'I don't care how good food scientists are at their job, it is not possible to design a processed food with the complex antioxidant capabilities of a plant.'

Low Glycaemic Load* *Carbs You Can Eat*

Pumpernickel bread, plain steel-cut oatmeal, wholemeal rye bread, spelt multigrain bread, All Bran cereal, muesli, Ryvita, lentils, beans, apples, cherries, grapefruit, kiwi, oranges and tomato juice.
* Note: glycaemic load is below 10.

extra sugar to make up for the loss in flavour from fat. This sets up a situation in which two scoops of full-fat ice cream carry a lower glycaemic load (registering 6.1) than a typical cup of low-fat yogurt (registering 8.5 on the GL scale). The ice cream has a lower GL because fat slows absorption of sugar, although this doesn't make ice cream a health food. Mind you, both a serving of ice cream and of yogurt have a fraction of the glycaemic load of a plain bagel (which racks up a whopping 25 points on the GL scale). Indeed, we get a high percentage of our daily sugar intake from baked goods. Hidden sources of sugar are also found in all manner of nutrition drinks and bars, some of which deliver a mother lode of sugar. It's also high in foods such as tinned soups, baked beans, breakfast cereals and ready meals, as well as many 'savoury' snacks and meals. The spike in blood sugar created by these everyday foods not only creates sugar ageing, it also raises your body fat composition – as all sugars not immediately used for energy are stored as fat. And a spike in blood sugar inevitably takes a bite out of your energy supply.

When you eat a high glycaemic load food, for example a doughnut, you quickly produce (and just as quickly lose) a lot of energy – and you generate a lot of internal pollution in the process. Not a reasonable fuel, a doughnut will overtax the cell's ability to handle the excess rush of sugar without providing the co-factors necessary to make energy efficiently or to clean up the toxic by-products of your natural combustion. A complex carbohydrate (such as lentils or brown rice) generates a slow-burning flame that cleans up what little smoke it creates, whereas a refined carbohydrate (such as a plain bagel) produces a flash fire that dies down quickly and throws off all sorts of damaging by-products that cannot be removed without depleting your cells of nutrients they need for other processes.

> ### The Skinny on Bars and Shakes
> *Judging from the almost £100 million that will be spent this year on meal replacement bars and shakes, people are willing to sacrifice taste for convenience. While I always prefer whole foods (a handful of trail mix is perfect in a pinch), some meal replacement choices are better than others. My primary concern is sugar. Many of the bestselling meal replacement drinks contain a lot of sugar and other carbohydrates (like sugar alcohols that don't raise insulin but do contribute to calories). Original Slimfast Meal Bars and Shakes contain 25 and 40 grams of carbohydrates respectively, which is too much to process at one sitting. Making matters worse, the drinks do not contain fibre to slow down sugar absorption. If you must have a liquid meal, go for one of the higher protein formulas, which tend to have less sugar. For my money, the bars are a better bet because they contain complex carbohydrates with fibre. Even so, keep an eye on the sugar content, and beware of saturated fats, which are mixed into bars to give better mouth feel. Look for bars made with all natural plant ingredients with less than 12 grams of sugar, at least 6 grams of protein, and less than 6 grams of fat (with maximum 2 grams saturated fat). The best bars are made from whole foods; look on the ingredient label for nuts and seeds, whole grain fibre, and natural sweeteners such as honey and fruit juice – some bars even have dehydrated fruits and vegetables, which I consider to be a bonus.*

Hidden Allergies

There are three problems with foods in terms of reactivity and sensitivity. *Immediate* food allergies are often swift and severe, as with peanuts and prawns, and most people are acutely aware of these inflammatory triggers. *Delayed* food allergies are difficult to recognize because their symptoms can appear up to three days after exposure, in the form of rash, headache and joint soreness among others. They can often be the source of constant fatigue. A third category is food chemical *sensitivities*. These are not true allergies, but are inflammatory reactions to chemical compounds in foods, such as lactose intolerance and insensitivity to caffeine or fermented foods.

Classic food allergies (like an anaphylactic allergic reaction to peanuts or prawns) and subtle food allergies (such as irritable bowel or eczema stemming from a subtle wheat or egg allergy) are both based on an immune system malfunction. White blood cells produce antibodies (IgE and IgG) that attack the food, often creating energy-draining and symptom-producing inflammation and oxidation in the process. The difference is in the type of immune antibody involved. A classic allergy is the result of an immediate IgE antibody reaction; a subtle allergy is the result of a delayed IgG antibody reaction. Classic and subtle allergies have very different symptoms. The IgE response occurs quickly, resulting from an instant release of histamine and other chemicals and inflammatory cells that cause redness, itching, swelling, hives or shortness of breath. The IgG response is slower to develop and harder to recognize, involving antibodies that can appear 2 to 3 days after exposure, causing myriad symptoms that often seem mysterious to people because they take so long to appear.

It's important to diagnose subtle allergies and sensitivities because they cause such an array of problems that often go unrecognized. While tests can be helpful for identifying delayed allergies, the gold standard for diagnosing hidden food reactivity (both allergic and sensitivity) is the elimination diet. For one month you stop eating the most common allergens such as wheat, dairy, peanuts, shellfish, soya, citrus fruit, nuts/seeds, chocolate, coffee and fermented foods (yeast, alcohol, soy sauce, pickles and cheese). I also cut out foods that people say they crave or eat a lot of because those often turn out to be offenders. After the month you add back the foods one at a time for two to three days, eating enough of each (usually twice per day) to challenge the system to cause symptoms if that food is a problem. (When an allergy produces a delayed reaction, eating a small amount of the trigger may not cause noticeable symptoms.) With a strictly enforced elimination protocol (the 21-Day Plan can be a starting point for this) you can pinpoint the cause of even subtle allergies (as well as other food reactions) with considerable accuracy.

Bottom Line: Trouble Foods to Avoid

Let me finish up this guide to energy drains with the list of what not to eat. Your goal is to avoid the three damaging inflammatory processes and to stop your body from wasting energy on repairing and cleaning up from foods that harm your cells. Here is what to eliminate, along with a quick look at healthier substitutes. The 21-Day Plan offers practical, complete menus and recipes for avoiding these trouble-makers.

Red Meat: With apologies to your local butcher, for the next 21 days I'd like you to take a break from eating red meat (beef, pork, lamb and veal). It causes inflammation by promoting the formation of unhealthy fatty acids, oxidation by introducing free radicals, and (if non-organic) possible exposure to toxins from antibiotics, growth hormones and pesticide residues. Replace red meat with healthier protein options. After your 21-day abstention, eat meat only sparingly if you must.

Transfats: Primarily found in packaged baked goods and margarine (fortunately, home-baked goods do not contain transfats), these cause premature ageing of the circulatory system, accumulation of fat in the midsection, and damage to the DNA. Use a smidgen of butter and olive oil, and avoid transfats for life.

Refined Carbohydrates: White flour, white rice, potatoes and sweets are too quickly converted to sugar – draining energy, promoting inflammation and glycation, and producing free radicals. Refined carbs are also easily converted to midsection fat. Swap with whole grains and unrefined sweeteners like honey.

Wheat: So many people have become sensitized to the 'New World' wheat that pervades our food supply. It can be a major source of inflammation and refined carbohydrates. Swap this form of wheat for 'Old World' wheat (spelt and kamut). For the 1 to 2 per cent of the population who are gluten intolerant, none of these grains is acceptable.

Cow's Milk Protein: Another common allergen and sensitizer, cow's milk also contains saturated fat, which causes inflammation, and is a potential source of antibiotics and growth hormones, which your body has to work to remove. For 21 days eliminate cow's milk (opt for soya or rice milk). For many people non-fat yogurt from cows is OK, but for those with true milk allergies there are other forms of yogurt from sheep, goat or soya that may be better choices.

> ### *The Ideal Balance*
> *Keep in mind my ideal balance: 40 per cent complex carbohydrates; 30 per cent lean protein; 30 per cent healthy fats. In my experience most people eat either too much protein, too many saturated fats or too many carbohydrates. Get accustomed to loading your plate with vegetables (have a vegetable and salad with dinner). Take a small peach-sized portion of carbohydrates, and consume less protein than you're used to.*

Coffee: Overstimulates your nervous system and sets you up for a crash. Wean yourself off coffee. Eliminate coffee for 21 days or at the very least drink half your current dose; substituting with more calming green tea or at least decaf coffee is even better.

Alcohol: By taking a break from alcohol you allow your detox mechanisms, especially in your liver, to work less hard and free up energy for repair.

Power Foods to Enjoy

Finally, here's what I want you to *eat* with gusto. Power foods will create the new, vital you. They'll provide all of the good stuff: sustained release of sugar with complex carbohydrates balanced by fibre and lean protein; a high level of nutrients to create energy and repair damage; substances that promote detoxification; and defensive superstars that fight inflammation and oxidation. When you eat these foods daily, you will absolutely renew your cells, increase your life force and feel younger and more energized. Follow the recipes in the 21-Day Plan. The foods in the plan are by no means confined to the superstars in the Power Foods chart on the following page. All vegetables, whole grains, pulses, fish, nuts and seeds can and should be welcomed into your world and prepared with a generous helping of TLC.

Naturally, if you're accustomed to eating a meat-rich diet, these foods may not appeal to you at first glance, but I suggest you try our recipes because it's very likely you've had one or more of these items improperly prepared. Most people overcook food, leaving the greens wilted and sour; the garlic and oil burned and bitter; the beans and lentils soggy and heavy on the stomach or causing too much gas. Instead of boiling broccoli, I brown it in the oven with fresh olive oil and garlic. To rid fish of its fishy smell it's always washed first with lemon and salt, then rinsed under water before cooking. Poultry is always cooked with aromatic spices to impart flavour. The 21-Day Plan offers many recipes to energize your kitchen.

POWER FOODS

	Complex Carb	Lean Protein	Soluble Fibre	Good Fats	Energy Nutrients	Fights Free Radicals	Anti-inflammatory	Promotes Detox
Salmon, trout		****		****	**		****	
Halibut/flounder/sole		****		**	**		**	
Eggs (poached or boiled)		****			****			
Soya	***	***	***	**	**	**	**	**
Yogurt (plain is best)	*	***			***	**	****	
Whey protein powder		****	**		**		***	****
Almonds/almond butter	*	**	**	***	**	**	***	
Walnuts	*	**		***	**		***	
Lentils	****	***	***	*	*		*	
Beans (red, black)	****	**	***	*	**	**	*	*
Wheat germ	**		**	**	****	***	**	**
Quinoa/spelt/kamut	****	*	****		**	**	**	**
Flax seeds	***			****	**	**	****	*
Olive oil				****	**	**	****	
Grapeseed oil				****	**	**	****	**
Spinach/kale	**		***		***			
Swiss chard	**		***		***	***		**
Broccoli/Brussels sprouts	**		***		***	***	**	****
Watercress, rocket	*		**		**	**		****
Avocado				****	**	**	***	
Sea vegetables			*	*	****	***	**	***
Shitake/reishi			**		***	***	***	**
Fresh veggie juice	*		*/***		***	***	***	***
Onions					**	***	**	****
Garlic				*	***	***	***	****
Blueberries	*		**		**	****	**	***
Kiwi	*		**		****	****	**	**
Papaya	*		**		***	***	***	**
Grapefruit	*		**		**	**	**	**
Apples	**		**		***	**	**	**
Red grapes	**		*		**	***	*	*
Turmeric					***	***	****	***
Cinnamon/ginger					***	***	***	***
Green tea						****	***	**
Vinegar							**	**
Unfiltered honey						***	*	
Dark chocolate (70%)						****	*	
Red wine (moderate)						***	***	

'In our former agricultural society, when people had to catch their own fish or raise their own animals, protein was eaten sparingly and with great appreciation – I recommend that we all reconnect with that perspective.'

If you want to lose weight, watch your intake of fats and carbohydrates, and eat more steamed fish and veggies. While the fats in my plan are healthy, they do add calories. When you're trying to slim down, the trick is to eat foods that contain a lot of water and fibre with minimal calories, such as spring greens, kale, celery, lettuce and fish. If you, like most people, are accustomed to carbohydrate-dense snacks, you will lose weight simply by following the 21-day meal plan. If you are the kind of person who operates on coffee and anything you can gobble as you run out the door, you'll find that eating this new way will calm your nervous system and give you tremendous endurance. If you tend to panic when you feel hungry, you'll also do just fine, because these foods have ample fibre and a reasonable amount of healthy fats, both of which are satiating. You simply have nothing to lose by eating the Power Foods way.

A Matter of Convenience

By no means should you give up and have a cheeseburger if you can't get salmon and Swiss chard for dinner. Most cities and even villages now have food shops and delis, and even restaurants that both prepare healthy meals and deliver. The goal is to eat lean protein, complex carbohydrates and vegetables, preferably fresh, but frozen is certainly acceptable too (freezing actually preserves the nutrients in food that can be lost while it travels across the country or the globe, sits in a warehouse and then on the supermarket shelf). A tin of wild caught salmon prepared with lemon or a touch of low-fat mayo and a salad is a perfectly acceptable lunch. I am a big fan of frozen organic fruits and vegetables in a pinch, and also recommend keeping fully cooked, organic (where possible) frozen meals in the freezer, and stocking your pantry with organic (low-salt) tinned lentil and bean soups.

When you're in a hurry, good intentions tend to go out the window. But this sets up a cycle of energy depletion just when you need it most. Whether you take an hour preparing a meal or five minutes, make sure that what you eat sends an energetic message to every cell in your body.

Supplements: When Good Food is Not Enough

Many people come to me with bags full of supplements – they've got megavitamins, antioxidants, high doses of obscure nutrients, herbs from remote corners of the planet, 'natural' hormones from their latest nutrition guru, and all manner of proprietary formulas for everything from energy to sexual potency. They come looking for guidance, and sometimes even for more tablets, and I almost always disappoint by telling them to throw most of it away. So often healthfood shop assistants and 'alternative' newsletters and websites take a one-size-fits-all approach to supplements, causing people to purchase and consume tablets they don't need. Some alternative practitioners push their pet magic bullets as heavily as conventional doctors push the latest pharmaceuticals, but I am not a big fan of taking a lot of supplements regularly. I believe that most people can and should get the nutrients they need from food. If after significant changes to lifestyle and diet there are still deficiencies, or if there is a disease process that requires a supplement, I will recommend one, but my goal is to use supplements only to jump-start a treatment and recovery protocol. I aim to avoid daily use of all but the most absolutely necessary supplements, which for many people is simply a quality multiple vitamin.

'When you think you don't have time to eat well, take a deep breath and realize that supportive nourishment may very well be the one thing that actually pulls you through a big challenge.'

One compelling reason for my reluctance to supplement is that because nutritional science is fairly new, researchers have only begun to unlock the compounds (most of them found in plants) that are beneficial to your health. Plus there are inherent risks in using too much of any one extract or supplement. Ten years ago, most doctors and scientists didn't appreciate there is more than one type of vitamin E; now we know there are at least six types (tocopherols and tocotrienols), and some of them are more powerful at fighting free radicals, and even tumours, than others. The same can be said of subclasses of carotenes (the vitamin A family). When the entire carotene family is used together as it is found naturally in foods it strengthens the immune system and reduces the risk of cancers, but when a single member of the family, beta-carotene, is used alone it can actually cause lung cancer to spread more rapidly. Folic acid can help prevent heart disease and some cancers and birth defects, but may increase the risk of colon cancer. Selenium can protect the prostate from cancer and the heart from arteriosclerosis, but it can increase the risk of developing skin cancer. This is just a fraction of the cross-reactions and side-effects of vitamins and minerals. Appropriate use of supplements, especially with the megavitamin doses found in many healthfood shop products, can be extremely complicated.

Herbs for Health?

Understanding one vitamin or mineral, though, is child's play compared to analysing any one herb, which entails discovering which of the hundreds of compounds found in a plant benefits health without producing side-effects. When you look at what's on the shelves for just one herb, say echinacea, you don't know if the capsule contains the powerful leaf and root components, or relatively worthless stem parts. In the UK and the EU, herbal remedies must be made to assured standards of safety and quality and must be licenced – although until 2011 not every product will have been subject to scrutiny. Imported US herbal products are subject to almost no quality control at present. It is therefore important that you carefully research anything you plan to take. American products should carry a label saying GMP, which means the manufacturer is complying with good manufacturing principles. You can also check www.consumerlabs.com for information. In the UK, you can visit www.mhra.gov.uk to view reports on all registered herbal products.

My recommendation is to complete the first 14 days of the 21-Day Plan, following the balanced, nutrient-dense menus and recipes. In the third week of the plan, if you want to try a supplement specifically to increase energy, I've listed some here that I have often found useful for jump-starting energy. The key is to try only one new supplement at a time so that you can determine its effects, if any. I usually give a supplement for at least a week before evaluating its impact on a patient's health and sense of energy (some take up to six weeks to have a notable effect). Naturally, if a supplement makes you feel poorly or even just a little strange, stop taking it immediately. Everyone's metabolism and nutritional profile is different, so it's im-

It Ain't Easy Being Green

If you've ever set foot in a healthfood shop, or browsed the internet for health-boosting foods and nutrients, you'll know that the market for products promising that elusive fountain of youth of abundant vital energy is flooded with 'green' drinks (also in powder form). These are nutrient-dense powders made from plant – primarily seaweed – compounds such as chlorella, spirulina, blue-green algae and wheat grass, and mixed with other whole food ingredients. If you don't like to eat your veggies (optimally eight or nine servings a day), these drinks are not a bad idea because they deliver a bounty of vitamins, minerals, antioxidants and other nutrients in a whole food form. These concentrated powders may even have benefits beyond the typical land vegetable in helping remove heavy metals from the gut. You can find green drinks in combination with berry extracts (for extra antioxidants) and sometimes with herbs like Siberian ginseng or probiotics for strengthening your intestinal tract.

possible to predict how any one nutrient or formula of nutrients will affect you. My mantra with supplements is to err on the side of caution, and see your doctor before taking new supplements if you are being treated for a medical condition.

Co-enzyme Q10 (Ubiquinone): CoQ10 is an essential critically important nutrient, occurring naturally in the human body, required for the mitochondria to make ATP (your energy currency) and also as a necessary antioxidant for neutralizing the large number of free radicals generated as a by-product of creating ATP. Occasionally your body cannot supply enough CoQ10 for optimum energy. For example, the statin drugs, Lipitor (atorvastatin) and Zocor (simvastatin) may deplete CoQ10; if you take a statin you might consider supplementing with CoQ10, especially during periods when there are heavy demands on your energy. It has been shown to help post-exercise recovery in more highly trained athletes. This nutrient also has been shown to improve cardiac function in people with cardiac disease. CoQ10 goes right to the mitochondria to make the machinery more efficient. It's safe to use long-term, for example if you're taking statins, but not everyone needs it. If you're not deficient, taking CoQ10 won't give you more energy. (Rarely, a side-effect can be cognitive changes – feeling 'foggy': if this happens, stop CoQ10 and the symptoms should clear quickly.)

L-carnitine: Carnitine is an amino acid that has many beneficial uses in the body. One of these is to facilitate the uptake of fatty acids into the mitochondria. Fatty acids not only help stabilize the mitochondrial membrane and provide some anti-inflammatory protection, but are sometimes used as a back-up fuel source in the mitochondria – bypassing the usual glucose mechanism. This could be useful when one's glucose stores are low – during endurance athletic activities – and for people with chronic debilitating illnesses (including current ongoing research studies on fatigue in cancer). (Side-effects are unlikely – as with many supplements, occasional stomach upset may occur if too much is taken on an empty stomach.)

Krebs Cycle Nutrient Co-Factors: Many people have insufficient stores of the critical vitamin and mineral co-factors needed for the mitochondria to produce energy. Inadequate diets, stress, toxic loads and chronic health conditions can all deplete the body of essential nutrients. To help rebalance this, taking a targeted multivitamin/mineral supplement can help put you back on the road to being able to produce more energy. The most important nutrients to look for, which can be found isolated in some 'mitochondrial formulations', are B complex, copper, zinc and magnesium. Iron can be tricky; while it's an important nutrient co-factor, there are contraindications (for example, some men have high-normal haemoglobin counts and should not take iron supplements). Note: while higher doses of water soluble B vitamins are quite safe, minerals and other vitamins have a greater potential for harm, so make sure to check with your doctor before using these nutrients.

Adaptogens

Adaptogens are an important group of herbs that can help the body to maintain energy. Studies show that adaptogens can strengthen the immune system, act as antioxidants, support the adrenal gland's ability to regulate cortisol, and help the body maintain muscle mass. Adaptogens do not simply increase energy, they also help maintain the balance between the body's energy-producing and -consuming mechanisms. Which herb works best is very idiosyncratic; it's like feeling a difference between aspirin and ibuprofen. People who have serious medical conditions or take medications should check with their doctor before taking any herb or supplement.

Cordyceps *(cordyceps sinensis)*: One of my favourite herbs, cordyceps is a mushroom that particularly excels at supporting the adrenal gland. It was originally used in China, where it remains popular, but is manufactured to pharmaceutical standards today in the West. Studies show that it makes cells more efficient at using cortisol, so the adrenal gland can produce less cortisol and not work as hard. Cordyceps has been shown to be an excellent antioxidant, to increase cellular lifespan, to strengthen the immune system, improve the ability of the cell to metabolize sugar, help the liver detoxify more effectively, and increase sexual function and energy.

Ashwaganda *(withania somnifera)*: This is a powerful, balancing Ayurvedic tonic, another of my favourites. Its use as an energy herb originated in India. While its mechanisms of action are quite different from cordyceps and ginseng, its end result is similar: ashwaganda improves the utilization of cortisol and metabolism of sugar, strengthens the immune system, and is both anti-inflammatory and antioxidant. Ashwaganda has the added benefit of reducing the effects of stress – while stimulating the processes that enhance energy production, and it also has a calming effect on the nervous system.

Russian Arctic Root *(rhodiola rosea)*: Russian rhodiola has been used for decades by Russian cosmonauts and athletes to increase energy, and especially to increase stamina for endurance activities. Extensive research in Russia (and some good research in the United States and Germany) has shown that rhodiola can improve cognitive function (particularly under stress) and elevate mood by facilitating production of serotonin. It is thought to reduce stress by helping the body use cortisol more efficiently and dampening the autonomic nervous system's production of excess adrenalin. It is both an antioxidant and anti-inflammatory agent. Unlike ashwaganda and cordyceps, rhodiola can be overly excitatory. I recommend starting with a low dose of 100mg in the morning. If you take it at night it might keep you awake.

Ginseng: Similar to cordyceps, ginseng has been used for thousands of years in China as a universal remedy for balancing energy, stress, mood and immunity. In studies it's been shown to improve exercise performance and stamina, and reduce fatigue. Like cordyceps, ginseng reduces the need for the adrenals to produce cortisol, and also allows the body to utilize sugar more effectively. Ginseng is also an antioxidant. You will typically find two non-Siberian forms of ginseng in healthfood shops: *panax* (Asian) and *panax quinquefolium* (American). These two varieties can affect individuals differently. I have had patients who only get results from Asian ginseng and others who say only American works for them. Like rhodiola it can be excitatory, so start at a low dose.

Siberian ginseng *(eleutherococcus)*: Not related at all to the true ginseng family (other than bearing a passing physical resemblance), eleutherococcus is one of the most widely used adaptogens. Research has shown it can increase stamina and energy without overstimulating the nervous system. As a balancing herb, Siberian ginseng is excellent for helping you adapt to environmental, physical or emotional changes.

Shizandra *(shizandra Chinensis)*: This Chinese herb is much less known in the West, but has been highly respected in Asia for millennia as a powerful adaptogen. It has been shown to improve energy, stamina, athletic performance and recovery, as well as enhancing cognitive performance, particularly under stressful conditions. Historically it was used as one ingredient in multi-ingredient traditional Asian formulas, but more recently its powerful effect as a single herb has been recognized. As with many other adaptogens, it helps support the liver's ability to detoxify.

Liquorice root: In my four years of medical school, liquorice was one of the few herbs ever mentioned – and we were warned *not* to use it because of its known ability to raise blood pressure. While bad for hypertensives, this makes liquorice root particularly well suited for people with low energy and *low* blood pressure. While technically not classified a true adaptogen, liquorice can be very effective in supporting the adrenal gland's functions. Most people who think they have eaten liquorice have actually had a commercial preparation of aniseed-flavoured sugar gel, with no (or minimal) flavouring from liquorice. Liquorice root comes in both chewable and capsule form.

Chapter 3

Power Detox, Remove Toxins, Increase Vitality

CASE STUDY
NEVER GETTING BETTER

SAM, aged thirty-two, came to me as a last resort. A lifelong asthmatic and allergy sufferer, he had been on maximal medications for years (nasal and lung steroid inhalers, bronchodilator inhalers, anti-histamines, anti-inflammatories, expectorants, with frequent rounds of antibiotics and oral steroids) but didn't feel that he was ever heal-ing. 'It's like I'm walking on eggshells, always afraid of a flare-up. My energy is constantly low because of worry and the medications.'

His fears had come true one day a month prior to his first visit with me. He arrived at his office on a Monday morning where new carpet had been laid the previous Friday evening, and began having difficulty breathing. Within twenty-four hours he was on a respirator in the intensive care unit (ICU) with life-threatening asthma. Since then he had been placed on a number of different prescription medications for asthma. With no end to the drug regimen in sight, the approach felt to him like a plaster, not a cure.

As with most sufferers, his asthma was highly susceptible to all sorts of environmental triggers, such as dust, mould and pollen, and the bout in the ICU had shown that he was also highly chemi-cally sensitive (specially to volatile organic compound [VOCs] such as carpet adhesive and solvents). I immediately began a two-fold approach to reducing his immune system's tendency to overreact. First we worked together to remove triggers, and then I developed a treatment plan to build up his body's ability to process any unavoid-able exposure to internal and environmental triggers. I ordered further tests to determine whether he had vitamin or mineral deficiencies, subtle food allergies, an overabundance of the immune system's inflammatory messengers, or possible organ (especially digestive) dysfunction – all of which could disrupt his body's ability to process environmental toxins. He tested abnormal in all of the above areas, which meant that taking a comprehensive approach to improving his overall health – rather than just treating his symptoms – would do his asthma a world of good.

We worked on rigorously cleaning his environment, with ad-vanced HEPA filters at home and work, removal of caustic chemical cleaners, plastic shower curtains, dust mites, mould and carpet ad-hesives – the list was extensive, but he was highly motivated after his bout at the ICU. I took him off many foods he was allergic to and put him on a more plant-based diet, removing animal products that cause inflammation. He began to take a number of supplements (includ-ing omega-3 fatty acids, magnesium, the spice turmeric, medicinal mushrooms and probiotics for intestinal flora) to reduce inflamma-tion, strengthen his ability to remove toxins and support his immune system. I gave him acupuncture, initially twice weekly, then weekly to reduce inflammation and stress hormones. We included relaxation and imagery exercises combined with biofeedback breath training (see page 46) because anxiety can make asthma worse.

Within the first week he felt stronger, and after a month we be-gan to slowly taper some of his medications. Now, two years later, he has remained symptom-free, using only occasional bronchial inhalers and seasonal allergy pills. He has maintained his healthier lifestyle, and says that he feels more energetic and 'alive' than ever. He told me that he had thought before coming to me that he'd never heal, and that his healing journey had truly started when he realized there was a lot he could do to alter his frail condition.

Internal Detoxification

You have an extraordinary ability to neutralize toxins. Unlike frogs and bees and many other endangered creatures, you have elaborate mechanisms throughout your body, headquartered in the liver, for removing stuff that doesn't belong inside you and that can harm you in many different ways. This is the system that you're depending on when you're waiting for a hangover to go away or recovering from a bout of food poisoning.

But not all detox systems are equal. The strength of your internal detox abilities depends on many variables. The amount of toxins you are exposed to, your vitamin, mineral and nutrient levels, how much alcohol you drink, the amount of fibre you eat, how much exercise you get, your hydration levels, and even how much you sweat can affect your ability to isolate and excrete chemical compounds that don't belong – whether they are natural by-products of your own metabolism like free radicals, natural chemicals you've intentionally ingested like alcohol or caffeine, or one of the many industrial chemicals you are exposed to every day from air, water and food. While almost everyone is built to clean up after their own metabolism, people today have a storehouse of industrial chemicals that have accumulated over a lifetime of exposure, which makes bolstering your internal detox a high priority. In my experience, strengthening your detox mechanisms, releasing chemicals stored in your body and reducing the continual onslaught of chemicals makes a huge difference in health and energy – as it did for Sam.

Even before there was such a thing as a lab, humans evolved a sophisticated detox system. This was meant to handle the by-products of normal metabolism such as the free radicals generated by energy production that damage cells. Your cells basically have a built-in combustion engine that needs constant pollution control. The detox mechanism also evolved to remove potentially harmful, naturally occurring chemicals in plant and animal foods. With industrialization we have significantly added to the list of substances the body must neutralize.

Multiple Chemicals

There are many unknowns about the long-term effects of having multiple industrial chemicals stored in your organs, fat tissues and bloodstream. A national study commisioned by WWF-UK found a highly toxic cocktail of chemicals in every one of the 155 people it tested. In another study, an average of 75 chemicals were found in blood samples of families across the UK. The many negative ways in which the 100,000 commercial chemicals now approved for use interact with your genes and interfere with how DNA directs cellular operations and maintains health are exceedingly difficult – almost impossible – for scientists to demonstrate. Unfortunately, there are so many chemicals in our environment with the potential to affect our health in so many different ways that it's difficult to determine which ones should be removed from use. Even so, I am optimistic that you can make changes to better cope with what is known as the body-burden of industrial chemicals.

A growing body of solid scientific evidence (much of it gleaned from studying how pharmaceuticals are metabolized) shows that we do process and excrete environmental toxins, and that we can make our detox system more efficient. This is the sweet spot of my interest in environmental medicine, and it is one of the new frontiers of medicine.

'Diet, lifestyle, allergies, the health of your digestive tract, genetics, and medical history all play a role in determining how well your body handles your extensive exposure to the man-made chemicals that are a defining characteristic of modern life.'

Global warming is only half the picture of what's become of all the industrial chemicals introduced since the 19th century; the accumulation of toxic chemicals in our food and water supply and the consequent increase in the body burden of toxins is the other half. For many years I have researched methods to help my patients clean up their internal toxic load – it's a sort of Kyoto protocol for your body. With the 21-Day Plan

I will teach you how to use the latest research to improve your ability to detoxify, freeing up your resources to create energy rather than clearing out debris.

Chemicals and Your Environment

First, let's take a look at what we're up against. In the UK, over 222,000 million kilograms of pollutants are released each year, a good proportion of thesm toxic. In addition to this massive release of toxins into the air, water and soil from industrial sites, chemicals enter your body directly from chemically treated and enhanced food and the dizzying array of man-made substances you come into contact with on a daily basis. Everything from car exhaust and plastic by products to lawn fertilizers to pesticides on produce, drug residues in meats and milk, volatile organic compounds (VOCs) in paints and adhesives, cosmetics that penetrate the skin, and even pharmaceuticals and the capsules they are in randomly leave behind residues – modern chemical footprints in the human body. The fact that we've survived our collective pillaging and disruption of the environment is a testament to the resilience of the human body. No one has studied the effects of this sort of low-level exposure to multiple chemicals over time, but it has been established that combinations of toxins have additive, or synergistic, effects, meaning that the presence of one toxin can magnify the effect of another. For example, it's been demonstrated that low doses of lead and mercury – low enough to be harmless to lab animals – can become fatal when the two are administered together. Linking chemical exposures to a specific disease [in a research study] is extremely difficult, partly because the exposures are vast and uncontrolled – they occur to millions of people over great distances – and partly because the human detox enzyme system is so complex and individualized – your system may be different from your

'The mitochondrial DNA inside your cells is responsible for creating energy and is very vunerable to toxins.'

mother's, sister's or daughter's. Of course, there's also precious little research funding (from government or industry) available to analyse the problem.

One thing is certain: when toxins are present in your body they cause excess energy expenditure that can lead to fatigue and disease. All toxins can damage DNA, both directly and via free radical generation. As cells cope with contaminants, they require additional energy (known as ATP) in order to package off and remove the toxins presented. On top of that, they also need energy to fix any cellular sabotage that occurred as a result of the exposure. The liver's role as master detox mechanism also requires additional energy for each additional toxin it's presented with. All of this explains why my programme, which improves the efficiency of the detox system and reduces exposure to toxins, also helps your own energy.

Humans clearly can and do co-exist with enormous quantities of industrial chemicals (many people contain toxins in their bodies for decades without apparent harm), but in spite of the many obstacles to research, scientists have begun to make associations between pollution and many diseases – including various cancers, diabetes, obesity, asthma, reproductive disorders, cardiovascular and autoimmune diseases, and neurological development syndromes. In a review of research by the Silent Spring Institute in the US, researchers identified 216 chemicals that were linked (in at least one animal study) just to breast cancer. These included pesticides, dyes, pharmaceuticals and hormones.

The Health and Environment Alliance suggests that at least 300 toxic, man-made chemicals have been found in human blood and tissue – some of which have been banned for years. Others continue to be produced, entering our bodies through our water, the air, in consumer products or in food. What's more, a survey carried out by the UK branch of Pesticide Action Network found 80 pesticides in foods, and the survey concluded that 52 of these 'have been designated by the international authorities as having harmful effects on health'. These included 33 identified by the WHO as actually toxic, and 28 considered to be carcinogenic. In the UK, one study links

500 man-made chemicals with breast cancer; these are thought to disrupt the hormones in our bodies, and mimic the role of oestrogen – the hormone closely linked with the development of breast cancer. The ubiquitous presence of such chemicals should be reason enough for you to make an effort in shoring up your own natural detox mechanisms.

Perhaps even more disturbing was a study conducted on the umbilical cords of newborn babies. In a small study conducted by the non-profit Environmental Working Group, researchers analysed umbilical cord blood collected at birth from a random selection of infants in the United States and found that it was laced with an average of 200 industrial chemicals that entered the umbilical cord from the mother's body. Some of these substances were in concentrations that were six times those found in the mother. After birth the problem for many continues; breast milk is one method the body uses to expel fat-based toxins that it stores in the breast tissue. There's increasing evidence that women in the West produce breast milk that contains residues of industrial chemicals. I actively encourage women to breastfeed – it's nature's healthiest food – but women of child-bearing years need to be particularly careful about avoiding toxins and following the programme in the second half of this chapter for removing toxins before they get pregnant. Nobody can say for sure how these industrial chemicals – known carcinogens and nervous system toxins among them – affect your baby's earliest stages of development. No regulatory action can be taken without proof of cause and effect. But in the meantime research is beginning to hint at irreparable damage to nervous and reproductive systems.

You don't need to wait for the proverbial smoking gun to take steps to lower your body burden of toxins. In my practice, which is focused particularly on preventing illness, reducing exposure to chemicals and making sure people are neutralizing them efficiently is a universal goal – it reduces the likelihood that you will develop a disease and it frees up energy otherwise occupied in keeping your body's detox mechanisms operating on overdrive.

Your Natural Detox System: How It Works

As indelicate as this may sound, here is one of the keys to survival in the 21st century: your body has the ability to identify toxins and remove them by way of your urine, your breath, your bowel movements and even through the pores of your skin. You have a large roster of enzymes and antioxidants that can defuse toxins and flush them out before they cause damage. These systems are present in every cell, but your gut and liver are specially high-powered detox machines. The gut and liver regularly identify and package toxins to ship them out of your body on the scale of the post office at tax time. If you eat conventional, non-organic produce your urine contains a steady stream of pesticide metabolites (or residues). If you apply sunscreen, some of the chemicals in the sunscreen will be absorbed through your skin and found in your urine days later. Industrial chemicals can be detected in people's sweat. All of this is due to your natural detox system working to remove the toxins.

My goal for every patient is to improve the body's natural detox system. At the end of this chapter, and in the 21-Day Plan, you will find my step-by-step programme for boosting your body's detox mechanisms. But first, a quick primer on how your body does it, which will help you understand how the detox plan works and why it is so crucial to health and energy.

Your Gut's Instinct

Your body processes more than 25 tons of food over a lifetime, placing your gut on the frontlines of pollution control. Your intestinal tract can both absorb beneficial nutrients from food and drink and prevent absorption of harmful substances from food and drink. Unfortunately, the gut too often allows absorption of industrial chemicals and other harmful substances (like natural toxins in foods) on a regular

'The body is not a perfect detox machine; some of the chemicals are left behind in your bloodstream and stored, particularly in your fat cells.'

basis, either because it does not recognize them as harmful or it is simply too overwhelmed or damaged to
reject them all. The 6-metre/20-foot
expanse of mucus, cells, connective
tissue and muscle that constitutes
your gut ejects toxins in four ways.
First, fibre in your gut can absorb

'Evolution hasn't caught
up to pollution, and
the gut simply isn't
equipped to keep up
with all the toxins we
dump into it now.'

toxins and carry them away. Second, substances excreted into the inside of the gut by the cells lining it can try to neutralize toxins. Third,
the intestinal cells forming the wall of your gut try to reject and neutralize the toxins attempting to be absorbed through them. And finally, the cells try to stick closely together using adhesive molecules
between cells – forming a Maginot Line if you will – to prevent offenders from sneaking in between the cells out of the intestines and
into the surrounding tissues and bloodstream. And if all the above
systems within the gut fail – either because the gut is damaged or
'leaky' or the cells don't even recognize the toxins as a threat and
allow them to waltz on through – there's yet another line of defence
just beyond the intestinal wall: the immune system, composed of
your lymphatic system with its white blood cells and drainage chan-
nels. Even with all the above defensive systems, however, toxins still
escape through the gut into the rest of your body on a regular basis.

Sadly, the modern world hasn't been very good to your gut:
medication piled upon medication; ever more powerful germs; damaging levels of stress with no relief; and the abysmal contemporary
diet loaded with unnatural chemicals have all breached, and in some
cases even shattered, the gut's defences.

The gut has a limited ability to recognize and neutralize mercury, for example. After toxins like mercury or PCBs or organo-
phosphate pesticides have made it past the gut, the next stop is your
liver, where once again you're left with what evolution has given you,
which in the case of the liver is a pretty sophisticated, but often overwhelmed detox system.

Your Liver: Gatekeeper and Detox Machine

While the liver's function includes making cholesterol and processing fats, proteins and carbohydrates, much of its energy is expended
detoxifying your body. All food absorbed by the intestines is shunted
first to the liver before the body will allow it into the general circulation. Likewise, inhaled and topical agents can wind up in the liver for
detox. Once the liver receives any chemical it must decide whether or
not a substance gets a green light (beneficial nutrients pass through
untouched); a yellow light (substances like triglycerides get tagged for
reprocessing); or a red light (toxic substances from industrial chemicals to cigarette smoke get red-flagged for detox and elimination).

The liver's job goes far beyond identifying toxins; it is also able
to transform the vast array of harmful molecules your body encounters (including alcohol, pollution, food additives, pharmaceuticals or
even flu viruses) into harmless molecules that can be easily sent out
of the body as waste. (In its spare time it also produces 80 per cent of
the body's cholesterol needs, stores glucose in the form of glycogen,
processes extra calories into triglycerides and other fats, and has an
internal immune system.) Fortunately with this huge list of critical
responsibilities, the liver is constantly renewing itself – it is one of
the body's fastest regenerating organs.

The liver accomplishes its remarkably precise clean-up in two
phases that even a Comet repairman could admire. First, it employs
a large family of enzymes, called *cytochromes*, to turn specific toxins into general free radicals – this is known as *Phase I liver detox*.
Secondly, the resulting free radicals (called toxic intermediaries) are
then neutralized by the liver's highly sophisticated army of free radical fighting *conjugators* – this is known as *Phase II liver detox*. If you
think of your liver as your internal washing machine, the liver enzymes of Phase I are the laundry pre-treatment – they are a kind of
Vanish for your bloodstream. Once the enzymes have removed the
'stains', the Phase II conjugators step in as a sort of all-purpose Persil
for your bloodstream. Working together, the two phases of detox are
able to remove toxins from your body.

There are lots of molecular players in both phases of liver detox. During Phase I detox at least 120 members of the enzyme family known as cytochrome P450s pretreat the hundreds of thousands of toxins that your body encounters every day. Exactly which member of the liver enzyme family is involved in taming a particular toxin depends on the substance that's being neutralized. For example, caffeine, certain pesticides, some of the carcinogens found in cigarettes, and the polyaromatic amines found in charbroiled beef are all detoxified by the activity of one cytochrome known as CYP1A2. Certain antibiotics like erythromycin require a different cytochrome, CYP3A4, to be metabolized. The abilities of a particular cytochrome to properly detox a range of molecules can vary significantly from individual to individual, and this is often what accounts for different people's threshold of tolerance to different chemicals.

Idiosyncrasies in the cleaning power of a particular enzyme can be largely genetic, which is a white-hot area of scientific research at the moment. For example, when it comes to digesting caffeine, which is metabolized through your Phase I detox pathway, there are two types of people in the world – rapid caffeine metabolizers and slow caffeine metabolizers. The difference is due to a slight variation in the gene code for CYP1A2 (called a genetic polymorphism). About half of all Caucasians have the slow variant of the gene code, which means caffeine hangs around in their systems longer, versus only 14 per cent of Asians. In one fascinating study of 2,014 men and women published in *The Journal of the American Medical Association (JAMA)* in 2006, being a slow caffeine metabolizer was associated with a dramatically increased risk of heart attack for subjects who drank more than four cups of coffee per day, whereas fast caffeine metabolizers drinking more than four cups per day had a reduced risk of heart attack compared to the control group. Drinking one cup a day had no effect, regardless of your genetic makeup. That's a significant difference in heart attack risk for heavy coffee drinkers based solely on

'If caffeine easily gives you the jitters, drinking more than one cup a day could be deleterious to your health.'

how your liver is genetically programmed to detoxify caffeine!

This study demonstrates how the activity of your liver's Phase I enzyme detox system can have a profound effect not only on how you feel, but also on your overall health and energy. As the science of genomic medicine advances, researchers are continually discovering more about the body's various detox enzyme systems. For example, a European study published in the *Journal of the US National Institute of Environmental Health* established that for men, an individual's gene code for Phase I detox of the industrial pollutant PCBs (found commonly in oily fish) determined whether or not the presence of PCBs in the bloodstream caused a decrease in sperm count. Your liver's ability to detoxify can even affect your sperm count! One exciting result of the latest research is that simple blood tests are becoming available that allow your doctor to measure many of these cytochrome detox capabilities, and doctors can use this information to better individualize dosages for drug therapies.

How Busy Is Your Liver?

Beyond genetics, the other variable that affects how well your liver's Phase I cytochromes work is how busy they are. The more substances they have to face, the less chance there is that they will be able to fully detoxify all the substances they are responsible for. This is why, for example, grapefruit juice can affect drug dosages. Compounds in grapefruit juice inhibit the ability of specific members of the cytochrome P450 family of enzymes to metabolize certain drugs. This allows the drugs to build up in the body, a process that can be very harmful, yet has also been used therapeutically. For example, certain drugs (such as the potentially heart-toxic chemotherapy drug adriamycin) can be given in one-half to one-third the normal dosage when the patient drinks one glass of grapefruit juice a day. By monopolizing a Phase I detox system, grapefruit juice causes the drugs to hang around longer in the bloodstream.

This can be the case with any Phase I detox enzyme system. Any substance, for example a specific chemical in cigarette smoke, can monopolize a Phase I cytochrome and cause another substance, such as a specific pesticide, to hang around longer in your bloodstream, leaving the body no choice but to store it in your fat cells. In this way, overloading your detox enzyme system can cause chemicals to build up in your body as they wait their turn to be detoxified. This toxin gridlock can have a damaging effect on your health including disrupting your hormone balance, your nervous system, your immune system and even your reproductive system. Because your Phase I detox system has this limited capacity, it's critically important to reduce your exposure to toxins.

Sometimes the opposite problem can arise: your Phase I detox system is going great guns and your Phase II system cannot keep up the pace – usually due to a dearth of raw materials (nutrients) from food needed to get the job done. Think of using a lot of Vanish on a stain and then not washing the shirt. You're left with a disgusting shirt. Well, it's the same with your internal washing machine; if your Phase I system is working away and Phase II is inadequate, then you're going to feel disgusting – generally you'll have a hungover feeling that won't go away.

Taming Toxins

As I pointed out at the beginning of this section, Phase II relies on an army of free radical-fighting antioxidants called conjugators. Conjugators are amino acids that specifically target free radical compounds from Phase I; they efficiently neutralize the compounds and allow them to be eliminated. These conjugators are continually made by your body, and they all can come from key nutrients that you must eat. Problems arise when either your Phase II conjugators are depleted or your Phase I system is on overdrive. When this happens you get a build-up of free radicals – you're oxidized or rusty! And you need more free-

'A detox programme that reduces the toxic load presented to Phase I and is rich in food substances that increase Phase II detox can bring back vital energy.'

radical fighters fast. For tips on how to improve Phase II see the programme at the end of this chapter.

The importance of maintaining balance between the two phases of the liver's detoxification processes is a critical open secret, but
many doctors are clueless about it. Too many toxins/drugs/chemi-
cals can overwhelm Phase I and lead to toxin build-up in the body,
with resultant low energy and ill health. The flip side of this is that
it is not uncommon for people to have normally functioning Phase
I systems, but poorly functioning Phase II systems, thus setting up
a situation of *oxidative stress* – with a build-up of large quantities of
unquenched free radicals from Phase I that can also lead to illness
and low energy. I often suspect that the liver's detox phases are out
of whack when people tell me they feel like they've got a constant
hangover – or, like Sam, when they're waking up fatigued and feeling
like they never have quite enough energy.

You will learn how to build a better detox system in the last section of this chapter, 'Boost Your Detox System'.

The Solutions: Zap Toxins and Build a Better Detox System
Reduce Your Exposure

At the risk of sounding like Dr Strangelove, I have to emphasize that
toxins do have a remarkable talent for getting into your body, and
the first step in any good detox programme is to slow the flow. Consider the ways in which toxins can make their way into your cells:

- Chemicals can drift in through your nose and mouth as volatile organic
  compounds (VOCs) like paints and solvents, or simply as fine particles
  like most air pollution from car exhaust and industrial smokestacks.
- Toxins can be absorbed through your skin, as is the case with
  thousands of chemicals used in cosmetics (some of which are known
  carcinogens). Chemicals used in sunscreens (on average 4 per cent
  of what's applied to the skin) have been found in people's urine up
  to five days after application – to get there they had to pass through

multiple skin layers and into the bloodstream, potentially depositing some molecules for storage in fat cells, before being shuffled off to the liver for detox and excretion. For this reason, researchers recommend that infants (whose detox systems are not fully developed) be protected with non-toxic sunscreens specially formulated for them.

- Contaminants can enter with the water you drink – modern water-treatment plants are not designed to remove most industrial chemicals including pharmaceuticals. A report by the UK's Royal Society of Chemistry (RSC) found that synthetic chemicals from consumer and healthcare products bypass filters at water purification plants. The list includes phthalates, a family of 120 chemicals linked to reproductive problems in men, and parabens, preservatives with a suspected link to breast cancer.

- A 2008 report by the Drinking Water Inspectorate (DWI) found that pharmaceuticals including cancer and psychiatric drugs, are finding their way into the UK water supply. Visit their website for details of all chemicals that can appear in our water and what's being done about it: www.dwi.gov.uk.

- Our food supply is laced with chemicals: some, like PCBs and DDT, have been banned for years, but never leave the environment and are ubiquitously present at low levels – even in whole organic milk. Other toxins are still in use: just last year Teflon (used for non-stick cookware and even clothes and carpets) was identified as a 'probable human carcinogen' and inventer and manufacturer Du Pont has agreed to stop using it (though not until 2015). Hundreds of new chemicals are introduced every year for use in farming and food manufacture.

Unlike the film *Dr Strangelove*, this chemical horror story is not a product of anyone's imagination – it's public information, although you may have to dig deep to find it. Between your respiratory system, your skin and your digestive tract, your body is an open door to every conceivable toxin. With this cumulative load of chemicals in so many aspects of your life, it is essential to make a concerted effort to reduce exposure in any possible way. Here's how I would prioritize the project to zap toxins.

Eat Organics

Let's begin in a realm that has the greatest impact on toxic load and lends itself to maximum control: the food you eat. Food can deliver a toxic punch to your system in a number of ways. Almost any food can carry bacteria such as salmonella or E. coli; *conventional produce* – grown using agricultural chemicals such as pesticides and herbicides – can carry toxic residues; and any processed food – packaged in jars, tins, bottles, cartons and plastic containers and made at an industrial facility by a food producer – can contain additives, preservatives, colourings, thickeners, dough conditioners, flavourings or any one of the thousands of chemicals approved for use in commercial food preparation. More than 12,000 ingredients end up in the food supply of the average Western nation as a result of processing and curing according to Ruth Winters in her marvellously detailed book, *A Consumer's Dictionary of Food Additives.* To give you more perspective on the chemical load in your food, UK manufacturers spend millions of pounds each year on flavourings and flavour enhancers alone – just a fraction of many, many additives. It's not only the ingredients in processed food, but also packaging that can leach substances into the food. The food industry has a lot of technical data to convince you these chemicals are safe to eat for a lifetime. But I'd rather you fill your stomach with the marvellous vitamins, minerals, fibre, phytochemicals and beneficial oils that plants have to offer, especially because scientists are constantly discovering new important functions these wonderful natural food constituents perform.

'Eating organics – food grown with old-fashioned methods such as soil composting and non-toxic pest management – is the best way I know of imbibing nature's bounty with minimal interference from synthetic chemicals.'

That said, it would be nearly impossible to buy only organic foods and, depending on where you live, this could also be an expensive proposition. But you can prioritize your organic food choices.

Beware of Pesticide Loads
Buy organic versions of these fruits and veggies, whose
conventionally grown versions have been found to have the
highest pesticide loads:

Peas	Cherries	Apples	Lettuce
Grapes	Celery	Pears	Nectarines
Spinach	Strawberries	Potatoes	Peaches

Produce: The Pesticide Action Network, a campaign group working to eliminate toxic pesticides, tested a range of fruit, vegetables and other food stuffs for pesticide residues. Among the worst offenders were flour and bread, potatoes, apples, strawberries, pre-packed salads and tomatoes. Another study found peaches, apples, peppers, celery, nectarines and strawberries to have the heaviest toxic loads – one conventional apple can carry as many as 14 different pesticides! Above is a list of the dozen most polluted fruits and vegetables; I recommend that you bring this list to the supermarket and commit to buying organics for these items. You get a break on onions, asparagus, mangoes and avocados, which have been shown to carry the least amount of chemicals. A good general rule of thumb is: the thicker the skin (for example, bananas, citrus fruit and avocados), the lower the amount of chemicals that have been absorbed into the flesh that you eat. Careful washing (especially with a safe citrus-based produce wash) is still in order, however, to prevent chemical residues on the produce skin from contaminating what's inside.

I recommend avoiding foods grown with pesticides whenever possible. It's never too late to change: just five days of an organic food diet was enough to dramatically decrease the levels of pesticides measured in the urine of children in a convincing study conducted in 2006 at the Rollins School of Public Health, Emory University in the US. In their conclusions, the study's authors wrote, 'We were able to

The Problem with Pesticides

Most people ask me, 'Well, what's so bad about pesticides?'
Let's start with how most pesticides work – they are mostly
neurotoxins built to fatally damage a pest's nervous system. In
animal studies, many pesticides appear to target the dopamine-
producing neurons in the brain involved in coordinating
movement. At the very least, it's advisable not to ingest even
minute amounts of known neurotoxins on a regular basis.
On another level, many pesticides have been shown to disrupt
the body's hormone signalling mechanisms – altering levels
of thyroid and oestrogen among other deleterious effects. In
fact, scientists now place the majority of pesticides in a class of
environmental pollutants known as hormone disruptors. (In
high doses, pesticides kill by being neurotoxins, but in relatively
small doses with long-term exposure they can produce adverse
reactions such as hormone disruption.) Such chemicals are
implicated in epidemiological trends toward reproductive
disorders (such as infertility) and hormone-based cancers
like prostate and breast cancer. Finally, many pesticides are
carcinogenic and others are tumour promoters. There are only
a limited number of studies that evaluate the cancer risk for
individual pesticides, though, and much more work is required
before detailed assessments can be made.

demonstrate that an organic diet provides a dramatic and immediate
protective effect against exposures to organophosphorus pesticides.'
And for my money, that's reason enough to switch to organics.

Processed Foods: Any food that's prepared and packaged for you
is 'processed', and just about everything in a package – salad dressings, frankfurters, biscuits, milk, bread, cereal – is processed. Getting
those products to the supermarket where they can sit on a shelf and

look pretty requires food engineering, which for the most part involves industrial chemicals.

From the point of view of convenience, processed foods give people what they are often looking for – quick, cheap calories with a flavour punch. Processed foods also give the major food companies what they are looking for – revenue. The processed food industry is one of the largest manufacturing sectors in the UK.

The problem is that, when you eat a processed food, for the most part you don't know what you're eating! The inclusion of potentially carcinogenic nitrates in processed meats is one example. Another is the widespread use in processed foods of ingredients made from genetically modified (GMO) crops. I was shocked to learn that 60 per cent of processed foods contain GMO ingredients (on the other hand, no organic foods with a British or EU organic kitemark contains GMOs). Processed foods routinely include corn and soya products made from GMO crops. The long-term health effects of eating foods that contain GMOs are unknown, but I have some concerns. For example, GMO corn is engineered specifically to tolerate more Roundup weed killer. The result has been an increase with GMOs in the use of Roundup. Other GMOs have the ability to produce their own pesticides built into the plant's DNA. None of this has been studied for long-term health effects. By avoiding processed foods you also avoid eating GMOs – which from my perspective is a very good idea.

Genetically mutated plants are only one of the unsavoury ingredients you might encounter in a processed food. A bottle of popular French salad dressing contains 18 ingredients (not including water). There is absolutely no healthy reason that a dish you can make at home with two ingredients – oil and vinegar (plus maybe a pinch of salt and a squeeze of lemon juice or teaspoon of mustard) – should contain 18 ingredients, including sugar, colourings, xanthan gum, calcium disodium EDTA, maize (corn) starch and tartaric acid. You don't need that junk, especially not on top of your beautiful organic vegetable salad!

I want you to buy your food one ingredient at a time – fish,

> ### Processed Meats and Bacon
> *Studies demonstrate a connection between consumption of processed meats and stomach cancer, colon cancer and bladder cancer. Processed meats (including sausages, bacon, frankfurters and processed hams) often contain nitrite or nitrate and N-nitroso compounds, which are potent carcinogens that can induce tumours in animal species. Processed meats also usually contain high amounts of salt, which can irritate the stomach lining and enhance the carcinogenic effects of compounds. Recent studies detailing these connections with more than 100,000 subjects are considered preliminary. Until there's further direct evidence of deleterious effects, food companies can continue to sell meats processed with nitrates and salt. But you don't have to eat them!*

broccoli, onions, garlic, olive oil, lettuce, apples, walnuts – you get the picture. I realize how difficult it is to avoid those long stretches of processed food aisles in the typical supermarket, but it's crucial that you do. My nutrition superhero, Marion Nestle, renowned nutritionist and professor of nutrition, food studies and public health at New York University, puts it succinctly: 'My rule of thumb is to never buy foods that have more than five ingredients. The more processed a food is, the more ingredients it is likely to have and the lower the nutritional quality.' And I would add that the more synthetic ingredients in a food, the higher the chance that you are eating something bad for you that requires more energy to metabolize.

Milk and Red Meat: The value of buying organic milk is a subject of heated debate, though when you look at the facts it's pretty clear that buying organic milk is a no-brainer. The crux of the matter is in how farmers get cows to produce more milk. In her book *What To Eat*, Marion Nestle points out that in an attempt to cut costs and meet demand over the past thirty years the dairy industry has doubled the amount of milk obtained from each cow in the US, mostly by injecting the animals with hormones – and in particular BST. While BST has been banned in the UK and EU, and the use of growth hormones prohibited, pesticides in animal feed, as well as antibiotics, GMOs and other chemicals do make their way into meat and milk. What's more, the current surge in the US of resistant E. coli infections in meat is partly the result of using suboptimal doses of antibiotics that select out for highly resistant bacteria. In the 21-Day Plan I recommend reducing your dairy intake and eliminating red meat altogether because I want you to avoid saturated fat as well as potential toxins.

Chicken: A lot of my patients, when asked to switch from red meat, start eating more chicken. Chicken is a pretty decent meat alternative: lower in saturated fat and associated arachadonic acid, especially if cooked with the skin off, which is where most of the saturated fat resides in chickens. But conventional chickens can be polluted. Extensive use of antibiotics in conventional poultry farming in the US has resulted in an increase in antibiotic resistant bacteria, especially salmonella. Birds sold under organic labels cannot legally be given routine antibiotics and vaccinations can only be used if there is known disease that cannot be controlled by any other means. And because their feed is higher quality, they usually taste better.

Buying Chicken: A chicken can only be as healthy as its upbringing, and the only way to determine that is to look behind the claims being made on the label. Problem is, it's hard to separate the hype from reality. The list overleaf explains what the labels mean in the UK marketplace.

'A recent survey by the UK's RSPCA reveals that 73 per cent of consumers now buy higher welfare chicken since learning about the conditions in which standard chickens are farmed.'

- The 'Red Tractor' symbol is part of a voluntary scheme. Birds with the symbol meet assurance standards, guaranteeing the health of the flocks and food safety. Red Tractor chickens have been reared to a minimum welfare standard. These are conditions for 'standard' chickens and already exceed the EU welfare rules being introduced in 2012. Worth paying extra for.
- 'Extensive indoor' or 'barn-reared': these chickens mustn't be packed more than 15 to a square metre of living space (and not more than 25kg per square metre in combined weight); they shouldn't be slaughtered before they are 56 days old.
- 'Free range': the maximum indoor stocking density is 13 birds per square metre (and not more than 27.5kg per square metre); in addition, each bird, for at least half its life, should have continuous daytime access to open-air runs with a maximum density of one bird per square metre.
- 'Traditional free-range': the maximum indoor stocking density is 12 birds per square metre (and not more than 25kg per square metre); continuous daytime access to open-air runs should be given from the age of six weeks, and these runs should allow at least 2 square metres per chicken; poultry houses shouldn't contain more than 4,800 chickens. Slow-growing varieties of chicken should be used, with a minimum slaughter age of 81 days.
- 'Free-range – Total Freedom': in addition to the criteria for 'traditional free-range' chickens, these birds should have open-air runs of unlimited area.
- 'Organic' chickens are free-range and slower grown. They are slaughtered at 81 days, given organic feed (containing no GMOs) and no routine antibiotics. They are kept in smaller flocks, with more space to move about inside and out.
- Freedom Food is the scheme for animals reared to the RSPCA's welfare standards. Chickens are more slowly grown and stocking densities are lower, though they are not necessarily free-range birds.

Fish: Fish provides the marvellous omega-3 fatty acids that we can't get enough of, yet paradoxically the fat that is so healthy for us is also the main repository in fish for storing environmental toxins – primarily mercury and PCBs, but also dioxin and pesticides (especially in farmed varieties). What's the problem with this stuff?

- **Mercury is a non-biodegradable (it lasts forever) heavy metal, released into the air primarily from industrial sources (especially from coal-burning plants), that falls in rain and snow into the planet's water supplies. Industries have also disposed of it by dumping into the ocean, into migratory paths of fish. According to the Environmental Protection Agency in the US, mercury concentrations in fish can be 1 to 10 million times its concentration in water due to 'biomagnification' (when small fish with low mercury levels get eaten by bigger fish – like swordfish and tuna – the predator's mercury increases exponentially). When people eat mercury it targets the nervous system and the kidneys. The developing brain and nervous system of a foetus are most vulnerable, but adults are also at risk. In my practice, 80 per cent of people eating fish (which is often tuna) frequently have mercury levels above limits deemed acceptable by government regulatory bodies (which allow concentrations of mercury in food up to 1 part per million, which is more mercury than I'm comfortable with eating on a regular basis). Symptoms include numbness, fatigue, irritability and loss of memory. Fortunately most of us can clear lower levels of mercury from our bodies within a month of two if we discontinue eating foods contaminated with it.**
- **PCBs (polychlorinated biphenyls) are industrial pollutants used in a number of different ways including engine coolants, flame retardants and in carbonless copy paper. PCBs were banned from use in the UK over thirty years ago, but, like DDT, still persist in the environment and accumulate in fatty foods, especially fish. PCB exposure regularly affects the brain and the nervous and hormone systems. It can damage the immune and reproductive systems, and has been linked to cancer as well as increased rates of allergies.**
- **Dioxins persist in the environment as a result of industrial processes, such as the production of certain herbicides and disinfectants, waste incineration and chlorine bleaching of pulp at paper mills (small**

amounts of dioxins are also produced naturally during forest fires and volcanic eruptions). Dioxin has a destructive effect on the immune system that caused the World Health Organisation to label it a 'known human carcinogen'. It also affects the reproductive, endocrine, circulatory and nervous systems.

Fish are not the only sources of exposure for these contaminants, but they are the source of heaviest exposure. In addition to environmental exposure, the fishing industry does not have tough standards for pesticide use in farming. While some farm-raised fish are relatively toxin free (notably prawns and tilapia), farm-raised fish can be treated with a combination of parasiticides and antibiotics and, in the case of farm-raised salmon, even food colouring to make its flesh look pinker. What's more, they can be fed corn or other grain, which reduces the amount of beneficial omega-3 fatty acids that come from the typical wild algae-based diet. And the overcrowded conditions in which farmed fish live are not only inhumane, but increasingly breed disease, foul the nearby waters and endanger indigenous fish species. Because of the problem with pollution I strongly recommend you make careful choices in the fish you eat.

The following table comes from my favourite source of data on the health of the world's fish populations, the non-profit Environmental Defense Fund website, www.edf.org. This organization continually monitors health advisories from more than 120 government and scientific databases to come up with an overall safety rating for each type of fish. Scientists at Environmental Defense Fund calculate recommended consumption levels based on methodology developed by the EPA in the US. I like the way EDF works with the data, telling you how many meals you can eat per month. Their assumptions are based on weight and portion size (which I've detailed below), so you can find a mix that's right for you. Mercury is particularly toxic to foetuses and young children, so the women's category is more conservative. In the UK, pregnant women are advised to eat no more than two portions of oily fish per week, and shark, swordfish and marlin should be off the menu. I'd take that one step further and suggest that pregnant women should avoid fish altogether.

Your Monthly Fish Allotment: A Numbers Game

The number of times per month *you can eat fish depends on what fish you're eating – if you stay within the 4+, you can have at least four meals,* total, per month.* *Exposure is cumulative: eating fish from a highly contaminated group (0 to 3) reduces the number of meals you can have overall.*

FISH	MEALS PER MONTH		HEALTH
	Women**	Men**	RISK
Wild Alaskan salmon	4+	4+	Low Level
Crab	4+	4+	Mercury
Monkfish	4+	4	Mercury
English Sole	4+	4+	PCBs
Snapper	4+	4+	Mercury
Atlantic mackerel	4+	4+	Low Level
Prawns	4+	4+	Low Level
Tilapia	4+	4+	Low Level
Farmed rainbow trout	4+	4+	Low Level
Clams	4+	4+	Low Level
Farmed oysters	4+	4+	Low Level
Black sea bass	4+	4+	Mercury
Canned light tuna	4+	4+	Mercury
Mahi mahi	4+	4+	Mercury
Skate	4+	4+	Mercury
Halibut	4+	4+	Mercury
Yellowfin tuna	4	3	Mercury
Eel	3	3	Mercury
Wild oysters	3	3	PCBs
RockFish	2	2	Mercury, PCBs
Mackerel	2	2	Mercury
Flounder	1	1	PCBs
Atlantic salmon	1	1	PCBs
Swordfish	0	1	Mercury
Bluefin tuna (sushi)	0	0	Mercury, PCBs

* Source: environmentaldefensefund.org at www.edf.org
** Note: Assumes 65kg/144lb woman and a 170g/6oz portion; and 78kg/172lb man and a 230g/8oz portion. Children have a lower threshold of tolerance and should eat less fish. I suggest that pregnant women should *not* eat fish.

The Air You Breathe

What sent my patient Sam to the intensive care unit was exposure to the volatile organic compounds (VOCs) in carpet adhesive. VOCs are petroleum-based chemical compounds that readily evaporate – becoming caustic airborne toxins – from a vast array of products including paints and lacquers, paint strippers, cleaning supplies, pesticides, building materials and furnishings, office equipment such as copiers and printers, correction fluids, adhesives, permanent felt-tips, nail varnish and fuel. VOCs are consistently higher indoors (up to ten times higher) than outdoors and the EPA in the US admits VOCs may have short- and long-term adverse health effects. In comparison to other pollutants, the monitoring of VOCs in the UK is not yet well developed and there is no long-term database of information. However, there is in place an EU directive that limits the maximum level of VOCs that can be contained in decorative paints, stains and varnishes. According to several studies, including one by ALSPAC (Avon Longitudinal Study of Parents and Children) short-term exposure to 'cocktails' of VOCs can aggravate symptoms of fatigue, headaches, dizziness, eye and skin irritation within 8 hours of use. Long-term exposure has been linked to the development of cancer, respiratory disease, immune system suppression, birth defects and even genetic changes.

A growing variety of building materials and household prod-

Non-toxic is Chic

Interior designers often prefer the following for their natural look, but I like them because they are healthier for you. Ask for these when you renovate:

Soya-based paint remover	*Milk and clay paints*
Zero VOC paints	*Venetian (polished) plasters*
Beeswax polish & wood finisher	*Natural clay plaster finishes*
Low VOC glazes, lacquer and sealants	

VOC Labelling

More than ten voluntary labels are used in Europe for many low-emission products. In the UK, VOC labels are used and indicate the content of VOCs using one of five classifications: Minimal (0 – 0.29 per cent), Low, Medium, High and Very High (VOC content greater than 50 per cent).

ucts emit low or no VOCs, and it's worth doing your homework to track down these healthy alternatives.

If low-VOC paints haven't hit your local DIY shop you might want to point out to them that occupation as a painter has consistently been associated with a 40 per cent increased risk of lung cancer. Conventional paints are typically loaded with VOCs that fly out of the tin and enter your respiratory system, wreaking havoc on your DNA. The DIY industry has been quietly acknowledging the health hazards in paint, and a number of companies have begun to offer healthier options. One of my favourite brands is Auro decorating products, which stand out among manufacturers of natural paints and wood finishes because they are totally committed and uncompromising in their environmental aims and standards. A good range of other non-VOC paints is now on the market – take the time to find them.

Another major source of VOCs, carpet offgassing, can include a mix of up to two hundred different chemicals including the probable carcinogen formaldehyde. The source of chemicals can be the carpet fibres, the backing, or the adhesives used at installation. While offgassing can last for weeks according to environmental scientists who measure such things, there are also long-term concerns. Fitted carpets can harbour environmental toxins including fungal spores, bacteria and dust-mite droppings (researchers have found an average of 67 grams of dust per square metre of carpet). There are numerous solutions:

- First and foremost, use area rugs whenever possible.
- Go for natural fibres – the rug itself should be cotton or wool (though beware of wools treated with mothproofing).
- Check the backing – latex and backing that's glued on, rather than sewn, can offgas a multitude of chemicals. Look for carpets with jute or other natural backings sewn on.
- If you must have fitted carpets make sure the installers are using tacks, not adhesives. If they must use adhesive, ask for a non-toxic type such as Tremco or STK.
- Last but not least, buy a high-quality vacuum cleaner with a certified HEPA filter to capture small particles rather than bringing them up from the floor then spewing them out the back end. Use it often.

The Way You Clean: Cleaning is an important way to reduce environmental toxins, but all too often it simply adds to the chemical burden. It's a good idea to evaluate all of your cleaning products and habits for potential VOC exposure. The rule of thumb is to start with those products you're most in contact with – hand soap, laundry detergent and softener, shampoo, body wash and body lotion, work surface and other cleaners – all can be sources of toxic chemicals.

Take a good look at the hand soap you use every day. I am opposed to antibacterial soaps. First of all, studies have shown it's primarily the length of time you scrub under running water that determines how clean your hands get (the amount of time it takes to get through one verse of the Happy Birthday song is just about right for a good handwashing). Second, there's mounting evidence that the antibacterial compound triclocarbon (called triclosan on most labels) is a hormone disruptor that may be linked to rises in reproductive problems – and this chemical is not removed from the environment by water treatment plants. If you really need to sterilize your hands, use a 70-plus per cent alcohol product, or a reputable name such as Dettol, Carex or AHS.

Bottom line: buy a simple handsoap without chemical or antibiotic additives. I'm also a big believer in using non-biological, scent- and dye-free laundry detergent (residues of which can stay

'Be aware that cleaning products are known to contain carcinogens, reproductive system toxins, allergens and neurotoxic substances. Luckily, every day there seem to be new, gentler and safer products on the market for keeping your house and your environment clean.'

in contact with your skin all day and night). In general, stay hyper-vigilant about the products you are using at home. (A good place to look for such products is www.ecohip.org, which lists and sells some of the best possible natural, organic and eco-friendly products. Another site to try is Green Essentials: www.greenessentials.co.uk.) Learn about these cleaners of the future and start using them; you will no doubt notice, as have I, that these healthier products smell better than their more toxic counterparts, and they tend to energize – as they sanitize – your environment.

A Word About Plastics

I predict you'll be hearing a lot more about the hazards of plastics in coming years. It is estimated that UK consumers use more than 13.1 billion plastic bottles per year! A growing number of scientists are concluding that certain plastics can expose people to harmful chemicals – especially when used for storing and serving food. Of major concern is a basic ingredient in many plastics called *bisphenol A* (BPA). Historically used to make polycarbonate tableware, water and wine bottles, baby bottles and food tin linings, plastics that contain bisphenol-A are not yet labelled in the UK, as they are in Canada and the US, despite calls from numerous health pressure groups such as the National Childbirth Trust. BPA has been found to leach from bottles into babies' milk; from tin liners into foods; and from bottles into soft drinks and water. Scientists have identified BPA as a hormone disruptor, and have begun to establish a link between low levels of this chemical and some diseases on the rise in the West, specifically obesity and diabetes. In Japan, plastics manufacturers voluntarily discontinued using BPA, the Canadian equivalent of the US Food and Drug Administration classified BPA as a dangerous substance, and manufacturers in the US are beginning to discontinue its use as well. Some, but by no means all, UK manufacturers plan to follow suit. At present, the European Food Safety Authority (EFSA) has concluded thet the current tolerable daily intake (TDI) of 0.05mg/kg of body weight per day remains valid. This may not be good news for concerned consumers.

Yet another ingredient in plastics, called *phthalates*, may be an even bigger problem. The United States is one of the few developed

Safer Plastics

Follow these recommendations for reducing exposure to toxins in plastics.

- *Seek out glass, ceramic, stoneware, wood and stainless steel materials for kitchen equipment and food storage.*
- *Avoid storing fatty foods, such as meat and cheese, in plastic containers or cling film.*
- *Use stainless steel or wooden utensils for cooking.*
- *Check recycling codes and look for safer plastics such as 2HDPE, 4LDPE and 5PP.*
- *Avoid plastics that have been shown to leak hazardous materials into food: 3PVC, 6PS and 7.*
- *Avoid putting plastic in the dishwasher.*
- *Throw away plastics with cracks or cloudiness.*
- *Use glass baby bottles or plastic bag inserts that are polypropylene or polyethyelene (number 5).*
- *Do not microwave foods in plastic containers.*
- *Do not allow cling film to come in contact with hot food.*
- *Follow expiration dates on tinned foods, which typically employ plastic liners.*

countries to permit the import of plastic toys made with this poly-vinyl chloride (PVC) additive. This is a concern that's very well explained by author Mark Schapiro in his terrific book, *Exposed: The Toxic Chemistry of Everyday Products and What's at Stake for American Power.* He writes, 'In the average home phthalates are everywhere – in shower curtains, shampoo bottles and even raincoats. A component of that distinct "new car smell" comes from phthalates in the dashboard. It's been found in umbilical cord and breast milk. Phthalates when ingested can impede the production of LH, a hormone responsible for triggering cells in the testes to produce testosterone, and for the normal menstrual cycle.' Phthalates were banned in toys and childcare articles sold in Europe eight years ago, although in the UK this only extends to toys and items that are put in a baby or child's mouth. You should try to avoid them. Here are my suggestions for reducing your exposure to plastic residues.

Aeroplanes and Cars

Aeroplane and car interiors can be full of pollutants primarily due to the materials used for the interior finishes, which are made of plastics that outgas (particularly when temperatures rise), circulating particles of the plasticizers known as phthalates, which are known hormone disruptors (see above). In addition, by virtue of travelling at or above 30,000 feet in the atmosphere, aeroplane cabin air can contain high levels of ozone (in particular, narrow-bodied planes rarely have ozone control systems). Ozone is a known respiratory system irritant (it's been shown that the more overweight a person is, the more likely it is that ozone will cause breathing problems). In one fascinating study in the journal *Environmental Science and Technology* researchers demonstrated that oils on your skin and hair can react with ozone, magnifying its deleterious effects. The take-home message of that study was that if you shower before a flight you may feel better afterwards. For all these reasons – and because of the numerous cleaning products used in between flights – aeroplane cabin air can be particularly challenging for people with allergic, asthmatic and other respiratory conditions.

If you have to fly every week for a living or spend a lot of time in your car, short of wearing a gas mask, you will want to follow the detox programme at the end of this chapter and in the 21-Day Plan, include as many organics in your diet as possible, and make sure you reduce toxins in the other parts of your life that you have more control over.

Cosmetics

Mercury in mascara, lead in lipstick, coal tar (a known human carcinogen) in toothpaste and mouthwash. Killer cosmetics may be the least of your health worries, but they present a hazard indeed. In fact, cosmetics present enough of a hazard that the European Union has taken steps to limit toxic chemicals in personal products. In January 2003 the EU banned the use of chemicals that are known or strongly suspected of causing cancer, mutation or birth defects.

There are, however, other chemicals that routinely feature in cosmetics and personal hygiene products, which have not been banned in the EU and which may pose a risk to health. Short of going completely au naturel, there are steps you can take to reduce dangerous exposures. Carefully evaluate your sources of greatest exposure; products that you use over a large surface of your body – such as moisturizing lotion or bubble bath. Lipstick, toothpaste and mouthwash, of course, come in direct contact with your mouth and gums, where they can be readily absorbed. On the following page there is a list of ingredients to avoid – check the labels... it's all about choices. In the UK, visit www.safecosmetics.org.uk for details of the safest personal care products.

'The main systems responsible for maintaining energy – nervous and cardiovascular systems and the mitochondrial respiratory chain – are damaged by heavy metals.'

Cosmetics Not to Die For

Here is a list of cosmetic ingredients that contain potential health hazards. I'd avoid them. For more information on other potentially dangerous ingredients in cosmetics and personal care products, visit the Women's Environmental Network at www.wen.org.uk.

Ingredient	Might Be Found In . . .	Potential Health Hazard
Triclosan	Antibacterial soap	Hormone disruptor
Coal tar FD&C Blue 1 and Green 3	Dandruff shampoo, anti-itch cream, toothpaste, mouthwash	Probable carcinogen
Diethanolamine (DEA)	Moisturizers, bath products	Hormone disruptor, possibly carcinogenic
Toluene	Nail varnish	Nervous and reproductive system toxin
1, 4 Dioxane (PEG)	Bath products	Carcinogen
Formaldehyde	Shower gel, nail varnish, hair dye	Immune and respiratory system toxin
Artificial fragrance	Multiple products	Hormone disruptor
Parabens	Multiple products	Hormone disruptor
P-Phenylenediamine	Hair dye, foot powder	Nervous system toxin, allergen
Lead	Hair colour creams	Nervous and reproductive system toxin
Hydroquinone	Skin lightener, moisturizer	Probable carcinogen
Phthalates	Nail varnish	Hormone disruptor
Quaternium-15	Moisturizers, haircare products	Immune toxin

Source: Environmental Working Group's Skin Deep database, www.cosmeticsdatabase.com.

Heavy Metals

Poisonous elements – mercury, lead, cadmium and aluminium – that are ubiquitous in nature (though in infinitesimal amounts), heavy metals have accumulated to significant concentrations in the environment as a by-product of industrial manufacturing processes. The EPA in the US and European Food Safety Authority and the EU Commission Regulation have determined that all of us are able to have low levels of these heavy metals inside of us without damage. But, as is the case with so many pollutants, those studies have not taken into account cumulative industrial exposure to multiple chemicals (which everyone alive today has experienced), nor have the regulatory authorities taken into account individual differences in the body's heavy metal detox mechanism.

Toxic effects in the nervous system include growth and developmental delays, reduction in cognitive functioning and diminished function of the cardiovascular system. They also interfere with the generation of antioxidant and detoxifying molecules. The ability to excrete these toxins, particularly mercury, is highly individual. Most people's natural detox mechanisms can clear slightly elevated levels of mercury. For higher levels of mercury, a prescription chelating agent may be needed. I routinely test for heavy metals for anyone who is experiencing unexplained fatigue – and I recommend you do so too.

TAP INTO THE SOURCE

Boost Your Detox System

My detox programme consists of the following key elements:

- Reduce exposure to toxins.
- Increase detox foods that support the body's natural detox mechanisms.
- Nutritional supplements (when indicated) to boost the body's natural detox.

- Saunas to release toxins stored in fat tissue.
- One-day juice cleanse to clean the slate.
- Consume more clean water to mobilize toxins.
- Gut rehabilitation (when indicated) to Improve the gut's detox ability.

I. Food

In Chapter 2 we covered many Power Foods that are maximally beneficial for healing the body and generating energy; a crucial part of helping your body generate more energy is helping it spend less time and effort detoxifying. Some of the most important foods that help make the job of detoxifying more efficient are:

- The brassica family (cruciferous vegetables): broccoli, cauliflower, kale and Brussels sprouts. Yes, this incredibly powerful vegetable family, which we all know is good for us but everybody loves to hate, also happens to be important for detox. Just take one member, broccoli, as an example; these little green trees (as my eleven-year-old daughter likes to call them) contain numerous potent phytochemicals: *Indole-3-carbinol, sulphurophanes* and *glucosinolates* to name some of the biggies. Indole-3-carbinol (which is only formed after crushing or during cooking) helps the liver break down old oestrogen into harmless forms that can be eliminated. The harmful oestrogen metabolites have been identified by researchers (Eleanor Rogan and others) as a major factor in stimulating the breast's oestrogen receptors, predisposing women to breast cancer. Cruciferi's *sulphurophanes* increase Phase II detoxifying conjugators in the liver and elsewhere as well as performing tumour-destroying functions. That's a lot of power from little green trees and their knobbly cousins.
- The allium family (sulphurous vegetables): onions, leeks, chives, garlic and shallots. Think of this as the vegetable underground working (in a highly complex way) to liberate your body from toxins. These members of the allium family (which happen to be lilies) are rich in sulphur, a major component of detoxifying conjugators. The family name comes from allicin, released by crushing or cutting the garlic

bulb (which loses its beneficial properties within hours of exposure). Onions also have quercetin, one of the most powerful phytochemical antioxidants: it quenches free radicals and acts like a natural antihistamine for people with allergies.

- The thistle family: artichokes, dandelions and burdock. Ancient and ubiquitous healing plants, members of the thistle family have been shown in research to enhance the flow of bile, thus aiding in liver detox. Milk thistle in particular has been shown to help protect the liver from food-bourne toxins (including poisonous mushrooms). Both artichokes and dandelion contain inulin, which helps regulate blood sugar.
- Green tea. As discussed in Chapter 2, green tea is a Power Food: it is one of nature's best antioxidants. Green tea also has been shown to induce Phase I and Phase II detox enzymes and conjugators, thus lending a powerful hand to your body's detox mechanism.
- Fibre. Speeds removal of toxins from the gut by binding them and preventing them from being absorbed in the first place.
- Nuts/seeds. Provide essential fatty acids to reduce inflammation that produces toxic by-products requiring extra energy to neutralize. Pecans and walnuts also contain beneficial ellagic acid (see red berries).
- Seaweed: arame, hijiki, kombu, wakame. In addition to numerous vitamins and minerals, seaweed contains alginic acid, which is thought to bind heavy metals in the intestines and cause them to be eliminated.
- Spices: turmeric, ginger. These potent antioxidants and anti-inflammatories also enhance Phase II liver detoxification.
- Herbs: rosemary, oregano, parsley. These herbs are powerful antioxidants with antimicrobial properties as well.
- Red berries: Among the numerous benefits of berries is ellagic acid – found in many red berries, particularly raspberries, and some nuts (see above). Ellagic acid has been shown in research to increase Phase II liver enzyme activities, enhancing their ability to target so-called reactive intermediaries, lending crucial support to the liver's detox mechanisms.
- Yogurt. Yogurt is terrific for gut health, helping to reset the immune system. The lactobacillus culture in yogurt has also been found to be

highly protective against the toxic effects of the carcinogens found in fried meat.

- **Red wine.** Resveratrol in wine and dark grape skins has been shown to inhibit damage caused by the heavy metal cadmium. In addition to inhibiting many other cell-damaging free radicals, it may be one of the most important anti-ageing phytochemicals.
- **Whole grains.** In addition to many health benefits bestowed by the critical nutrients in the grain's germ, whole grain (higher fibre) diets increase elimination and decrease absorption of environmental toxins compared to refined flour diets.
- **Citrus fruits.** In addition to copious amounts of vitamin C and antioxidants, citrus oils contain limonene, which is said to increase the level of glutathione S-transferase, one of the most important Phase II conjugators.
- **Water.** The simplest way to help your body flush toxic by-products is to drink copious amounts of clean, filtered water that will allow the kidneys to better eliminate the detoxified conjugated products of Phase II detoxification. Lack of water – dehydration – also makes it harder for both nutrients and toxins to move through the ground substance that is in between cells – such as that area between the gut cells and the blood vessels that all absorbed substances need to traverse.

II. Nutritional Supplements

There are important supplements to consider taking to help support the liver's – and nearly every cell's – ability to identify, detoxify and remove toxins. All of these have beneficial effects on many functions in the body. The table overleaf is a guide to which nutrients are most beneficial, based not only on their importance for detoxification support but also on their ability to help with other health issues – and on their ability to reduce energy expenditures (increasing net energy) by freeing up resources from detoxifying. These supplements should not be taken all together. Usually one or two at a time will suffice. The selection depends on your global health issues and general nutritional and detoxifying needs. It is important to discuss

Nutritional Supplements for Natural Detox

Function	Name	Why should you consider taking this?
Liver detox	B Vitamins	If you need support for your nervous system in addition to your liver
	Minerals (copper, zinc, selenium)	To increase the body's ability to make its own natural antioxidants, and increase efficiency of energy-generating processes
	Antioxidant vitamins (C, E, carotenoids)	If you are exposed to a lot of toxins or if you do not eat a wide range of fruits and vegetables
	NAC (N-acetyl-cysteine)	If you have heavy metal exposure or breathing problems
	SAMe (S-Adensyl -Methionine)	If in addition to needing help detoxing the liver, you have depression issues or joint inflammation
	MSM (Methyl-sulf-methane)	Present in sulphurous foods, but you need more to help not only with the liver, but with general inflammation, especially joint problems
	Glycine	Critical amino acid for Phase II detox, improves recovery of the liver after alcohol-induced damage
	Lipoic acid	Helps support circulation (especially in diabetics) in addition to the liver
	Milk thistle	Supports the liver, protective against both natural food-bourne and industrial toxins
	Bitters	Promotes better digestion in addition to increasing flow of bile and enzymes within the liver
	Schizandra	Ancient Chinese remedy for detoxifying, especially within the liver; often combined with other Chinese herbs for broader use
Gut Repair	Prebiotics (Beta -Glucan, Inulin, Fructo-Oligo-Saccharides)	If you are having intestinal problems and you are taking probiotics: supports growth of beneficial bacteria and helps inhibit pathologic ones
	Probiotics (acidophilus, bifidophilus)	Helps digestion, intestinal function in general, and the immune surveillance within the intestines
	L-glutamine	Supports repair of the intestinal lining: also critical for nervous system protection
Heavy Metal	NAC/glutathione	Important nutrient for helping remove heavy metals once they are within the body

with your doctor or practitioner the best combination of activities, foods and supplements for you. Note that some very important nutrients (such as the omega-3 fatty acids from fish oil and flax) are not on this section's list as they are not specific for detox (see Chapter 2 for these).

III. Saunas

Used historically in many indigenous cultures (Roman, Russian, Scandinavian, Turkish, Mayan, Inuit and Native American) for literally thousands of years, the use of saunas as a detox tool has recently caught the attention of scientific researchers – particularly since the 9/11 disaster at the World Trade Center left so many people loaded with industrial toxins. While every cell and especially your liver and gut are designed to remove circulating toxins, the more serious long-term problem with toxic body burden is that chemicals tend to set up long-term housekeeping in your fat cells, which are very slow to detoxify – if they ever do. These unwelcome visitors then become

The Safety of Saunas

The jury is still out on whether or not saunas enhance the release of toxins from interior fat cells. The practice is not harmful for healthy (non-pregnant) people, though, and has other benefits such as stress reduction, improving circulation (lowering blood pressure) and muscle relaxation. I recommend a good sauna whenever possible, but your doctor needs to give you the OK before considering sauna for regular therapeutic use. There are precautions to consider, including health issues that may prohibit their use, such as severe chronic disease, pregnancy, heart disease and while using certain medications. And because saunas naturally dehydrate, proper hydration and electrolyte balance are essential before going in.

'Scientists have been able to determine that mercury, dioxin, antibiotics, and even heroin and cocaine can leave the body through your sweat glands – but that doesn't tell us whether or not those toxins have been liberated from fat cells.'

like the neighbours from hell, causing all manner of damage to DNA. The hope – one that is beginning to be borne out by research – is that taking a sauna can help move toxins out of fat cells.

The idea is to raise the core body temperature, and basically to sweat out the gunk. In some interesting research on PCBs, scientists have demonstrated that concentrations of PCBs in fat tissue were reduced with saunas. An additional study suggests that the skin's sebaceous (oil) glands – which discharge when you perspire – are an excellent excretory system for PCBs – which argues heavily in favour of having a good sweat.

Overall, I think saunas will be found to be increasingly helpful in detox programmes. In the meantime – if your health allows it (which is the case for most of us) – take saunas regularly and enjoy.

IV. Fasting

My basic rule of fasting is *never water alone.* You need nutrients to aid in detox; which is why I refer to the day without solid food in the 21-Day Plan as a *Cleanse.*

'This is not a fast that denies your body nutrients and caloric energy, but rather it allows your digestive tract to rest while providing maximal nutrients, minimal sugars, sufficient calories and zero pollutants.'

Convincing Evidence

In one series of highly convincing studies conducted in Scandinavia, patients with severe rheumatoid arthritis were placed on a supervised juice fast for one week, followed by a vegetarian diet for a month. By the end of the period, patients had dramatic improvements in every parameter measured for their illness – there was a decrease in pain, stiffness and use of medications along with a sense of improved energy and overall well-being. Even more astounding, the measurable improvements lasted for up to six months, even after patients went back to their former less healthy diets. In a different kind of study, researchers looked at the effects on heart health of the religious practice (in this case Mormon) of fasting for a day every month by evaluating 515 elderly people in Utah in the US. Those who reported fasting once a month were 39 per cent more likely than non-fasters to have a healthy heart. One theory for the beneficial effect, which is backed by animal studies, is that periodic withdrawal of food might resensitize the insulin-producing beta cells. By improving insulin metabolism fasting may have an effect on better heart health.

Important new research by British gerontologist Alan R. Hipkiss and others highlights one of the key mechanisms by which periodic fasting may not only protect your DNA but also improve your ability to generate energy and increase life span. This happens by the activity of internal anti-ageing molecules of the family called sirtuins (SIRT 1–7). While most of the initial research has been conducted with animals, the mechanisms relate closely to the same processes and chemicals occurring in humans. Episodic fasting not only improved the ability of the mitochondria to withstand damage and more efficiently generate energy, but facilitated other mechanisms that significantly extended the life of the cell.

Like saunas, periodic, brief fasts have been used beneficially for thousands of years in indigenous health systems, and I recommend them, having reviewed the research and experienced a number of different fasts. The most basic beneficial outcome of fasting is in starting with a clean slate. Not only does fasting rest your overworked gut, but especially if you introduce maximally healthy nutrients (with vegetable juices, probiotics, fibre etc.) fasts can promote detoxification, reduce inflammation, improve overall health and dramatically increase energy.

For this programme, I ask you to follow the juice regimen for just a single day, but juice cleanses have been shown to be effective and safe for as many as three days.

TAP INTO THE SOURCE

Liquid Lunch

The key to a successful cleanse is in providing essential nutrients (including calories) and drinking sufficient fluids. Providing nutrients with freshly made juices is a key to maintaining energy levels and providing support for your body's detox mechanisms. One of the biological processes of fasting is mobilization of substances for detox in the liver and throughout the body. This vigorously activates Phase I liver detox, producing many oxidative (free-radicalized) intermediary by-products. This then necessitates a highly active Phase II to clear the toxic by-products. If you don't drink juices to provide abundant phytochemicals rich in antioxidants and key nutrients for making Phase II conjugators – and particularly if you start out nutrient depleted – a fast can actually make you feel toxic as Phase I buildup overwhelms Phase II. Because the Phase II conjugates need extra replenishing during a cleanse, I recommend fresh juice every two to three hours made from a rainbow of vegetables and fruits, with an emphasis on dark greens, including the deeply detoxifying brassica family (see my juice recipes in Part Three). Drinking water or other non-caffeinated, minimally sweetened beverages in between these juice 'meals' aids in flushing out neutralized toxins, staving off hunger and preventing blood pressure drop.

The pay-off of the one-day juice cleanse usually comes the next morning when you wake up feeling more energetic and 'clear'. It is essential to make careful choices as you transition back onto solid food. If you are suffering from severe chronic disease, diabetes or are pregnant, consult your doctor before undertaking the juice cleanse.

V. Gut Optimization

As we've discussed, your gut is your first line of defence against most toxins. Just about everyone can treat his or her gut better, but particularly if you suffer from irritable bowel or other digestive systems, here's what you do: chew better; eat mostly vegetables, fruit and fibre; provide healthy bacteria such as the probiotic cultures found in yogurt. You chew your food better so that the gut has to do less work breaking down food; and certainly eating fibre is a simple solution – the more fibre you eat the easier it is for the gut to clean itself. But encouraging the growth of healthy bacteria is a bit more complex.

Recently, scientists have confirmed that having an abundance of unhealthy bacteria produces inefficient digestion, and can release toxins that inflame the intestinal wall and leak into the general circulation, causing fatigue and other symptoms (including worsening inflammatory conditions such as rheumatoid arthritis). Most recently, scientists have uncovered evidence connecting specific species of bacteria in the gut to being overweight: certain bacterial species are able to extract calories from otherwise indigestible food, and are thought to be one link to the obesity dilemma. Establishing healthy gut bacteria also strengthens the immune system and helps keep the intestinal wall barrier system intact.

'The healthier your gut bacteria, the healthier you will be overall – this is a maxim understood for centuries by many cultures that have cultivated the making of yogurt as a sort of art and medicine.'

So how do you get the good bacteria? Eating yogurt loaded with sugars and additives (as are the majority of yogurts sold in supermarkets) will not help. Regularly eating plain, unsweetened yogurt, preferably organic, or taking a probiotic supplement (acidophilus or bifidophilus) are important ways to build your gut's flora. You can add a touch of honey if you like. Some people who suffer from milk allergies can tolerate goat's yogurt, now widely available. I also love my yogurt with a little cucumber and some walnuts or flax meal. As your gut begins to feel better, and you wean yourself off sugary varieties of yogurt, you will start to understand why plain yogurt has been considered a part of good nutrition around the globe for many thousands of years.

What Not to Do

Colonics: There is no published information that colonics aid in detoxifying the body, though you will often see them included as part of non-medical detox regimes in health spas. A colonic removes over a metre of stool from the large intestines, which can result in a feeling of relief – of course it would, since you are lighter with an empty colon when you finish. But within a couple of days the colon fills up again. Since the small intestines – not the colon – are primarily responsible for removing toxins, extracting the contents of the colon really cannot reduce your toxin burden. Cleansing can only happen from altering what you put into your body, and fine-tuning your detox mechanisms with food and supplements – not from a colonic flushing out the lower portion of your intestines.

Purges (emptying the digestive tract): A purge should only be conducted under medical supervision, for example, in preparation for a colonoscopy. While healthy people who experience temporary constipation can take an occasional laxative, they are not meant for regular use. Chemical laxatives (including herbal senna and cascara) result in dependence. A full purge (removing every piece of matter from mouth to anus – forgive the graphic description) can be occasionally helpful. Some of my patients report that precolonoscopy purges result in improvements in bowel problems. The detox regime in this programme can do the job without the purge.

Coffee enemas: Yes, you read that correctly. Coffee enemas are used in many so-called detox clinics around the world. They are purported to help the liver detoxify. I would steer clear of them. While recent scientific literature does give some support for coffee's ability to enhance the liver's detox mechanism, there are many other foods, practices, nutrients and herbs that can do the job without hooking yourself up to an espresso machine – or as in the case with coffee enemas, introducing coffee into your rectum.

Chapter 4

Power Exercise, the Energy Factory

CASE STUDY
TOO TIRED TO MOVE

PATRICK had been a highly motivated, productive construction manager in his late twenties, but had spent the last four months battling a difficult viral infection. For several weeks tests had shown that the virus had completely abated and that he was in a prolonged recovery phase, but he continued to complain of fatigue and uncharacteristic sluggishness.

Through this period he had remained mostly sedentary, afraid to exercise for fear the energy he would expend while working out would somehow reactivate his illness. Formerly lackadaisical about his personal health habits, the illness had brought Patrick to a new awareness of the importance of leading a healthy lifestyle – except that he was still avoiding exercise.

While excessive exercise (pushing yourself to exhaustion) can suppress the immune system, moderate exercise actually strengthens the immune system and helps the body generate energy. I finally convinced Patrick to start a cautious exercise programme. He started with light aerobic walking and 30 crunches every other day. Within only one week he had more energy than he had had in months, and within two weeks he felt, for the first time, that he was putting the illness behind him. A month later he was more invigorated than he had ever been, with his new-found love of exercise.

NOTHING RAISES YOUR ENERGY faster and more effectively than exercise. The simple act of moving can jump-start your metabolic machinery and boost your energy levels. Primary school teachers have known this for years, but now even the top medical researchers have shown on a molecular level that exercise – just a moderate, brief bout – increases the level of energy-producing chemicals in your cellular energy factory, the mitochondria. This power surge happens everywhere in your body from your biceps to your heart to the parts of your brain that control memory and intelligence. When you exercise, you're not just training your muscles, you are also training your DNA. That's an amazing thought – that you can actually change the DNA that you inherited – and in such a simple way. Studies show that, with moderate exercise, the mitochondria literally grow in size and become more efficient – it's like trading up your batteries from triple AAA to lithium. This all means that the more you move, the more energy your body will make – that's why movement was a key factor in Patrick's recovery.

Don't Join the Club

I hate even to use the word exercise because so many people feel they've heard it all before – and that they've tried and failed. Statistically, most gym memberships are dropped after the first two months – you join for the New Year and then quit going when you simultaneously get the flu and have to do a last-minute rush job. But being fit is not about weights and fancy treadmills. It is not a club you join and abandon. Moving your body to a point of raising your heart rate is a fundamental aspect of physical and mental well-being, one of the most efficient methods your body has of generat-

'Recent research shows that exercise has a direct, immediate effect on energy – if you do nothing more right now than stand up and hop up and down for three minutes you will feel a surge of energy and you will feel more alive.'

'Forget everything you think you know about exercise. I want you to see physical activity as a means to reconnect with your body as it was meant to be – a wellspring of pure energy.'

ing energy. There are many ways to exercise, from simple walking to dancing to yoga or whatever else activates your body and raises your heart rate. What matters most is not *how* you work your muscles and raise your heart rate but that you do so *consistently*.

The human body is like a self-winding watch – it's designed to generate energy when you move. When you activate your muscles, everything is geared toward revving up your molecular machinery. Oxygen utilization becomes more efficient; sugar is processed better; fat and calories burn faster; brain cells regenerate quicker; you think more clearly; your heart gets bigger and stronger; the balance of your nervous system shifts toward the calming aspect (parasympathetic); and your emotional happy switch gets turned on by the release of neurotransmitters like serotonin and endorphins.

To be blunt: you shouldn't be sedentary until you're six feet under. If you need motivation, watch the group that leads the New York City marathon every year – they are wheelchair athletes paralysed from the waist down but they have incredibly powerful upper bodies. If they can train for and finish a 26.2 mile (42-kilometre) race using only a fraction of their muscles to propel their bodies, you can start to move too! My simple programme of basic movement and core training, along with specific energy exercises and a dose of sports psychology, is designed to give your body exactly the activity level it needs to achieve optimal energy. It works best if you just take it one step at a time.

How Exercise Generates Energy

The ancient Greeks were the first certifiably exercise-obsessed Western culture, but scientists of all eras have recognized that humans were designed to be continuously on the move. Your genome is the same as your hunter-gatherer ancestors', whose active lifestyle of roaming around procuring (then later harvesting) food dominated human history up until the 20th century. The sedentary lifestyle that's causing so many health problems today began to take hold with the advent of commercial farming and mass-produced cars; then television came along to keep us glued to our seats; and now we're up against a vicious triumvirate with the rise of computers, the Internet and games consoles. I know people feel they're exercising with their Nintendo Wii games, but waving your arms in front of your TV set is not exactly the same as taking a brisk constitutional in fresh air.

Quite simply, you are not designed for a life without exercise; humans are supposed to move every day – whether that means walking for twenty minutes, pulling weeds or going to the gym. This is not at all unique to people; most animals traverse vast distances daily relative to their size. Research from the Salk Institute showed that if you put a running wheel in a mouse's cage it will run 4 to 5 kilometres every night, and will eventually become a better problem solver than its neighbour without a wheel. The reason for this need to move is complex it's certainly a genetic imperative that insures

The O₂ Factor

The O_2 Factor

Oxygen is a crucial raw material of energy production. And the extraordinary ability of exercise to increase the oxygen supply to your cells makes exercise the OPEC of your body's energy needs – when you exercise the raw material of energy floods the market. With exercise your lungs become more efficient at extracting oxygen from air; the heart pumps more blood and blood vessels dilate, which increases oxygen delivery; haemoglobin releases a considerable quantity of reserved oxygen when body temperatures rise; and with time new capillaries actually grow. When you don't exercise, you're practically suffocating your cells – you're not maximizing your oxygen reserves or your energy supply.

finding food, but energy creation also seems to be at the molecular heart of the issue. By this measure, exercise is like plugging into the grid – it creates energy (as long as you don't overdo it).

'As little as 30 minutes of brisk walking causes measurable increases in the production of energy-generating substances, in the transport of energy within the cell, and in the transmission of energy between cells.'

Exercise Prescription

Some of the most groundbreaking – yet elegantly simple – science on the biology and benefits of exercise has come from a *brain research* lab at University of California at Los Angeles. The director of the UCLA Neurotrophic Lab, Dr Fernando Gomez-Pinilla, has been leading methodical studies about the influences of exercise and diet on the brain – specifically on how those lifestyle factors can aid in recovery from spinal cord and brain injuries as well as help reverse Alzheimer's and even the negative effects of a diet high in saturated fat. Gomez-Pinilla's research has led deep into the fundamental mechanisms of exercise physiology, which in turn has allowed his team to unlock some of the secrets of energy creation.

Since the early 1990s scientists have known that the body's ability to generate energy (in the form of the molecule ATP) nearly doubles within five to ten days of starting a training routine, but it took the ingenious scientists at UCLA to begin to understand why this is true. In 2006, they were able to demonstrate that exercise significantly stimulated genes to produce more of the energy-balancing factor (mitochondrial uncoupling protein 2) responsible for producing energy (or ATP) as well as for reducing the free-radical by-products of energy production. Their research showed that moderate exercise can both turn on the energy switch and clean up the pollution generated by energy production. This happens throughout the body.

But they went even further and demonstrated that the same

energy-balancing mechanism switched on by exercise also activates proteins responsible for making the brain better able to think, via a mechanism called synaptic plasticity (synapses are the connections between brain cells and when they're plastic, it means that they can grow and improve). Exercise accomplishes this by boosting brain-derived neurotrophic factor (BDNF), a molecule responsible for shaping the old grey matter or brain cells. Exercise is so powerful, researchers found, that BDNF can be elevated for a full day following a session of moderate exercise.

With exercise, as in all aspects of your life, what begins at an energy level – with thought or intention – translates to the molecular level and then reverberates throughout your body. When you exercise, you make more energy-generating mitochondria and they work better; you also train your muscles to burn more sugar calories for the same amount of effort and to produce more enzymes that metabolize fat – like a lot of little Pacmen zipping around eating up flab. As muscle grows and fat begins to dissipate, your cardiovascular endurance and energy levels rise and it becomes easier to exercise.

Deeper breathing makes an important contribution to the exercise-energy equation. Intriguing research from Alan R. Hipkiss, a pioneering anti-ageing researcher, demonstrates that aerobic exercise regenerates the principal enzyme (NAD) responsible for both supporting the basic operation of mitochondria and retarding mitochondrial ageing. The studies suggest that aerobic breathing regenerates this crucial mitochondrial enzyme by reducing reactive oxygen species (free radicals).

In other words, a moderate aerobic workout – that doesn't overstress the respiratory system – renews energy-generating mitochondrial structures and can even reverse some of the effects of ageing discussed in Chapter 2 – not all bad for a 'therapy' that's absolutely free and helps you lose weight to boot!

'Exercise would be considered a miracle drug if you could bottle and sell it, but it's right at the tips of your toes. Just take a brisk walk, and this miracle cure is yours.'

Tired Muscles?

For years we thought muscle fatigue and soreness were due to lactic acid build-up, but it turns out an entirely different mechanism may be at work. Investigators at Columbia University recently identified calcium leakage as the culprit. It's long been known that muscle contraction occurs when calcium enters into the muscle cell; when the calcium moves back out, the muscles relax. The latest research reveals calcium is actually stored in tiny packets in the space between cells and released when the muscles need to contract. However, for some people the packets of calcium start to leak. When this occurs, the calcium's effect is diminished. Without fully loaded calcium packets, the muscles get less calcium when they need it and they contract less efficiently. Making matters worse, the escaped calcium builds up around the muscle causing an enzyme to be released that actually damages muscle tissue. This is basic research; we don't yet have firm recommendations about how to plug the leaks, but because the findings have exciting implications for heart muscle fatigue many scientists are searching for more answers. Stay tuned.

The Depression Connection

A growing body of research points to exercise as a spectacular energizer when fatigue stems from depression. The runner's high is a widely recognized phenomenon, but even I was surprised with the latest findings from investigators at Duke University. The study pitted moderate exercise against the antidepressant Lustral for beating depression – and exercise won hands down! In a cohort of older patients with major depression, Lustral initially worked faster than exercise to relieve symptoms, but at the 10-month follow-up the group that walked or jogged on a treadmill for 90 minutes a week was significantly less depressed than the medicated group. Exercise elevates all of the same neurotransmitters targeted by antidepressant medications (serotonin, dopamine and noradrenaline), but this and other studies support the use of exercise instead of prescription antidepressants for many people. This is cheering news, indeed, given that exercise is a 'therapy' with few side-effects – especially if you keep it moderate enough to avoid injury.

Many studies show that treating depression improves your energy-generating capabilities. While there are certainly people who do need psychotropic medications to stabilize their emotional lives, for many people mood dictates their energy levels, and a sure, healthy path to a better mood is regular exercise. In my experience, many people ready to come off antidepressants have succeeded by incorporating a regular exercise programme (along with other healthy lifestyle changes) into their tapering-off schedule. (A note of caution: chronic overexercising to the point of exhaustion can make depression worse, and individuals on antidepressants should not taper or stop their use without a doctor's supervision.)

How Much Is Enough?

'If anyone is compelled by any movement to breathe more, that movement becomes exercise for him.'

GREEK PHYSICIAN GALEN, C. AD166

This isn't the first time I've looked to the past for healing wisdom, but it really is incredible to me how perceptive Galen's comment was almost 2,000 years ago. He was speaking at that time about what we now call aerobic exercise, which is increasing oxygen supply to your cells and revving up your metabolism through movement and breath work. In reality, the question of how much is enough depends on your goals. In my practice, the bar is set atop two pillars: prevention and energy generation. With exercise I want you to prevent chronic illness and increase your energy supply. This requires three aspects of activity:

1. **Revving up your metabolic machinery with movement and deep breathing.**
2. **Activating your core muscles with attention to your posture.**
3. **Increasing your strength.**

You can achieve these goals in a number of ways without becoming a gym junkie. In this chapter and the 21-Day Plan I offer a foolproof method for getting in touch with your inner athlete. At the very least we will jog your genetic memory back to a time when you had to move to survive!

Revving Up the Machinery

After reviewing most of the literature and working for decades with patients, I clearly see that the simplest and best remedy for fatigue is a straightforward prescription of aerobic activity. You need 90 minutes a week of movement that raises your heart rate to 70 per cent of its maximum capacity (60 per cent if you're unfit). If you move your body to the extent that your heart beats noticeably faster, your breathing is more rapid, *and you can still hold a conversation*, then you are in the right zone. I'll even settle for you to commit to cumulative 10-minute bouts of this kind of activity that adds up to 30 minutes in a day, three days a week. Dancing like crazy to iTunes for 10 minutes at a time will do it. I'd be very happy if you were to do a continuous, 30-minute, aerobically active workout – if you can sustain that routine over the long term. The key is for you to come up with a heart rate-elevating activity (or range of activities) that you can – and will want to – perform for 90 minutes a week for the rest of your life.

Any movement (even parking further from the shopping centre entrance and walking the few extra steps) will improve your health, but you must raise your heart and respiratory rates in order to challenge your mitochondria to produce more ATP and to increase your energy.

Walking briskly (at the pace of a jog without the pounding) is enough, whether you're on a pavement, a treadmill or a nature path in the woods. Cycling (free or stationary) is great, swimming, jumping rope, walking stairs, doing star jumps to your favourite song, running gently in place – all of the above are acceptable ways to rev up your machinery and generate energy molecules. What matters to me and almost all the exercise experts in the world is that you reach your magic number for producing results: 70 per cent of your maximum heart rate, which is 220 minus your age multiplied by 70 per cent (see 21-Day Plan, Day 5 for more details). That's somewhere between walking at a normal pace on a flat surface and running so that your heart is pounding and you can't catch your breath.

'The difference between regular motion and motion that will create more energy is the difference between strolling up the supermarket aisle and walking at a brisk pace up a gentle hill.'

Getting Results

The beauty for novices is they are guaranteed to get results. Studies of sedentary middle-aged men with heart disease showed that measures of fitness improved by 50 per cent when they began a fitness routine, while similar training in normally active, healthy adults improved by only 10 to 15 per cent over the same period. One patient of mine is a restaurant owner who has had a very tough time with weight. He and his wife had been exercise averse for years. Then one year a friend gave them a Christmas present of two weeks with a trainer, a gift he told me about initially with an attitude of disdain. I didn't see them again for six months until one day I ran into them in the park in their exercise clothes. They told me they were too cheap to waste the gift – and knew their friend would find out if they didn't use it. So in January they took the plunge. After their first half-hour walk they passed up a crème brûlée that night. After the second walk

they invested in good trainers. In the end the two weeks were a rev-
elation to them. He said, 'I noticed the difference in my energy right
away, and almost felt sad for the years I'd spent depriving my body
of what it needed.' Six months after that, at his next check-up, he had
shed three stone and said he felt 'like an eighteen-year-old again'. The
key here is that your best motivation is going to be the real results
you will experience almost immediately.

Moving to the Next Level

Once the 70 per cent target heart rate begins to feel too easy, you
have two choices for upping the ante – lengthen your workout or increase your intensity. The smart move is to increase the target gradually, say, to 75 per cent for one week, then 80 per cent the next week.
(Athletes can push their target heart rate to 90 per cent of maximum,
but regular folks shouldn't.) If you're a walker, one simple way for
you to increase target intensity is to add ankle weights, which can increase the energy expenditure of walking to values usually observed
for running (handheld weights also increase the intensity, but pose
a downside risk of raising blood pressure and putting a strain on
posture). Taking a hill or the stairs a little faster will do the same, but with
less consistency than ankle weights.

'It's documented that too much exercise with inadequate rest increases susceptibility to infections, decreases the body's ability to heal, alters sleep and hormonal patterns, and increases circulating levels of the stress hormone cortisol.'

It's often tempting to just keep on trucking for longer and longer
periods, but that's not the most ef-
ficient way to intensify a workout.
Some elite athletes train by running
up to a couple of hundred kilometres a week, but unless you're
looking for a new full-time job as a
runner, I give you permission to stop
an aerobic workout after 30 minutes.
Adding an interval training session
to your aerobic routine dramatically
increases your metabolism for hours

Overtraining

It is possible to get too much of a good thing. Jacqueline had been coming to me for years, always complaining of low energy and susceptibility to colds. She slept only five or six hours a night and kept an intense job as an ad executive. Six days a week she started her day at 5am with 90 minutes of intense exercise. For years I had been nearly begging her to reduce her exercise level and get more rest. She felt that it was only the exercise that kept her going, and was mortified at the idea of putting on a pound with less exercise. Finally she had to travel to Canada for two weeks, staying in a small town with a hotel that had no gym, and it snowed heavily nearly the whole time she was there. A couple of days she got outside to run early, but after a few days gave up and slept more – and felt an immediate difference in her energy. I got a call a month later to tell me that she had not had such high energy in years. Upon returning home she tried my advice, exercising moderately (down to 60 minutes four days a week), and felt terrific. Thank goodness for inclement weather.

A subset of my patients, like Jacqueline, overexercise and suffer fatigue as a result. If you get up too early and exercise too much, or you don't take enough rest days in between exercise sessions, it's possible that you're overtraining. Rather than rejuvenating you and increasing your energy, too much exercise can produce a state of energy depletion and unwellness. Over-exercising also produces way too many cell- and mitochondrial-damaging free radicals. It depletes the body's energy-reserve (glycogen) stores, leading to anaerobic (without oxygen) rather than aerobic (with oxygen) metabolism – which is very energy inefficient. These processes lead to a degradation of the cells' ability to function and create energy.

Studies show that overtraining actually undermines performance. If you've been pushing yourself hard and feel you've hit a wall in terms of your performance abilities, try getting more rest: it's what overtrainers need most. You may find that your fitness miraculously improves – even as you sleep!

after a workout. With interval training (short bursts of exhaustive activity separated by brief rest), you burn more fat than you would by just lengthening your jog or brisk walk. A good interval workout – if your joints can handle it – is to sprint all-out for 45 seconds, then rest for 60 seconds and repeat three or four times. With interval training you can rapidly improve your aerobic capacity, and you will find you're able to carry on a conversation while exercising at a much more vigorous pace than you were able to before challenging yourself with intervals.

Activating the Core

Raising your heart rate is the nuts and bolts of energy-generating movement. Then there's what I consider to be the more intellectual part of the package – core training. Core training – that is, strengthening and engaging the muscles of your abdomen and torso – has become something of a fitness fad in the past decade.

You may have been in a yoga session and heard the instructor holding forth on the second and third chakras (according to Ayurvedic medicine these energy centres are in the general vicinity of your lower abdomen and solar plexus). This area is the seat of the core muscles, which are coordinated by a collection of nerves that stretch the length of the spine from the chest down, with powerful connections throughout the body. The core includes the deepest muscle in your abdomen, the grandly named transversus abdominis. The TA is like a weight belt: it attaches at your lower back on either side of your spine and wraps around your abdomen, clinging to your rib cage at its uppermost edge and to your pelvis at its lowermost edge. This is the muscle that characteristically atrophies with a sedentary lifestyle (and stretches

'Core work is essential, and it's a wonderful way to combine conditioning with raising vital energy – or a deep sense of inner strength – which Eastern traditions refer to as Qi or prana.'

with pregnancy), resulting in a pro-truding stomach and an aching back. Sitting on top of the transverse ab-dominis is the rectus abdominis, the muscle stretching across the front of the abdomen, which in peak condi-tion is the 'six-pack' that power lift-ers strive for and elite athletes natu-rally develop by logging training time. Engaging the full core is what allows seemingly miraculous athletic performance.

> 'When you move with a properly engaged core, it's like igniting the spark of energy that comes from completing an electrical circuit.'

Swing with Your Core

Tiger Woods doesn't swing the golf club with his arms alone; he swings with his core. Same thing can be said for a Wimbledon champ. And the same should be said for each one of us. When you sit, stand or walk, you should engage your core to support your back and take chronic, energy-draining strain out of your everyday activities.

You can can do this formally with yoga, Pilates, tai chi or, in the case of my programme, crunches and push ups along with at-tention to the core during any activity. (See the 21-Day Plan, Day 2 for the best way to do a crunch.) Say hello to your core when you lean over the sink to brush your teeth or put away groceries – hold in your stomach muscles, engage your transversus abdominis, breathe deeply and slowly, and feel the energy rising from your solar plexus.

You don't have to call it Qi or a chakra, but you will see that finding and activating your core gives more power to your activity and to your life. In addition, developing core skills – whether or not you go to the extent of becoming a yoga or Pilates devotee – provides the balance that centres the spine, protecting you from lower back and neck injuries that can become truly debilitating over time.

Increasing Your Strength

In my experience, strength training inhabits the absolute lowest realm of most people's exercise existence, and yet it's a key anti-ageing activity that is easy for you to perform.

'Strength training is an ideal way to realize the potential your body has for creating energy. By building muscle, you build more energy factories.'

Regularly giving your muscles a resistance challenge is crucial for avoiding chronic musculoskeletal problems, and it allows you to burn more calories per kilo – it keeps your metabolism physically young. Strength training also builds healthy bones throughout life, and – along with core work – helps stop you from ageing into a hunchback. Most people think of bone as an inert, steel-like structure forged in childhood, but this fails to recognize the secret life of your skeleton. Bone is a dynamic, living part of you – it's composed of connective tissue, cells and blood vessels within a calcium matrix. Your body needs constantly to deposit layers of calcium to maintain the integrity of your skeletal matrix, and the best way to encourage continual re-modelling is to apply the healthy stress of weight-bearing exercise.

The marvellous thing about strength training is that beginners have the most dramatic results. In general, previously sedentary people can improve muscular strength by 40 per cent, while an elite athlete would only improve strength by 2 per cent in the same period (of course they're starting at a much higher level). It is entirely possible to double the size of your muscles with intensive strength training. (This increases the size and number of mitochondria, both increasing your energy generation, as well as allowing you to burn more calories, since muscles are highly active metabolically and more muscles than fat means better ability to use calories from food.) Bottom line: your muscles are starving for attention, and they respond relatively quickly when you give them a challenge.

Strength training doesn't have to be pumping iron. It can also be part of your core workout, or the central focus of, say, a yoga session. In my programme, both push-ups and core crunches accomplish strength training together with core work. The key to getting stronger is to provide gradually more intense challenges so that your last lift is the most difficult of the day – for example do

Hollywood's Secret Core

Excellent posture is one factor that separates the gods and goddesses who walk the red carpet on Oscar night from the rest of us. But film stars are usually not born, they are made. They learn to engage their core – often with the help of countless yoga or Pilates classes or by studying the Alexander Technique, a system developed by a Shakespearean actor in the 1920s. Alexander technicians describe their mission as reducing unnecessary muscular force applied to the body. I like to think of good posture as taking the strain off your spine – banishing the dreaded shoulder slump with your neck flexed forward, vulture-like. When you stand, your neck and spine should be in a straight line at a 90-degree angle to the ground; visualize your body as hanging from a string attached to the crown of your head. The best way to achieve such stellar alignment is to engage your core. Get a grip on your abdominal muscles; use your diaphragm to initiate breaths; tuck your butt slightly under your pelvis; move your shoulders back by pinching your shoulder blades closer and downwards; and feel that string pulling your head upward.

Here's a good exercise that will help reshape your body in the mould of a softer version of an RAF sergeant or red-carpet diva. While sitting (you can do this periodically at your desk or anywhere), straighten your spine.

- *Hold your arms straight down, palms facing forward so that you are forced to bring your shoulders back and down. Now twist gently at your waist, keeping your shoulders and chest in a horizontal line while your neck remains in a straight vertical line with your spine.*
- *Breathe from your diaphragm, not your chest. Practising in front of a mirror is a powerful help. Most of us have no idea what our posture looks like, which also separates us from movie stars, who have to endure seeing themselves on the big screen.*

bent-knee push-ups, but make the last a full push-up; or do tricep pulls with a 500-gram weight, and on the very last one use a two-kilogram weight. But make sure to allow your muscles to fully recover after a session. Every time you do a weight-bearing exercise you are producing slight, microscopic injury to the muscle tissue. The process of repair is what actually thickens and strengthens the tissue. A day or two of rest for each muscle group is essential for allowing the remodeling process that produces stronger muscles.

As you progress – on the road to mini-Mr or -Ms Universe status – it is increasingly important to vary your routine. There are so many muscles in the body that working only a few eventually creates imbalances and injury. Once you've mastered the sit-ups and

Push-Up Reality Check

Research shows that strength builds quicker when you increase load *rather than repetition. If you have never been able to do more than a couple of push-ups at a time, here's how to get stronger. Increase the challenge throughout the session, with your last push being the hardest.*

- *For beginners, start your push-ups from a standing position.*
- *Place your toes about 60cm from a wall; place your hands flat against the wall with arms stretched straight out, and slowly bring your nose to the wall by bending your arms, keeping your core engaged, and body in a straight line like a plank.*
- *Now push away from the wall until your arms are straight again.*
- *Do this a dozen times; rest; then move onto the floor for two rounds of bent-knee push-ups – straight spine, core engaged.*
- *Finally, do one perfect all-out push-up, on your toes, body straight as a board.*
- *Next time, end with two perfect push-ups. Soon you'll be up to six or more.*

crunches of my programme, go ahead and explore other routines. While weight and circuit training are OK. I prefer exercises that utilize multiple muscle groups, mimicking normal daily activities. I glean terrific tips from the monthly magazine *Men's Health*, which has a regular 'Fitness' section with new ideas for strength training. But let's not get ahead of ourselves. First try to master six perfect push-ups at a go. Then you can entertain dreams of glory.

Gym Toys 101

If you've ever taken a peek at the strength-training section of a gym you've seen quite a few toys – it looks a bit like the polar bear cage at the zoo. While I'm not a big fan of buying stuff for exercise – most stationary cycles in people's homes turn mysteriously into clothing racks – some strength toys can be useful for working on those hard-to-reach and long-neglected muscle groups.

- **Bands:** Basically massive rubber bands that come in different tensile strengths to provide resistance. Hold the bands in front of you, core engaged, and stretch the ends of the bands in opposite directions to exercise the triceps and upper back muscles.
- **Balls:** You can pimp your push-ups with an exercise ball. Push up with your hands on the ball to improve balance, or with your feet on the ball and hands on the floor, core engaged, to really ratchet up the level of difficulty. Sitting on a ball and trying to remain stable while doing any exercise – such as moving hand weights – engages the core, improves proprioception balance, and intensifies any exercise.
- **Weights:** Handheld weights are still the standard for strength training. But I'm not taking about hulking up a 25kg weight, which is invariably done with horrendous postural adjustments. Simple 500g to 2kg hand weights are perfectly adequate training tools. I prefer exercises that mimic normal activities. Take a 1kg weight and, with your core fully engaged, simply go through the motions of loading the car with shopping – lift and reach – or of putting away a carry-on bag in the overhead compartment – lift the weights from shoulder height to up over your head.

- **Balance boards:** These add the element of balance to your strength training. New to the scene are micro-electric balance boards, which provide a nearly infinitesimal electric vibration that requires your nervous and muscular systems constantly to work for balance.
- **Skipping ropes:** The *sine qua non* of aerobic and resistance training – skipping provides aerobic, core, and upper body training. But skipping is extremely rigorous – most people new to aerobic training will be exhausted after a couple of minutes.

Why Are Ancient Martial Arts So Powerful?

Yoga, tai chi and other martial arts are the best means I know of for connecting your energy circuits. Such exercises have been developed by masters of these arts over thousands of years to gain access to energy sources – through mind, muscle and breath control. In the West, we love the fantasy of superhuman power in martial arts movies like *The Matrix* and *Crouching Tiger, Hidden Dragon* (or even Jackie Chan). These stories actually contain a seed of truth; while you're not likely to achieve wingless flight, martial arts challenge the body completely and yield results unlike any other exercise system. Also, learning the mysteries of martial arts almost always requires studying with a master – a situation that is both cinematic and conducive to getting better results. Working with ancient martial arts requires controlled breath work and focus – at their essence they are meditative and energy-generating movement exercises.

One of my favourite real-life martial arts tales comes from a Qi gong experience I had a number of years ago. A very dear friend of mine, a dedicated runner in her early thirties who'd always considered herself to be fit and regularly jogged a few miles around New York's Central Park reservoir, came with me to a rare class given by one of the great Qi gong masters visiting from China. We stood stock still, breathing, and occasionally lifting our arms – following the movements of a minute 85-year-old man wearing sweatpants and a T-shirt – for 45 minutes in a dingy little New York studio. I was fretting that my friend would find this typically subtle Chinese practice (similar to Tadasana, or the mountain posture, in yoga) to be unbearably tedious. I myself was struggling – muscles quivering, sweat pouring down my back – and trying to hide it, when all of a sudden the master stopped the class and abruptly told someone to sit down. I turned and saw that my friend was on the verge of passing out! The master chuckled softly and had her put her head between her legs until the dizziness passed. It turns out the seemingly mild practice of just a stationary Qi gong had been incredibly vigorous for this healthy young woman, who was reduced to a quivering pool of sweat while the elderly Master Wu stood there fresh as a daisy.

Eastern Energetics

Try as I have to find a scientific explanation for the vigour of these subtle practices, the research is incomplete. In any case, Western scientific experiments are not necessary in order to validate systems that have been practised successfully and with excellent health results in Asia for thousands of years. In Chapter 1, 'Power Mind', I detail some of the science that has examined the beneficial effects of Eastern practices like yoga (the most extensively studied of these practices). In one session, for instance, yoga has been shown to lower blood pressure, improve digestion, and reduce hostility, among other effects. Over the long term, yoga can reduce the time it takes your heart and vascular system to recover from stress, improve the way your cells respond to sugar, and activate a host of anti-anxiety and antidepressant neurotransmitters. From my observations as a scientist and practitioner, studies of the other martial arts like tai chi and Qi gong would likely yield similar results. In fact, they have already been shown definitively to improve balance in the elderly – which reduces their likelihood of falling and sustaining debilitating injuries that reduce their lifespan and enjoyment of life.

On a strictly physical level, practising the martial arts activates a vast range of mechanisms. They can involve the entire structural framework of the human body – bones, joints, ligaments, muscles, tendons and nerves, the cardiovascular, respiratory and digestive systems. They can also engage the mind in a deeper, more focused, and eventually contemplative state. You can derive enormous benefits from regular physical practices at the beginner's level.

TAP INTO THE SOURCE

Beginning Yoga or Martial Arts

- Find a teacher who closely monitors alignment: What shocks most people when they first try yoga is that it's a *weight-bearing* exercise requiring a tremendous amount of strength. The key is to practise with proper alignment so that the bones are in a correct position to carry the load, and the best way to ensure that is to take small classes or preferably private sessions when you first begin.
- Start simple: Unless you're a stretching fanatic, for most people the most difficult part of starting a yoga, tai chi or Qi gong is that they lack range of motion and balance. But every session will increase your range of motion and stability in joints such as shoulders, hips and knees by focusing first on seemingly simple postures. First you'll practise the basics before you begin to exert additional pressure on your joints and muscles with more challenging positions. Your teacher will proceed slowly with good reason.
- Go soft and slow: Postures that promote lengthening of muscles that have become chronically shortened because of high heels, sitting at your desk or on your sofa, or concentrating your exercise regime on walking or running, are a major cause of moaning and screaming among yoga and martial arts initiates. Classes that move too quickly and push too hard can exacerbate pain and tightness rather than help you work through them. On the bright side, muscles are relatively responsive and quick to strengthen and stretch with repeated gentle practice. The payoff: lengthening and strengthening also improves your balance and physical groundedness and centredness as your muscles begin to assert a more symmetrical pressure on the skeleton.
- Always engage the core muscles: The 'airbag' effect – contracting abdominal muscles on the exhale with exertion – is probably one of the most powerful secrets of martial arts (weightlifters use it, too).

- **Be prepared for exercise, not just relaxation:** A properly executed posture will combine the actions of muscles, tendons, joints, skeletal and nerve groups in ways that no other exercise can. This synergy is the key to a good workout. Yes, yoga definitely counts as exercise.
- **Breathe consciously:** No discussion of yoga or martial arts would be complete without mentioning the use of breath. A proper session will actively awaken control of the accessory (or helper) muscles of breathing – the muscles in the lower back, abdomen, shoulder blades, mid back, sternum and pectorals that make your ribcage work like a bellows to pull air into the lungs. By activating these muscle systems you draw more oxygen deeper into the body, which increases the oxygen supply in your blood and to all of your organs, and provides fuel for your cells to create more energy.
- **Focus your mind:** tai chi is derived from Qi gong, which is a set of purely meditative and healing exercises. Yoga is the same. Martial arts exercises – as should be the case with all exercise as well – should be done with your mind clear and focused only on the work you are doing. Mental tension and stress should melt away with exercise; with martial arts, achieving a meditative state is a key goal.

Martial arts fully involves mind, body and spirit. As part of my programme, I highly recommend you take some introductory courses in an Eastern physical art – whether yoga, tai chi, Qi gong or another system. You'll gain something from learning any of these techniques. You may find yourself connecting with a practice and decide to use some aspect of it for the rest of your life. For instance you may use the controlled breathing of tai chi at work, or the stretches of yoga as part of a warm-up or cool-down session. However deep you go, you will most certainly erase the element of boredom that can creep into the necessary human pursuit of a physically active life and significantly increase your energy.

Beyond Oxygen: The Benefits of Breath Work

When you begin to explore martial arts with a master, you will learn that breath work operates on a level far beyond the evident material or physical reality of each session. In almost every Eastern tradition breath work is spiritual work. In yoga, the most powerful type of breathing is called pranayama, and its practice seeks to unify body and mind. *Prana* is a Sanskrit word that translates roughly to life force and *ayama* translates roughly from Sanskrit to the storing and distribution of lifeforce or energy. Practitioners of pranayama consciously move energy by controlling their breath – as do tai chi and Qi gong practitioners.

Many people mistake breath work for deep breathing, but deep breathing implies a forced tensing of muscles. Pranayama-style breathing is the opposite of tension – it is a state in which the mind observes the smooth flow of inhalation and exhalation of air, with nothing to impede the flow – even though you hold your breath briefly in between the inhale and the exhale. The key, however, is that you retain the indrawn breath without straining to hold it. This retention is the point at which the energy or spirit of the breath is distributed, and it's a crucial moment in pranayama.

Don't Panic

People sometimes tell me they get a little panicky with breath work. This may be because they're so unused to breathing deeply or rhythmically outside of a stressful situation that they associate the initial efforts of breathing with fear and tension. I suspect they may also get tripped up by their expectations that they'll master the practice quickly or fear of failure that comes with attempting to learn something new. Helpful words of wisdom for the novice come directly from B.K.S. Iyengar, the great Indian-born yogi who developed Iyengar yoga, a healing system that is practised around the world. In his book *Yoga: The Path to Holistic Health*, Iyengar writes, 'If you fail after a few cycles be content with the knowledge that you have practised three or four cycles with awareness and attention. Do not turn away from failures. Accept them and learn from them.' In Western psychological parlance, Iyengar's tolerant perspective is known as suspending judgement – a practice I heartily endorse, especially when learning any new techniques. Allow yourself to learn and make mistakes. Allow yourself to feel uncertain and don't be afraid of this brief period of uncertainty. You will become more comfortable as you practise. You're learning a great tradition that will be good for you. Allow yourself to be a student of this new way of creating and managing your energy.

Think, Eat (and Be) Like an Athlete

I'd like to put to rest the myth of the buffed versus the not buffed that pervades society. We place our athletes on pedestals, creating legends around them and their regimes (and even their equipment!).

Everyone holds the potential for getting into shape. You can improve your fitness. If you're used to sitting all day, and tomorrow you walk a kilometre or so, you'll be fitter because of the activity and fitter to do it again. All of your activity contributes to your fitness, just as all of your inactivity contributes to being sedentary. Every extra step you take counts towards a more fit you. Some people are further along the fitness continuum, but the reality is we all have an inner athlete.

The crucial difference between you and, say, an Olympic rower – or even a film star getting ready for a part – is the amount of time spent working out. While athletes often have great incentives for working up a sweat, they're not all born with a burning desire to go to the gym. There are countless tricks for getting athletes to exercise more and perform better.

TAP INTO THE SOURCE

Get the Mindset

Creative visualization: Viewing yourself as athletic may very well be one of the most powerful tools you have for becoming athletic. All top athletes use visualization techniques before and during competition to enhance their performances, but only recently have neuroscientists begun to understand why this works. An intriguing study at the Cleveland Clinic in the US showed that thinking about exercise actually got people in better shape. Simply visualizing a muscle contraction – without actual exercise – strengthened muscles by as much as 35 per cent over a 12-week period of visualization. The muscles didn't actually grow in size, but the act of visualization strengthened the brain's signals to the muscles and signalling the muscles is an important first step in conditioning.

You can use this power of the mind to wake up your muscles to overcome whatever mental obstacles are stopping you from getting out and moving. The two keys are to make your imagery as realistic as possible, in full colour and detail – and to visualize in the present tense. Try this: before you go out for a walk, see yourself power-walking right down to the seams of your tracksuit bottoms, see your fine posture, your broad chest, your powerful strides, your arms swinging, your muscles rippling, and repeat an affirmation in the present tense: 'I am fit' or 'I am strong'. Now, go for your walk.

Tunes: Using music has been an open secret in sports psychology ever since Rocky Balboa ran up the steps of the Philadelphia Museum of Art to the chords of 'Gonna Fly Now'. Athletes still use that song to get themselves psyched up. The shrinking of MP3 players to lightweight, portable sizes has solidified the marriage of music and sports. So effective is music in enhancing performance that MP3 players have been officially banned from marathons by the sport's governing body in the US. Similarly, top swimmers commonly use tempo timers – basically waterproof metronomes that maintain the beat, more or less, of Justin Timberlake's 'SexyBack' – for training, but they are illegal in elite-level racing because the driving beat provides a competitive edge.

'Numerous studies confirm that people exercise longer and more vigorously to music.'

But of course you can use music to enhance and even jump-start your athletic performance. One of the most important elements is tempo, which research shows should be between 120 and 140 beats per minute – within the range of most people's target heart rate and most commercial dance music. Very conveniently, iTunes now has a Nike Sport Music section, which includes training playlists from athletes like Serena Williams and Lance Armstrong (who suggests working out to Weezer, Keane and Audioslave). There's even a new Nike + iPod that comes with a motion sensor that allows you to record, download and monitor the progress of your training sessions. Check it out. Or make your own action-packed song list. And know that absolutely nothing separates you from Rocky Balboa. Lance Armstrong, on the other hand, may in fact be from another planet.

Warm up: Have you ever had that feeling in the first five minutes of an exercise session that you can't possibly continue? That's because you haven't given your body a chance to warm up. You wouldn't think of starting your car on a freezing day and slamming the accelerator to the floor without first letting the engine warm up. It's the same thing with your body. When at rest your muscles are not at their most efficient; a full 70 per cent of the oxygen in your blood is unused and kept in reserve for strenuous activity. But blood flow does not adjust instantaneously to a sudden increase in effort. The ultimate risk is that people in poor cardiac health can trigger a life-threatening event by exercising too quickly before the metabolic machinery has been primed for action.

A gentle warm-up – even just lightly hopping up and down before starting a brisk walk – causes your body to begin to deliver blood and oxygen more efficiently. Haemoglobin releases oxygen more readily as your body temperature rises – it's like using a fuel injector to the carburetor in your car. Nerve transmission becomes faster as you warm up and the muscles utilize and create energy more efficiently as your metabolism quickens. All of these factors can explain why you may feel horrible at the beginning of a workout – or why you breathe so heavily if you suddenly sprint to catch a bus. But if you take a moment to warm up gently from your initial cold phase, you'll begin to allow the athletic you to emerge from the sedentary you. You'll see and feel the difference.

Nutrition

As all elite athletes can attest, your nutrient needs increase as your exercise increases. Most particularly, exercise uses B vitamins, anti-oxidants and carbohydrates in abundance. For the moderate exercise recommended in the 21-Day programme, a rainbow diet full of fruits and vegetables should be adequate, but if you fall short of that, a multivitamin may be a good idea.

Here are a few tips to ensure you don't use up your energy stores with exercise. First and foremost, be sure you are adequately hydrated before you exercise. Drink at least half a litre of water an hour before you exercise. Sugar-packed energy drinks are unnecessary except in extenuating circumstances, for example, if you're running a marathon or you have arrived from sea level to a 3,000-metre mountain and plan to hit the slopes hard. The way to get quick energy is to take it on board beforehand. Eat a primarily complex carbohydrate-based food one to four hours before exercise. Don't overeat – exercising on a full stomach is counterproductive to both your exercise performance and energy (not to mention digestion).

Supplements

When you start to significantly ramp up the intensity and duration of exercise to higher aerobic levels and greater resistance, there are specific supplements that may benefit energy and performance. If you are under a doctor's care for a medical condition, consult your doctor before taking new supplements.

Vitamins and minerals: As we have seen in Chapter 2, many vitamins and minerals are important for energy generation both to extract energy from sugar and to produce it in the mitochondria. Arguably the B vitamins are the most important with regard to exercise (B6, for example, supplies the central mitochondrial enzyme NAD), and calcium and magnesium are required for muscle recovery. A well-rounded plant-based diet can supply these, but for endurance and highly stressful events, taking a mixed vitamin/mineral supplement is a good idea.

Creatine: This is an important food nutrient for exercise performance. Creatine is a protein that is part of all muscle fibres and important as a building block for an energy reserve system in cells. Creatine supplements have been the subject of many studies, and it has been shown to improve performance and muscle strength at a dose of 20–30 grams (about one ounce). It can help decrease recovery time, increase lean body mass and strength, improve hydration of the cell and increase performance both for aerobic and resistance training. (Precautions include the risk of intestinal cramping and even muscle cramps with high doses and prolonged use. Inadequate hydration increases the risk of creatine side-effects. People with kidney disease and those taking kidney-stressing medications should not use creatine.)

D-Ribose: Ribose is one of the intermediate sugars created within the cell on the way to creating ATP from oxygen and glucose. Taking ribose (usually 20–30 grams) can provide a quick burst of energy. It minimally affects insulin levels. But it is not long lasting, and is probably best used only *during* a workout. (Precautions are minimal if used as recommended occasionally with exercise.)

Pyruvate: This simple sugar, like ribose, is an intermediate sugar downstream from glucose on the way to creating ATP. A number of research studies show that using it (at 5–10 grams/day) can help cells draw in glucose, increase glycogen stores and improve performance, especially in endurance events. Pyruvate's effect is roughly equivalent to carbohydrate loading before exercise, or using carbohydrates during exercise. (Precautions are minimal, as with ribose, and in the UK, it's usually combined with creatine.)

Citrate: Taking citrate (found as sodium, calcium or magnesium citrate) can reduce fatigue by reducing acidity, thereby reducing potassium accumulation inside cells. Another way to promote alkalinity is to eliminate fizzy drinks and adopt a more plant-based diet; that will naturally favour a more beneficial alkaline internal environment.

N-acetylcysteine (NAC): This amino acid discussed in Chapter 3 for detoxification also helps decrease the tendency for fatigue from exercise in two ways: first, NAC helps reduce free-radicals and clear toxins better; and second, it plays a role in decreasing potassium accumulation in muscles by helping produce more efficient ATP-driven pumps for balancing the cells' potassium and sodium levels.

Zinc: Low-level supplementation with this mineral can help increase exercise stamina, as shown in a 2005 study from the US. A small amount, 5mg (less than the daily recommended level of 11mg) was shown to reduce carbon dioxide build-up, help clear lactic acid and increase stamina. (Precaution: as with all minerals too much can be toxic. With zinc the safe intake level is set at a maximum 25mg/day. Studies with exercise have measured benefits with lower doses. Taking extra zinc may necessitate adding copper, as zinc inhibits copper absorption.)

Fenugreek seed: Surprisingly, this plant seed has been shown to increase the ability of the cell to replenish glycogen after exercise by up to 60 per cent. This is due to an amino acid not normally present in human muscles (4-hydroxyisoleucine) that is present in fenugreek. This amino acid may also be an important nutrient for regulating blood sugar and insulin. Dosage is 30 grams (about one ounce) per day. (Precautions: do not take fenugreek seed if you are taking anticoagulants – blood thinners. Also, fenugreek can lower blood sugar, so diabetics on medication and hypoglycaemic individuals should use this supplement only with close supervision by your doctor.)

Marine algae extract: This is also known as astaxanthin (a carotenoid in the same family as lycopene and beta-carotene). In multiple published studies from Japan, this sea plant extract has been shown to allow cells' metabolism to be more efficient – burning fatty acids for fuel more than glucose. By this, it also may help reduce body fat. It also has been shown to reduce damage from free radicals. This supplement illustrates the nutrient power of the seaweed and algae families that nutrition scientists are just beginning to explore. (Precautions include the need to know your source: algae is harvested from the sea and may contain some micro-contaminants such as other forms of algae. People with immune suppression, including AIDS, should avoid it.)

Eight Simple Energy-Generating Exercises

Brisk walk: If I had to choose one energy-generating activity to recommend above all, it is walking. Walk at a pace brisk enough to increase your heart and breath rates; maybe tackle a few flights of stairs while you are at it. As you walk, actively engage your core, monitor your posture, be aware of the range of motion in your hips and thighs, and breathe consciously, working your ribcage like a bellows. You might look a little strange to the casual observer, but you'll feel so much better when you are finished. With a little practice (and creative visualization), you may even give the impression to others that you are expert enough to be counted in the ranks of professional walkers – after all, racewalking is an Olympic sport.

Breath work: Inhale quietly and slowly, allowing your abdomen to rise, to the count of 4; pause holding the air lightly to the count of 4; exhale slowly, allowing your abdomen to contract, to the count of 6. Repeat four times. The simple act of slow, deep breathing can be incredibly energizing – and relaxing (see Breath Breaks in the 21-Day Plan).

Seated warrior (virasana): This is a very simple stretch and a phenomenal way to expand your breathing capacity (if you have trouble with your knees or back, do this sitting in a chair, not on the floor).

Kneel on the floor, shoulders back and down, neck and spine in a straight line perpendicular to the floor. Lower your buttocks to your feet. Raise your arms in front of you to shoulder level, then tightly interlock your fingers, palms facing you. Now rotate your wrists and forearms so that palms face out, fingers away. Maintain your posture. With fingers clasped and palms facing away, raise your arms until palms face the ceiling. Keep your shoulders pinched back, sternum lifted, chest expanded, relax throat and neck. Look straight ahead, body and neck in a straight line perpendicular to the ground – no tilting. Breathe evenly and hold the posture for one minute or as long as it's comfortable. With time you can extend this to five minutes. Bring your arms gently down to your sides. Place palms on the floor, kneel, stand up first with one leg, placing hands on knee for leverage.

Downward-facing dog (adhomukha svanasana): This simple yoga posture definitely gets your circulation going, but it's not recommended for individuals with high blood pressure, frequent headaches, or who are pregnant. Stand with your feet hip-distance apart, core engaged, head in a straight line with your spine. Take an abdominal breath. Bend from the waist until your palms touch the floor (it's OK to bend your knees). Place your right foot back about a metre or so from your hands. Now place your left foot alongside your right so that your butt is in the air, heels on the ground, and you are in an inverted 'V' position (again, it's OK to bend at the knees if it's uncomfortable to straighten your legs all the way). Straighten your spine (no hunching over). I like Rodney Yee's description in his book *Moving Toward Balance*: 'Practise with bent legs, emphasizing the lift of your sitting bones . . . Feel the integration between the length of the sides of your waist, the opening of your chest and the extension of your arms.' B.K.S. Iyengar further recommends tightening muscles at the top of the thighs and pulling in the kneecaps. Just hang out there for a moment, breathing quietly, arms and back straight, heels on the floor. Now bring your right foot back close to your hands, then your left foot, and slowly stand.

Qi gong energy ball: With this exercise, visualize yourself holding a large ball of energy, move slowly and focus on breathing – your arms should move with very little effort, almost as if they are moved by an invisible energetic force. Feet are parallel, knees slightly bent, butt tucked under, arms at your sides. Take a deep, abdominal breath in and out and continue to breathe consciously throughout the exercise. Begin by allowing your arms to float slowly up, shoulder-width apart, palms facing each other as though you're holding a giant beach ball of energy, waist high in front of you. Bend your arms at the elbows, bringing the imaginary ball closer to you. Now slowly rotate wrists to face palms away from your body and push the ball away until your arms are straight, stepping forward onto your left foot (knee remains slightly bent). Allow arms to float wide apart so that you make a T, bring arms gently down to sides with palms facing each other as you step left foot back to its original place. Float arms upward again, in front of you, holding the ball of energy. 'Lift' the ball over your head and let go. Now allow your arms to slowly float back down to your sides, breathing quietly, core engaged, butt tucked under, shoulders down and back. Repeat, this time stepping right foot forward.

Hopping: Skipping is the best, full-fitness, aerobic energy-generating exercise, but it's not always convenient to whip out a skipping rope. You can hop up and down just about anywhere – next to your desk, standing in line at the bank, waiting for a train. Hop 30 times; finish by standing for a moment with good posture and taking four slow abdominal breaths.

Push-ups and **core crunches** (see pages 156 and 251).

Rock out with your iPod: No explanation necessary. Freeform dancing is not only fun, but allows you to log an aerobic workout without the psychic pain.

Chapter 5

Power Rest, How to Recharge your Battery

CASE STUDY
STRESS-INDUCED INSOMNIA

FREDERICA came to see me feeling as though she 'could no longer function'. In her mid-forties she'd developed insomnia and had become so chronically exhausted it was beginning to ruin her life. She was exceedingly short-tempered with her family, had begun to develop headaches, indigestion and more frequent colds than ever before. As a result of her problems, however, she had tried to observe some good health habits – she had become more conscious of eating a well-balanced diet, exercised regularly (sometimes too intensely), and cut out any stimulants after noon. Even so, she was still exhausted by 8pm. Most nights she could fall asleep around midnight, but invariably woke up at 4 or 5am (sometimes known as the Hour of the Wolf, when our greatest fears tend to surface if we're awake). She would toss and turn, rarely going back to sleep. She was lucky if she got six hours of sleep on any night. It had become a vicious cycle, possibly accelerated by barely perceptible hormone shifts of middle age.

She had tried her regular doctor's prescription sleeping tablets (which he had given her only after he'd performed many batteries of tests to determine that she had no underlying illness), but they either left her feeling badly hungover, or they wore off after four hours. She reported that her doctor's attitude was, 'Hey, I'm more tired than you. Get over it.' Over-the-counter supplements and even prescription hormones seemed to have no effect whatsoever.

It was clear to me Frederica was suffering from stress-induced insomnia. This is the sleep problem I most commonly see. The cure would not be found in a sleeping pill, but in getting better control of her mind and thought processes, and in addressing possible underlying nutritional issues. I asked her to limit alcohol intake to one glass of wine with dinner (processing a heavier load of alcohol can cause early hour awakening), and placed her on a multivitamin with B-complex.

Frederica then began the real work of learning how to help her body sleep. I taught her how to do progressive relaxation exercises at bedtime: starting by contracting muscles in her neck and jaw, and gradually working her way down to her toes – focusing on the exercise and letting random thoughts go. This helped her drift off into a more peaceful sleep, and she didn't get stuck in her prior habit of allowing fears and anxieties to flood her mind just before falling asleep. When she woke up in the early hours of the morning, she practised dream remembrance. As soon as she was conscious of beginning to wake up she was immediately required to lock onto her dream. No matter how scary or weird the dream was, she had to stay in it in order to block the old habit of ruminating on her worries as soon as she woke up. More than half the time, she reported, this dream remembrance allowed her to go right back into the sleep cycle. If she lost the dream or awakened without memory of one, she immediately started either the progressive relaxation exercise or a breath-focused meditation. By the end of the first two weeks, she was clocking in seven or eight hours of sleep most days. Her energy soared.

FREDERICA'S STORY IS VERY COMMON – sleep deprivation is at epidemic proportions in the West – a recent study found that 71 per cent of Americans are sleep-deprived and get less than eight hours per night. In the UK, one third of adults gets five or fewer hours of sleep per night. Much of this sleep debt has been rung up by choice – people just don't want to turn out the lights. Before the electric light bulb was invented, people slept an average of 10 hours a day. Today we sleep less than seven hours on average, and a number of factors including stress, medications and habitual snoring often degrade the quality of that sleep. The incidence of insomnia, trouble falling or staying asleep, is rising (in part due to the ageing population – yes, older people tend to have more sleep issues). Clearly, it's time for people to start getting proper sleep.

Scientists have only recently begun to explain what every mother in the world knows: sleep plays an important role in overall health. Inadequate sleep is now associated with heart disease, diabetes and obesity among other chronic diseases. Recent investigations show that eight hours is optimum for proper healing and cellular rejuvenation, and that – even more surprising – the most powerful healing occurs between the eighth and ninth hours of sleep. Bottom line: just about everyone should make an effort to get more sleep, and more regenerative rest.

You probably don't have time to catch up with lost sleep by napping in the middle of the day – God bless the cultures that encourage a siesta – but you no doubt can make some adjustments in your habits to allow a better quantity and quality of regenerative rest at night. I'll share some very simple and practical – nonpharmaceutical – ways to improve your sleep in this chapter. As you start resting more, you will see that more and deeper sleep buys you considerable energy.

Healthy, Regenerative Rest

One of the comments I frequently hear in my office is, 'I don't need a lot of sleep'. A corollary of this is the oft-repeated phrase, 'I don't have enough time to sleep'. As gently as I can, I break the news that adequate, regenerative rest (there is such a thing as non-regenerative sleep, which I'll get to in a moment) is a critical foundation of health as well as an important source of abundant energy. Let's take a look at what science knows about sleep.

Why We Sleep

There are three main reasons to sleep: to conserve energy by slowing down metabolic processes, to regenerate tissue and to clear out toxins. Slumber is a time of semi-*hibernation*, when the body's neurological and hormonal systems operate mostly at low levels that conserve energy: body temperature is allowed to drop, so there's less work in generating heat; there's no new food to digest; blood pressure decreases; heart and breathing should be steady and slow for the majority of sleep time. This slowdown allows for *regeneration*; it gives time and resources for the cell's surface receptors and internal processes to recoup, repair and replace. Sleep is also a time of *detoxification*, when the body is able to clear out energy-draining molecular by-products that accumulate during the day as a result of high levels of activity.

By putting all systems on low power, sleep offers your body time and energy to carry out a full range of maintenance duties: rebalancing hormones (for example, replenishing cortisol and insulin supplies), strengthening the immune system, consolidating memory and repairing overworked areas of the body.

During the day, the natural ebb and flow of the body's processes create cell-damaging free radicals (by-products of normal metabolism) that tend to multiply in the presence of toxins such as heavy metals or excess sugar. Sleep's metabolic slowdown allows the body to clear out these harmful substances, preparing the detoxification systems for the demands of the next day's activities. Sleep improves cognitive functioning; both napping *and* a full eight hours of sleep have been shown to result in better performance on tests. Sleep may also actually help restore energy levels in the body by clearing the cells of a sleep-inducing

'While you slumber, your brain's immune cells get to work producing a crucial substance called interleukin 12, which is necessary for processing memory as well as for conferring immunity to disease.'

molecule in the brain called adenosine (see box).

Sleep makes you brighter, gives you energy and builds immunity. And those are just a few of its benefits.

The emotional repair that also occurs while you slumber rewards good sleepers with better energy. When you sleep, levels of serotonin, the emotion-regulating neurotransmitter, decline. This low level is not terrific if you wake up in the middle of the night, but the decline is felt to allow cell surface receptors of that happy molecule to resensitize and become better at keeping mood swings at bay the next day. This refreshing of chemical receptors in the brain explains why most people have a brighter outlook in the morning, and why you should try not to think worrying thoughts at night when your brain chemistry may be more vulnerable to dark scenarios. (Relaxation exercises help dissipate negative thoughts that tense your body and keep you awake.)

Going without sleep impairs a person's ability to integrate emotions with logic, which is a necessary skill for moral reasoning.

The Sleep-Energy Connection

Recently, scientists have begun to piece together a picture of sleep as an energy-restorative state. In a cunning bit of biological multi-tasking, a compound called adenosine – the backbone of the energy molecule adenosine triphosphate (ATP) – can put you to sleep when its levels rise in the brain. The accumulation of adenosine as a result of energy expenditure during the day is thought to trigger slow brainwaves that make you sleepy at night. The body actually prevents itself from overexertion by using a component of its energy-generating molecule to induce sleepiness. Then, when you sleep, your body gathers sleep-inducing adenosine from inside cells and in between cells, and uses it to replenish the energy. This molecular recycling routine is key to sleep's ability to rejuvenate your energy supply.

The good news is that having a high level of emotional intelligence prior to sleep deprivation helps when it comes to making moral decisions in a state of exhaustion. In one fascinating study, sleep deprivation resulted in an elevated expectation of a higher reward for risky behaviour

'Sleep deprivation has even been shown to have a profound effect on your ability to form moral judgments.'

in one part of the brain, and activity in the part of the brain having to do with expectation of loss was diminished. (You might want to enquire about your financial advisor's sleeping habits!)

Dreaming is not well understood, but it is another means by which sleep addresses emotional balance. In dreams, you try to work out the day's anxieties and stresses, another way in which sleep is a time for emotional repair.

All of the wonderful things sleep can do for you depend on getting a good night of it. As you'll see in the following section, good sleep is not only a function of quantity – how much you get – it is also a function of quality, or what kind of sleep you get.

What is a good night's sleep?

In the hundreds of sleep clinics around the world, where people's brains are wired to scanning machines and oxygen monitors while they dream of faraway places, researchers have learned that sleep is an incredibly dynamic operation. In healthy young adults – whose brainwave patterns have been used in sleep medicine as the model of what's normal – there are two states of sleep: *non-rapid eye movement* (NREM), which constitutes 75 to 80 per cent of overall sleep; and *rapid eye movement* (REM), which constitutes most of the remaining 20 to 25 per cent (brief periods of waking contribute about 5 per cent of sleep time). Sleep is *initiated* with the dominance of non-rapid eye movement, with its four distinct stages; and sleep *culminates* with a dominance of rapid eye movement, a mentally active form of sleep that allows you to wake up relatively alert (unlike reptiles, which are paralysed by a state of torpor upon awakening, which may sound eerily familiar to some). Throughout the night, the body cycles between the two states, and to get a good night's sleep you need enough of both, which is known in the medical business as having good sleep architecture.

Like a deep-sea diver, your consciousness descends through the stages of non-rapid eye movement toward the deepest and most restful fourth stage called *slow-wave sleep*. Then your brainwaves take the plunge into rapid eye movement – where the body is almost completely paralysed but the mind is active with *vivid dreaming* – before ascending back to the lighter stages.

As you alternate between the two states of sleep, your body alternates between two states of nervous system control. For the most part, NREM sleep produces slow alpha and delta brainwave activity on a brain scanner (electroencephalogram or EEG), and it is governed by the calming, parasympathetic portion of the nervous system that produces a steady heartbeat and breathing rate with low energy expenditure. By comparison, the vivid dreaming of REM sleep produces vigorous brainwaves – equal to and sometimes even more intense than waking daytime activity – and it is governed by the stimulating or sympathetic nervous system, which causes quickening of your heart and breathing rates as well as a rise in blood pressure and energy expenditure. For a good night's sleep sufficient to rejuvenate the mind and body and give you better energy for the next day, you need go to bed early enough to leave time for a full menu of both states of sleep.

'In eight hours of sleep, your brainwaves should submerge into vivid dreaming and then resurface again every 90 minutes – or about five times a night.'

Slow-wave sleep predominates in the first third of the night. At around 4am, when your circadian rhythm (your body's internal biological clock) brings your body temperature down to its lowest ebb, rapid eye movement begins to predominate; and the deepest stage of slow-wave sleep can fade away altogether. With a full night's sleep, as sleep time is extended the amount of vivid dreaming (REM) sleep increases. If you occasionally stay up until the early hours of the morning you will get short-changed on slow-wave sleep and have a less regenerative rest.

I like to think of non-rapid eye movement as the shutdown mode of your own personal software – it is the required first part of sleep. Rapid eye movement represents a shift to an altered state of dream-consciousness that usually follows

' When you go to sleep and *how long* you sleep determines whether or not you get a healthy, full run of all the states and stages of sleep – you need eight hours with more than half of that under your belt before 4am.'

the shutdown state, and thrives in the low body temperatures of the wee hours of the morning. Quite simply, sleep is a journey through different states and you need to take the time to fully realize that journey in all its states.

Unhealthy, Energy-draining Sleep

If it's true, as Tolstoy said, that unhappy families are each unhappy in their own way, then poor sleep is the unhappy family of the human genome – everyone seems to have his or her own unique way of not sleeping. There are, in fact, many causes of poor sleep, but by far the most common are stress and the normal changes of ageing. Many other functional problems, like sinus conditions or chronic pain, can destroy sleep, as can lifestyle choices like alcohol over-consumption. Making matters worse, poor sleep can magnify problems like chronic pain and stress, creating a vicious circle and wasting precious energy.

Over a period of about five years even sleep doctors were losing sleep over the definition of insomnia, which had been described traditionally as difficulty initiating or sustaining sleep, or early awakening. But there was a growing group of people with daytime complaints often associated with insomnia – fatigue, trouble concentrating and moodiness – who were not reporting that they had trouble with sleep. The sleep medicine community finally decided to include daytime symptoms that usually stem from sleep loss as part of insomnia, so now the realm of conditions related to trouble sleeping has expanded. You don't have to be lying awake counting sheep to qualify as having a bad night's sleep: your sleep can be very poor if it is constantly disturbed, for example, by heavy snoring. Below I cover a number of conditions that are known causes – but too often go unrecognized – of poor sleep. No matter how you miss out on sleep, however, your energy will be worse off.

The Heart of the Matter

Just take a moment to consider your heart. Thanks to the venerable Nurses Health Study (an ongoing multicentre investigation that's followed 122,000 nurses for more than 30 years), we've learned that getting just one less hour of sleep per night *(for example, shifting from eight to seven hours on a regular basis) significantly* increases *the risk of heart disease. A similarly significant study in Japan showed that a drop in sleep time from eight to five hours just two nights a week can help trigger a heart attack in people at risk for heart disease. Not only does a proper night's sleep protect your heart, even napping helps. I was encouraged to learn from a recent study of 23,000 people (at the Department of Epidemiology at the Harvard School of Public Health) that three half-hour midday naps per week dramatically reduced (by 37 per cent) the risk of suffering a heart attack and dying (as long as the nap doesn't come right after a big meal, which actually increases the risk of a heart attack)! Even the occasional catnap (just one or two a week) lowered the risk of heart-related death by 12 per cent. Who wouldn't trade a catnap for a heart attack if given the chance?*

The problem with sleep problems

The consequences of poor sleep range from total exhaustion to major health problems. With deprivation your body becomes inefficient at making energy: it dissipates a lot of energy as heat, resulting in a sort of energetic spinning of wheels. A protein in the energy manufacturing mitochondria is overproduced during sleep deprivation. This molecule disconnects the machinery within the mitochondria, forcing it to burn the nutrients within as heat rather than transforming them into other more useful forms of energy. It's the somnolent equivalent of burning the furniture when you start to run out of firewood!

Mounting evidence suggests that sleep problems are intimately related not only to lack of energy, but to illnesses such as breast cancer, obesity, diabetes, immune deficiencies and especially heart disease. In one fascinating study from the University of Chicago, sleep deprivation crippled the effectiveness of a flu shot! Sleeping for four hours a night for six days reduced healthy students' immune system response to flu vaccines by 50 per cent compared to volunteers who had normal sleep. Amazingly, it took between three and four weeks of normal sleep for the young volunteers to develop a healthy vaccine-conferred immunity to the flu after just one week of reduced shut eye. Never underestimate the value of good sleep habits!

Still not convinced you should give up late-night TV? Consider that a good eight hours' sleep is even thought to be important for weight control. In a recent highly publicized study, researchers at Columbia University analysed sleep habits and the body mass index (ratio of weight to height) of more than 9,500 people and found those who slept for only five hours each night were 60 per cent more likely to be obese than those who slept for seven or more hours per night. Scientists at the University of Chicago have produced a series of studies showing that sleep deprivation leaves its mark on metabolism and hormones, specifically leptin (released by fat cells and signals satiety) and ghrelin (produced by the stomach and signals hunger). In one study, after two sleep-deprived nights, participants' blood levels of leptin dropped by an average of 18 per cent and their ghrelin levels soared by 28 per cent, which helps explain why lack of sleep makes you eat and put on weight.

When you miss an entire night's sleep, your body goes into recovery sleep mode the following night, in which it makes up for lost sleep by spending lots of time in slow-wave sleep, sometimes skipping rapid eye movement altogether. If your sleep is disrupted frequently in a single night the body also tries to recover by increasing time spent in slow-wave sleep. But with a night of fitful rebound sleep you get short-changed on vivid dreaming sleep, and are likely to wake up groggy without the help of the REM phase to activate your brain cells.

Lagging behind

Jetlag is a study in rapid eye movement chaos. REM sleep depends on your circadian rhythms, and jet air travel across time zones is a sure way to wreak havoc on your body clock. To experience a full REM cycle you have to get significant sleep between 4 and 8am, when your circadian rhythms produce a 24-hour low in body temperature. When you fly east across time zones you start your day at a time when your body is supposed to be in the active dreaming cycle (for example your watch says 8am but your body clock says 5am). You get shortchanged on mentally active sleep and start your day straight out of slow-wave sleep, which feels quite sluggish. On the flip side, if you fly westward across time zones, you might fall asleep at the bottom of your circadian cycle when your body 'thinks' it's about 4am. In that case it's possible to go straight into vivid dreaming without passing through restful slow waves.

A jetlagged night of all REM or no REM can leave you feeling pretty strange. A walk in the morning sun at your destination can help reset your biological clock (see Light Therapy, below) so you don't feel as out of sync. Taking an extract of the body-clock regulating hormone melatonin (see Nutritional Supplements, below) two hours before bedtime in the new time zone has also been shown to help you dissipate the effects of nagging jetlag.

The body usually recovers on its own from the occasional bad night's sleep or trip across the Atlantic. Trouble starts, however, when the states and stages of sleep are chronically mixed up, or when you just don't get enough night after night.

Bad Sleep: The Causes and Cures

Poor sleep can be a function of inferior quality (having your sleep stages out of sync for any number of reasons) or inadequate quantity (getting too little sleep, which cuts off sleep stages), or it can be a function of both, which is absolutely the worst-case scenario. No matter what the cause, however, you can get your sleep problems under control and it is vitally important that you do so. I find that the best way to encourage my patients to practice better sleep habits is to let them know exactly what conditions and choices have a negative impact on sleep.

Ageing: It turns out that the definition of normal sleep goes out the window as we age. Much of the trouble has to do with shifting hormones at midlife – for men, too! – that affect the amount and type of rest you get. Chronic conditions that often come with age such as arthritis, sinus congestion and acid reflux can also disrupt sleep. With age, there is a decrease in growth hormone and evening elevations of the stress hormone cortisol as well as an increase of the immune system messengers – all of which negatively affect sleep and reduce the amount of time spent in the more restorative stages 3 and 4 of non-rapid eye movement.

Some of the trouble with ageing can be addressed with better stress management. By age forty, levels of the stress hormone cortisol tend to be elevated for most people, which scientists now believe may be a result of that hormone not reaching its low point at night. Managing stress during the day so that you are

'Older people are predisposed to have problems not only with sleep quantity but sleep quality – with inevitable consequences for both their health and energy.'

able to get to sleep earlier and sleep longer may promote beneficial declines in cortisol at night. In some cases sleeping more can be seen as an anti-ageing potion – circulating testosterone levels in healthy men are known to decline with advancing age, but when men sleep longer they are able to make more testosterone. Which just goes to show sleeping is not for sissies!

One of my favourite observations from sleep clinics is that people of a certain age (sixty-five and up) tend to believe that their sleep is *worse* than it actually is. Much of the trouble has to do with attitude. With meticulous psychological surveys, scientists have determined that whether a person views getting less sleep as insomnia or merely accepts it as a normal part of ageing depends largely on his individual attitude about growing old. One of my longtime patients who cruised into her seventies with abundant energy once told me that she had learned to accept getting less sleep as 'No big deal'. I'm not suggesting you ignore a sleep problem, but I am encouraging you not to become one of those folks of an advanced age who sit around complaining about sleep – that's a sure energy-draining activity.

Stress: Unbridled stress causes difficulty falling asleep as well as sleep disruption (waking in the middle of the night with trouble getting back to sleep). People wracked with stress can't turn off the worry: when they lay down their minds race; or when they wake up in the middle of the night, their worries take hold and keep them awake. Researchers have begun to follow the destructive path of the stress hormones and other biochemical messengers that keep your neuroendocrine system hyperactive, even into the middle of the night.

Stress per se doesn't necessarily keep you awake, but worrying about stressful things can keep you awake. And because sleep deprivation mimics the effects of stress by elevating stress hormone levels and activating anxiety-promoting areas of the brain, you set up a vicious circle: you're stressed so you can't sleep;

'Unremitting stress has also been shown to trigger nightmares, increasing demands on your nervous system.'

then the lack of sleep makes your stress worse. You quickly become perpetually exhausted. This is why I strongly recommend night-time relaxation exercises in the 21-Day Plan.

The many negative effects that unbridled stress produces in your nervous system can have serious consequences during sleep. The early morning between 4 and 8am – when rapid eye movement (REM) is at its peak – is the time of day with the highest incidence of heart attacks (and this doubles on Monday mornings). This is largely due to stress-induced declines in your heart's ability to handle the shift from the calming, parasympathetic nervous system dominance of non-REM sleep to the stimulating, sympathetic nervous system dominance of REM sleep. As your nervous system starts to wake up, a stressed heart sometimes just can't take it. Clearly, cardiovascular problems need to be diagnosed early and treated by a specialist. Along with proper treatment, a conscious stress-reduction programme coupled with regular moderate exercise will help to protect the heart during times like the early morning when nervous system shifts require healthy flexibility of the heart muscle.

One further caveat has to do with managing stress when you actually do wake up. If you wake up, jump out of bed and go straight into panic mode over your work responsibilities it can be tough on your ticker. This is why I strongly recommend you start your day with the two-minute meditation, the Early Morning Wake Up Call, detailed in the 21-Day Plan (see page 239). Starting your day with your stress under control will keep it in better control all day and give more consistent energy.

Sleep apnoea: Sleep apnoea is a condition in which breathing stops for at least 10 seconds at least 15 times per hour during sleep. It's often accompanied by loud snoring and is considered to be a major cause of exhaustion during the day. Short of your spouse guessing that you have the condition, daytime sleepiness is one of the biggest symptomatic tip-offs to sleep apnoea. At the extreme end, sleep apnoea can cause you to wake abruptly gasping for air. In some cases it does not wake you but continues to cause blood oxygen levels to decline – often significantly – throughout the night, suffocating the heart, the brain and all of the body's cells. Each spell sets off alarms (*take a breath!*) making it all but impossible to move beyond the very lightest stage of non-rapid eye movement sleep – forget about vivid dreaming! Studies of apnoea demonstrate that it's associated with dominance of the sympathetic nervous system, which places stress on the heart, too.

The causes of sleep apnoea are varied. It has a strong genetic component (if a parent has apnoea, you have a 40 per cent chance of getting it), most likely due to inherited traits in the anatomy of the neck and pharynx that make it harder to keep the airway open during sleep. It's more common in men and its frequency rises with age. Drinking alcohol and sleeping on your back can trigger the problem. By far the most common cause is obesity, which increases the risk of developing apnoea by more than 1,000 per cent! Excess body weight puts pressure on the throat and prevents it from opening enough to facilitate breathing. Up to 70 per cent of people with obesity have sleep apnoea. Having an underactive (hypo)thyroid can be a hidden cause of sleep apnoea, and when treated, sleep apnoea often also clears.

The symptoms of apnoea are pretty far-ranging, from frequent awakening, daytime exhaustion, poor memory and loud snoring (about 10 per cent of habitual snorers have apnoea). The health consequences can be devastating, including a significant increased risk of hypertension and heart attacks. For example, many people who have uncontrolled high blood pressure – for which medication seems not to work well – actually have sleep apnoea as the cause. A continuous lack of oxygen during sleep can precipitate an acute heart attack. If you have any of the symptoms of apnoea you should consider being evaluated by a sleep medicine specialist – hopefully before you have a heart attack.

If you have sleep apnoea, your doctor may be able to organize a continuous positive airway pressure device (CPAP). This device is placed over your nose and mouth and produces positive pressure (like a vacuum cleaner on reverse) that forces open your airway and causes more oxygen to flow into your upper airways and lungs. By stopping the drop in oxygen levels and frequent wakening, the device allows your body to pass through all the cycles of sleep. CPAP has been shown to conserve sleep energy and improve daytime energy levels. Oral appliances – which you can obtain from your dentist – to reposition the jaw muscle and tongue and increase the airwave space can be almost as effective as CPAP in moderate apnoea; and people tend to prefer the less invasive nature of an appliance compared to the CPAP device. Surgery should be the last option, and would only be useful for anatomical defects of genetic origin.

Preventing Sleep Apnoea and Snoring

Before going for these big-gun devices, however, there are a few changes you can make in your sleep habits that may reduce, or even resolve, sleep apnoea.

- *Lose weight. It is dramatically beneficial for sleep apnoea; a 10 per cent weight loss produces a 26 per cent reduction in apnoea.*
- *Reduce alcohol intake, especially later in the evening. Alcohol can over-relax the muscles in the throat and pharynx and contribute to their collapse.*
- *Elevate your head by 30 degrees (some bedding shops sell wedges to place under your head) to reduce the force of gravity on your throat.*
- *Switch to sleeping on your side instead of your back, again to avoid the forces of gravity. Use a pillow as a bolster to hold onto and help keep you in the side sleeping position.*
- *Use a sleep ball: tenacious back sleepers can try the sleep ball technique, in which you attach a tennis ball to the seat of your pyjamas to prevent you from sleeping on your back.*

Snoring: Scientists are undecided about the health consequences of general non-apnoea snoring. Light to moderate snoring is not caused by any abnormality, but rather originates from vibrations of tissue in the throat and air passageways. Your own snoring episodes can cause blood pressure to rise (not to mention what it does to your spouse), but snoring is not considered a cause of daytime hypertension (high blood pressure). My primary concern is what snoring does to your ability to get a good night's rest. The resistance that snoring produces in your airways can cause frequent arousal and fragmented sleep. It can throw off the normal balance of calming, parasympathetic nervous system domination during sleep. Snorers have an increase in stimulating sympathetic nervous system dominance during sleep, which consumes energy and can lead to daytime fatigue.

Snoring solutions are the same as for sleep apnoea. Try reducing alcohol intake and changing your sleep position before making the bigger financial and lifestyle commitment of obtaining a device like the CPAP. Sometimes helpful is a surgical procedure called a uvulectomy, removal of the small punching bag (uvula) that hangs at the back of the throat to prevent it from obstructing the airway.

Chronic sinus congestion: The common cold or chronic stuffiness from allergies can pose a real challenge to a good night's sleep and can even lead to sleep apnoea. You really do need the full cooperation of your nose to get adequate oxygen during sleep. A stuffy nose reduces the capacity of your major air passageway, and it forces you to work harder for air, which can make it easier for the back of the throat to collapse. Scientists even believe nasal congestion can block receptors in the nose that signal the brain that it needs air. A bout of a cold virus is not a big deal, but if you're routinely stuffy, I highly recommend working with an ear, nose and throat (ENT) doctor to determine the cause of chronic congestion and eliminate it. A 1998 study at Penn State University's Division of Allergy showed that targeted use of nasal steroids (like Nasonex) to quell inflammation improved sleep and reduced daytime fatigue for people with chronic sinus congestion. But there are remedies you can try short of using steroids.

Amazingly, the simple little device called a Breathe Right Strip – a stiff plaster that sits on the bridge of the nose and physically pulls the nostrils open – can be a big help for congested sleepers. More permanent remedies – such as identifying subtle food allergies – that target the source of congestion are key. By following the elimination diet of the 21-Day Plan, you may find that congestion starts to clear up, as wheat, dairy and other allergies can cause chronic sinus congestion. Getting acupuncture and chiropractic treatments from experienced practitioners can often help chronic sinus problems.

'A 2006 study at found that pain reduced the quality of sleep in 55 per cent of patients, poor sleep worsened the pain, and a poor-quality mattress magnified both problems.'

Gastro-oesophageal reflux disease: The reflux of stomach acid into the oesophagus – which is increasingly recognized as the cause of a wide range of problems including chronic sinusitis, asthma, bronchitis and chest pain – does much of its dirty work during sleep and can be a major factor in sleep apnoea. In a November 2007 study from Chicago Rush Medical Center, correcting the hyperacidity of gastro-oesophageal reflux significantly improved sleep apnoea, sleep quality and daytime fatigue for 70 per cent of patients.

The classic conventional remedy for gastro-oesophageal reflux disease is acid-blocking medications. These certainly work. I recommend using antacids to get the problem under control if it's bad, and then targetting the causes of acidity. If necessary, have an endoscopy by a gastrointestinal specialist or ENT doctor to rule out significant anatomic abnormalities. Remedies other than antacids include elevation of the pillow, so that by decreasing the force of gravity, stomach acid doesn't backflow into the oesophagus; and eliminating night-time acidic foods (especially tomatoes), spices, caffeine and alcohol.

Chronic pain: Chronic pain is a double-edged sleep sword: it can interrupt sleep, which degrades pain-inhibition processes in the brain, making pain worse the next day. Sleeping less doesn't affect pain as much as sleeping poorly does.

Evaluate your mattress (see below) and don't just live with pain. There are a number of avenues to explore including working with a pain specialist (often resulting in the use of stronger pain medications), physiotherapy, hypnosis, acupuncture and working to reduce inflammatory elements of the diet (see Chapter 2).

Inflammatory conditions: In conditions like arthritis, autoimmune diseases, multiple sclerosis, Lyme disease and even during a bout of flu, the balance between pro-inflammatory and anti-inflammatory chemicals produced by white blood cells of the immune system plays an essential role in regulating how well you sleep. These chemicals are produced during infections as important signalling messengers, but in chronic inflammation a steady stream of them can wreak havoc on your sleep and energy. In a study of elderly folks, higher evening levels of pro-inflammatory cytokines were related to getting less sleep. A very slight increase was associated with an increased waking time of about 20 minutes. Obesity also results in a chronic inflammatory state – fat is highly active in producing harmful cytokines that can interfere with sleep.

The single most important solution for reducing inflammation is lifestyle change: reduce weight and stress, exercise and sleep more, and eat an anti-inflammatory diet (see Chapter 2). Cut out sugar and processed foods especially, reduce meat consumption, and incorporate anti-inflammatory foods such as fish oils, spices and herbs.

Alcohol: If you're having problems with sleep or insomnia, you should consider cutting back on alcohol. When you drink alcohol as long as five hours before falling asleep, it can make sleep apnoea or snoring worse (even if you don't normally have those problems). Alcohol triples the tendency for restless limb movement that causes frequent awakening. When you drink, you can fall asleep quicker and get to a deeper, slow-wave sleep faster (you pass out), but as the alcohol is metabolized by the middle of the night (usually after the first two 90-minute sleep cycles), sympathetic nervous system activity increases, which produces fitful sleep (you wake up in the middle of the night with a parched mouth, feeling lousy). While a glass of wine with dinner is OK, for anyone having trouble sleeping, imbibing a couple of nightcaps is not the cure.

> 'Alcohol increases your deeper sleep at the beginning of the night and causes more restless sleep in the last portion of the night, so it can have an overall negative effect on sleep.'

Caffeine: Our favourite drug, the chemical stimulant caffeine can contribute to insomnia – even in your morning latte. The half-life of caffeine is three to six hours, meaning that if you have a cup at noon, a quarter cup's worth could still be in your system at midnight (as it could if you drink a larger dose, say, a two-cup-sized grande, at 6am). Caffeine has been shown to block the adenosine receptors. (As discussed in the box above, accumulating adenosine during daytime is one of the triggers for getting to sleep at night.) Studies have shown that caffeine blocks this mechanism and disturbs proper sleep. As with its distant cousin amphetamines, caffeine can cause significant withdrawal symptoms when eliminated – fatigue and headaches can develop after stopping even a single cup-a-day habit. If you have insomnia and consume daily caffeine, wean yourself off slowly and stop for two full weeks to see if you sleep better and have more overall energy. The Power Up! 21-Day Plan walks you through this process.

Medications: It is truly shocking when you look at the list of medication that negatively affects sleep. Drugs affect the chemicals called neurotransmitters, which govern brainwave activity. Pseudophedrine (in Sudafed and other cold medicines) is a good example of how medicines affect sleep; many people using it regularly suffer

> ### Nightmare Medications
> *Here's a short list of drugs shown in clinical studies or case reports to cause nightmares: antibiotics (such as Ciproxin and Zithromax/azithromycin), antidepressants (especially SSRIs like Prozac), cardiovascular drugs (especially certain beta-blockers like Inderal LA or Beta-prograne), and certain anti-inflammatories (like Synflex/naproxen). Bad dreams may be a small price to pay for curing a bad infection or stabilizing your heart rate, but just knowing these drugs can cause nightmares may help you feel less anxious when the boogie-man shows up in the wee hours.*

unwittingly from debilitating over-stimulation – including insomnia from even a small daytime dose of decongestants. Antihistamines in cold remedies, on the other hand, actually make you drowsy. Many of the most commonly prescribed medications are on the list of drugs that affect sleep (unbeknownst to patients and, usually, their doctors as well) including blood pressure medication, anti-seizure medication, antihistamines, decongestants and antidepressants. This is just one of many reasons that my goal for all patients is to reduce the number of medications they take by implementing lifestyle changes whenever possible.

Sleeping tablets: Sleeping tablets are useful when acute stress or health conditions occasionally interfere with falling or staying asleep. They can also be used to reset the circadian rhythms of your biological clock when you are travelling. They become a problem when people use them chronically. First of all, sleeping tablets do not guarantee healthy sleep architecture or complete elimination of daytime sleepiness. To do that, you need to treat the underlying condition and get to the source of the problem that causes insomnia (such as daytime anxiety). You will not get a magic, permanent fix from a tablet. The quick-fix mentality can actually lead to a worsening of the sleep problem over time and to the appearance of other problems related to lack of sleep. Polypharmacy – the prescribing of multiple medications, often for the same conditions – has been an increasing problem, occasionally with tragic consequences.

A brief synopsis of medicinal sleeping aids contains two broad categories: those that leave you drowsy in the morning and could become habit forming, and those that produce addiction and/or dependency. The former group includes soporific antidepressants (tricyclics such as Lofepramine and SSRIs such as Seroxat), the newer melatonin receptor agonist Rozerem (ramelteon, which is about to be launched in the UK), and OTC antihistamines (Sominex, Benadryl/cetirizine). The other group contains solely prescriptive sleeping medications that can be addictive – such as barbiturates (phenobarbital, Secobarbital), benzodiazepines (Dalmane, Valium, Rivotril), and narcotics (codeine, hydrocodone) – or can produce dependency such as Zolpidem and Sonata (Zaleplon).

I am not dismissing the use of prescription sleeping tablets: I prescribe them myself sometimes (though rarely compared with most other doctors). Judicious occasional use of these powerful medications can be helpful for acute distress or jetlag, and are necessary for others with more severe medical conditions or severe sleep disorders, especially when overseen by a sleep disorders specialist. But there are many other ways, detailed in the following section, that sleeping problems can and should be addressed.

'Insomnia is a commonly listed side-effect of numerous prescription and over-the-counter drugs; they can cause a wide variety of disruptions in the sleep cycle including nervous system overstimulation in the early stages of sleep and nightmares in the later stages.'

TAP INTO THE SOURCE

My Favourite Sleep Remedies

Make an effort to maintain a consistent pre-bedtime routine. This can include turning off stimulating activities (including electronic gadgets) at least an hour before sleep; utilizing relaxation rituals, such as breath work and progressive relaxation techniques (see below). Keep a regular, reasonable schedule – get to bed as close as possible to the same time every night (ideally by 10pm) and wake up at roughly the same reasonable time each morning. Sleep docs actually do call this consistency 'good sleep hygiene'. Of course, everyone knows that mothers are the best sleep hygienists in the world, but what follows are my best tips that *even* your mother may not know.

A good pillow: This is an easy change that can make a huge difference. The first thing I tell everyone to do is evaluate the pillow situation. A pillow is supposed to support your head so that your neck, airways and spine remain in a natural position with good alignment throughout the night. A very convincing 2001 German Sleep Medicine Lab study found that changing to a medium-firm pillow (the firmest was of no advantage) significantly improved both non-REM and REM sleep for people who have trouble sleeping without other underlying conditions or causes. Bottom line: a pillow should support your head, not bury it.

Pillows also frequently contribute to allergies, which is a big no-no when it comes to getting a good night's sleep. A crucial first step in improving sleep is to scrutinize your pillow for allergens, the source of which can be the filling (down and feather allergies are very common) or it can be dust mites inside the filling. I highly recommend that you examine the range of hypoallergenic foam pillows on the market and get one. When you find one that suits you, place it inside a dust-mite blocking pillow protector that goes under the pillow case (www.allergyuk.org is a great source for information on pillow allergies). But you also want to toss your pillow in the tumble dryer every few months to kill dust mites. Change your pillow every couple of years as its unwavering service of eight hours each night gives it a relatively short life span.

A better mattress: When it comes to mattresses, observe the Gold-ilocks imperative (not too hard and not too soft); medium-firm is your best bet. If a mattress is too hard it bites back and can cause pain and even numbness (limbs falling asleep) at pressure points; likewise, if a mattress is too soft it becomes more work to move around and can cause muscle and joint strains. The best mattresses support all of your body parts equally, even at the heaviest points, your hips and shoulders.

Unfortunately, couples often have different mattress prefer-ences, primarily because body weight is a big factor in mattress sup-port. Sometimes the issue can be resolved with a topper. You can actually have a firmer mattress with a soft feel by purchasing a bed with large quilting on the surface or by using a cushioned mattress pad. Because people over the age of forty lose elasticity in their skin, they have less tolerance for a firm mattress surface. Memory foams, the current darlings of the market, can bring harmony to the bed-room by adjusting for the individual body type, but many people find these mattresses to be exceptionally warm, which is especially unwelcome if you're suffering hot flushes.

Test Drive Your Mattress

Test driving in the store is important – after all, you're going to spend more time in your bed than you will in your car. In a terrific US survey, Consumer Reports *found that people who spent 15 minutes testing a bed in the shop – spending at least five minutes on each side, especially in their preferred sleeping position – were more satisfied with their ultimate choice than quicker testers. And they were as satisfied as people who were allowed to take the beds home for a test sleep!*

'You may want to take a look at spending priorities. Spending less on bedding and more on the mattress could be a sleep-inducing strategy.'

As much as I hate to break this news, a recent study from Oklahoma State University showed that price *does* make a difference. Changing from a cheaper to a moderately high-priced mattress significantly improves sleep quality. Another similarly rigorous study showed that by switching to a better mattress (in this case an adjustable air-spring/box-spring combination) a full 95 per cent of study participants with chronic lower-back pain reported reduction in pain, and 88 per cent reported a better night's sleep. This data was supported by a survey that found more than two-thirds of people with high-end mattresses were 'very or completely' satisfied with their purchase compared to one-third of conventional mattress owners.

Light therapy: You can use artificial full-spectrum lights in the morning to help reset the body clock so you can get to sleep at a more appropriate time in the evening. In the past decade, pioneering research lead by Columbia University investigator Dr Michael Terman, established that the circadian rhythms that help set your sleep patterns are highly susceptible to changes in exposure to light rays – whether from the sun or from bulbs that mimic the full-spectrum of sunlight. By exposing the eyes to specially designed full-spectrum lights (10,000 lux fluorescent bulbs) for 30 minutes in the early morning, scientists have helped people get to sleep earlier and stay asleep longer. It is thought that regular exposure to such light in the morning triggers a more advantageous nighttime release of melatonin, the hormone that governs your body clock, but the mechanisms are not fully understood. You may be more familiar with light therapy for its use in treating seasonal affective disorder (SAD), a type of depression that shows up in winter months and stems from sunlight deprivation.

Light therapy can truly work wonders for people who find it difficult to fall asleep before midnight and are sluggish in the morning. Rapid improvement in falling asleep earlier is often experienced after just a few days of 30 minutes of exposure to a light therapy box upon awakening in the morning (see www.allergymatters.com or www.patient.co.uk for more information on the boxes). For people (even teenagers) with more severe insomnia, who regularly stay awake until 1am or longer, shifting sleep patterns can involve sensitive timing. So while the procedure can be done at home, it is a better idea to work with a sleep specialist to devise the treatment programme for serious insomnia. The treatment also usually requires waking up a little earlier each morning, which takes real commitment. But if you are miserable from insomnia, it's worth trying.

'Studies have shown that a course of light therapy treatments can have a dramatically positive effect on both sleep and symptoms of depression.'

On the research forefront are special dawn-simulating sleep masks with embedded lights that turn on gradually four hours before the end of sleep. One might think leaving the curtains open would do the same thing, but bare windows raise the possibility that your bedroom will be flooded with ambient nighttime light, which poses its own set of problems that are conveniently the subject of the next discussion.

Dark Therapy: If exposing your eyes to light in the morning helps you fall asleep earlier and sleep longer, it should come as no surprise that blocking exposure to light at night can positively influence sleep. Scientists digging further into the sunlight-melatonin connection have discovered that the blue spectrum of light has the greatest impact on melatonin and circadian rhythms. If you are exposed to blue light late at night – from a computer or television screen or a digital clock near your bed – it can wreak havoc with your body clock, making it harder for you to get to sleep and to get up in the morning.

Interestingly, a 2008 study from the Corvallis Psychiatric Clinic in Oregon showed that using amber-tinted glasses blocked the excitatory blue spectrum of light commonly encountered during television and computer viewing. Using amber glasses during evening screen-watching time had a significant effect in inducing and promoting a good night's sleep. Amber sunglasses should do the trick.

Behavioural therapy: Here's the Catch-22 of sleep psychology: worrying about not getting enough sleep can stop you from getting enough sleep. Sleep docs have even developed a protocol of behavioural modification that's been shown to work 70 to 80 per cent of the time for people who can't sleep because of excessive preoccupation with, or apprehension about, falling sleep. Here's the drill:

- Go to bed only when sleepy.
- Get out of bed if you haven't fallen asleep in 20 minutes.
- Curtail all non-sleep activities in bed (no watching TV, eating, planning or problem solving).
- Arise at the same time every morning.
- Avoid daytime napping.
- Don't get attached to unreal expectations about getting a perfect sleep every night.
- Do not blame insomnia for all daytime problems.
- Do not catastrophize (imagine all the bad things that will happen as a result) after a poor night's sleep.
- Finally, if this chapter is making you worry too much about sleep, put it down and go out for a walk in the fresh air!

Relaxation exercises: Throughout the night, your brainwaves are continually cycling between slow-wave activity of non-rapid eye movement and fast-wave activity of rapid eye movement. Meditation and relaxation exercises can significantly help you get back into slow-wave activity if you are awakened in the middle of the night. For getting to sleep faster or for falling back to sleep in the middle of the night try meditation or relaxation exercises found in the 21-

Day Plan as a way of hopping onto the slow-wave sleep train that pulls you into the deepest stages of regenerative rest.

'Keep your room pitch dark at night, covering all digital clock or DVD player readouts.'

Acupuncture: Acupuncture, discussed in Chapter 1 as an aid to relaxation, is a helpful adjunct for treating insomnia. Thousands of research articles attest to the neurochemical effects of acupuncture, which significantly elevates endorphins to block pain pathways, promotes the production of chemicals that reduce inflammation, enhances circulation and reduces the activity of neuromuscular spasm. Inasmuch as acupuncture balances the nervous system and neurotransmitters, there's a logic for its use in promoting relaxation, which results in a better quality sleep. In China acupuncture has been used successfully for 2,000 years to treat sleep problems, though this effect has yet to be studied in controlled trials that are considered the gold standard in Western medicine. In my own practice I use acupuncture as part of a comprehensive approach to insomnia in conjunction with other treatments based on the underlying causes of the sleep problem.

Nutritional Supplements

'One pill will make you larger, and one pill will make you small, but the ones your mother gives you won't do anything at all.' People are always looking for the quick fix.

With sleep, lifestyle factors (proper diet, exercise, stress control, sleep hygiene etc.) are the most important means for successful long-term regenerative rest. Short-term prescriptions can be very helpful for acute insomnia that occurs in situations with great stress. While non-prescription nutritional supplements are generally less powerful than medication, they can provide a very helpful non-drug transitional aid to get you to sleep better until you can make lifestyle changes. If you are under a doctor's care for a medical condition, check with your doctor before taking any new supplements.

Melatonin

While many hormones affect circadian rhythms (your biological clock), the master hormone for regulation of the sleep cycle is melatonin. This hypothalamus-produced hormone rises just before you fall asleep and falls through the night, hitting bottom about two hours before you awaken. (It is also a powerful antioxidant that enhances the repairative function of sleep.) As mentioned above in Light Therapy, production of melatonin is very sensitive to sunlight and can be normalized by altering exposure patterns. Studies going back decades are very clear that ingesting melatonin extract can help reset the body clock and alleviate jetlag. Melatonin can also gradually help insomniacs feel sleepy at an earlier hour: take 1–3mg two to three hours before the desired sleep time. While melatonin can help normalize an out-of-whack sleep pattern, it is not a sleeping pill. Melatonin is not currently licensed for sale in UK pharmacies; however, it is available on prescription or over the counter in health-food shops.

Valerian (*valeriana officinalis*)

Valerian officinalis, a species of flowering plant in the valerian family, is the closest you can get to a herbal sleeping pill – its sedative powers far outstrip those of chamomile. Valerian would no doubt be more widely used in teas if it weren't for its particularly unpleasant odour. Research suggests that constituents of valerian root affect enzyme systems that control neurotransmitter levels responsible for sleepiness. In studies valerian capsules have even been used successfully to help people sleep during a period of withdrawal from Valium dependency. (Due to its sedative effect, valerian should not be taken before driving and operating machinery.)

L-Theanine

This amino acid, as discussed in Chapter 1, helps reduce tension and stress. I commonly recommend theanine as part of a comprehensive programme for insomnia.

Tryptophan/5-HTP (or, alternatively, warm milk)

The amino acid tryptophan has been well studied and used for decades to induce a drowsy state. It was banned in the US and UK because one contaminated batch from China caused serious lung problems 25 years ago but is now available by prescription and the FSA in the UK has agreed that some supplements can be marketed if the ingredient meets purity criteria. As a result of the confusion, some supplement companies sell 5-hydroxy-tryptophan (5HTP), a different form of the amino acid. 5HTP is less effective as a sleep aid than tryptophan. Warm milk is thought to increase tryptophan levels and is a natural way to use this amino acid to assist with sleep.

Passion Flower (passiflora incarnata)

Research has shown many active compounds in passiflora that lead to calming and sedating effects in the nervous system. Some studies have demonstrated this herb's utility as part of treatment for anxiety disorder and for patients coming off narcotics. Due to its mild potency, passion flower is most often found in combination with other calming herbs, particularly valerian. (It has some potential ud verse reactions, including dizziness; and people with cardiovascular disease should avoid passion flower because of certain potentially potent alkaloids.)

> ### A Cautionary Note on Kava Kava
> *Kava is a South Pacific herb used in ceremonies by indigenous cultures for its psychoactive properties, one of which induces a sleepy, dream-like state, which made it briefly popular as a sleep aid and anti-anxiety treatment. But I do not recommend kava for two reasons: (1) ingestion of kava capsules has resulted in cases of liver toxicity and even liver failure, and (2) its psychoactive properties can cause emotional disturbances, especially in people with psychological conditions. Try something else.*

Chapter 6

Power of Connection: Cultivate Spirit, Access Positive Energy

 CASE STUDY
A DEEPER CONNECTION

I hadn't seen David in five years. When I asked where he'd been, he told me this powerful story of spiritual rejuvenation.

David's soulmate from childhood and wife of twenty years died suddenly from an aneurysm. He was inconsolable in his grief. Depressed, he had developed back pain and headaches and was so fatigued that it became difficult for him to get out of bed. Knowing that grief was the source of his problem, he thought he could handle it on his own. But, after the second year of grieving, David went to his parents' house for the High Jewish Holidays, and by chance the family rabbi stopped by. The rabbi asked how David was and he reported feeling fine, but his family disagreed.

When his mother told the rabbi that David hadn't recovered from the loss, the rabbi asked only one question: 'Did David sit shiva for his wife?' (Shiva is the seven-day period of formal mourning after a funeral that is observed by Jews. During shiva, friends and relatives visit the home to offer condolences.) Having not participated in his religion since childhood, David initially scoffed at the idea.

After some persuasion, David agreed to undergo the ritual with the rabbi by his side, even though it was two years after his wife's death. For seven days David sat in his home as almost everyone who'd ever cared for him visited and sat with him. As he received their healing energy and thoughts, David became connected on a deeper level than ever with his friends and family – and also, he felt, with all of humanity.

At the end of that week, David felt a dramatic lifting of his spirits, and experienced waves of energy he had not felt since his loss. The powerful process of opening to the love and positive energy of others showed him how deeply his spiritual life could affect his health and vitality.

DAVID REGAINED HIS VITAL energy by connecting with his roots, with the healing power of a religious practice, and with a community of people who cared deeply about him and his family. David's spiritual healing, and the subject of this chapter, is about gaining access to a deeper, permanent, vital energy that works on a more profound level than the daily mechanics of a healthy lifestyle. It is necessary to recognize that you do not begin and end at your skin in order for you – and anyone – to recover your energy and health. Spirituality, connectedness and love – realizing that you are part of something universal and eternal, bigger than your flesh and blood – are vitally important for well-being.

Connection is important in my practice as a means for my patients to rebuild energy. I am not alone in this: connection has been increasingly recognized as enormously important in the practice of behavioural medicine, a field that includes doctors, psychiatrists, psychotherapists, research scientists and nurses concerned with social and behavioural factors that affect health. Connectivity can be achieved in many different ways. Western spirituality emphasizes a personal connection with God; Eastern and Native American spiritual philosophies place emphasis on a connection with all of nature and on being part of a greater whole that includes a universal energy or spirit.

Good Old-fashioned Listening

Until forty years ago, doctors cared for entire families; they knew who a person was within the family and within the context of their community – and they got insights into people's health based on what was going on in their lives. The old-fashioned family doc was much more attuned to the emotional and spiritual shifts that precede illness. It was not unusual for him to spend time chatting, inquiring about his patients' lives, before doing an exam. Today, (according to a study in *JAMA*, the Journal of the American Medical Association) the typical doctor interrupts a patient after just 23 seconds and steers the conversation in the direction he wants it to go – which may not lead to the deeper root of what's underlying a person's problems. While I appreciate the need for efficiency in healthcare, I maintain that the family doc was actually deepening his ability to make a diagnosis by taking the measure of his patients' spirit.

By emphasizing the role of spirit and connectedness I give my patients permission (which some of them feel they need in the face of the demands on their time) and encourage them to use the energy and practices of spiritual connectedness and community that allow them to heal themselves and to stay well. Sceptics might chalk the positive results up to elevated endorphins or decreased cortisol (anxiety hormone) levels, but I maintain that remarkable stories of the healing power of love, connectedness and spirituality are footprints of a deeper energetic process that is constantly at work within us and around us. And this energetic process is beyond what we can possibly understand with the gizmos and machines of scientific method.

'You can be connected through a relationship to the absolute or to your community or to nature or to music ... or to any greater energy or entity that transcends the nitty-gritty of daily life and gives meaning to your time here.'

This chapter will explain why you cannot afford to neglect the spirit when you are seeking increased energy in life and in your health. Cultivating connectedness is a joyous pursuit. There are so many ways to engage in a dance of energy with the universe. In the 21-Day Plan, I incorporate exercises for cultivating the 'Power of Connection', and you no doubt will invent many of your own as you begin to connect.

Connecting at Spirit Level

Behavioural researchers have mapped the landscape of spiritual connection and have shown that it includes:

- *frequent interaction with the transcendent as a fundamental part of life*
- *perceived divine love*
- *the perception that life consists of more than physical states, psychological feelings or social roles*
- *a sense of wholeness and internal integration*
- *a sense of inner harmony*
- *the experience of awe at the beauty of creation*
- *gratefulness*
- *compassion*
- *mercy*
- *spiritual longing – the desire to be closer or in union with the divine.*

In a fascinating study of spiritual experiences, researchers were able to measure with a survey whether an individual experiences God's love versus whether one just believes that God loves people as a whole. The investigators suggest that feeling loved is the key ingredient in making the link between spiritual issues and health outcomes. I have found in my own practice that it's vitally important to take the spiritual temperature of my patients, so to speak, in order to help them achieve total healing and optimum energy.

BEING CONNECTED

Even though it's difficult to subject spirituality and connectedness to scientific methods of analysis, researchers continue to try – and to make great headway. A wealth of studies demonstrates the importance of connectedness in numerous aspects of health: your nervous system, immune system, neuro-endocrine system, cardiovascular system and your very longevity all fare better when you have healthy connections to a deeper sense of self and to the world beyond yourself. In the sections that follow, I'll discuss the most important categories of connection that research and tens of thousands of years of empirical experience have shown to improve your health and increase your energy.

The Connected Body

Noted Duke University religion and spirituality researcher Dr Harold Koenig reviewed more than sixty studies published in peer-reviewed medical journals in the United States over a thirty-year period that established a causal link between immune and neuroendocrine system health. The key connectedness factors included spirituality, religion, social support and social participation. The following functions were all improved by being connected:

- *Immune response to vaccination*
- *Function of immune cells*
- *Antibody levels to latent viruses (indicator of immune system stress)*
- *Production of cytokines (molecular defenders of the immune system)*
- *Hypothalamic-Pituitary-Adrenal Axis Response (the stress hormone response)*
- *Production of pituitary hormone*

Spirituality

I have had the great privilege of taking care of a number of Tibetan Buddhist Rinpoches (pronounced RIN-po-chay) – these are the holiest monks in the Buddhist tradition. They embody the essence of Buddhism – compassion for others. Their most fundamental goal in life is to relieve the suffering of all creatures. Their deep spirituality doesn't give them immunity to physical illness – even the Dalai Lama gets a cold every once in a while – but their advanced spiritual work does give them a unique perspective on illness and a certain amount of control over their bodies. I was deeply moved by the sheer power of will of one Rinpoche, in whom, during one of his infrequent visits for a check-up, I discovered what I suspected to be a massive tumour in his lower abdomen that was causing his lower body to become hugely swollen. After consulting with an oncologist he decided to undergo chemotherapy and radiation. He had no fear of death, but he told me that his work was not complete, and he felt that he needed some more time. He decided to go to Washington DC for his treatment where he had followers who could look after him. There he would also be in the care of a wonderful oncologist with whom, it just so happened, I had worked with (and last seen) in Tanzania some twenty-five years earlier.

Three months after the move I received a call from his astonished oncologist: the tumour and all of the swelling had vanished, and tests could find no traces of the cancer! The doctors had never seen anyone come in with such extensive cancer, and achieve not just improvement but what seemed like a cure. With his body strong enough, the Rinpoche announced he would return to India to complete his work. I was sad to see him go, but elated at his recovery. Six months later I heard through a member of his community in India that he had decided his body was 'tired' and he needed a new one. (All Tibetan Buddhists believe in reincarnation.) He made preparations, and on a full moon of a Kalachakra Ceremony (a high holy day for Tibetan Buddhism) he left his body. I was a little broken-hearted, and also amazed at the power of his spirit; he couldn't beat the cancer, but he could set a schedule for it.

It is quite difficult to fathom the depths of spirituality of a Tibetan Rinpoche whose entire life is dedicated to cultivating compassion and wisdom. But on a more general level, spirituality has been increasingly recognized in medicine as a positive factor for health. Studies on the topic have been generated by top medical schools, many of which have concluded that spirituality should be recognized by the medical profession and caregivers as an important factor contributing to quality of life, which in general contributes significantly to better health outcomes.

This growing recognition of spirituality is a welcome development for most people. Studies both at Johns Hopkins and the University of Pennsylvania show that the majority of people don't mind being asked about their spirituality in a doctor's office, and more than 90 per cent of those surveyed felt that a spiritual outlook was important for physical well-being.

What is Spirituality?

One of the trickier aspects of studying spirituality is defining it. Researchers require standardized definitions. In order to put transcendence to the test, investigators commonly use questionnaires that thoroughly explore people's habits, values and attitudes towards spirituality. Intriguingly, one of the scales, the FACIT *Spiritual Well Being* scale, can tease out the differences in attitude between having faith versus having a sense of meaning and peace, which scientists have dubbed existential well-being. Another scale, the *Daily Spiritual Experience Scale*, is intended to measure a person's perception of the transcendent in daily life and his or her interaction or involvement with the transcendent in daily life. The idea is to measure experiences rather than beliefs or behaviours.

A recent joint study by researchers at Harvard Medical School's Massachusetts General Hospital and the University of California at San Diego used similar scales to study the effects of spirituality in twins, a subgroup of the population that helps scientists separate genetics out from behaviour. Investigators looked at the association between spiritual well-being and health outcomes in 345 pairs of male twins with an average age of 48 years from a national cohort known as the Vietnam Era Twin Registry (made up of twins who served in the US military between 1965 and 1975). Overall, spirituality was shown to be associated with better general health, vitality and social functioning.

Spirituality and Mood

Some of the power of spirituality can be attributed to its effect on mood. We know that spiritual practices such as meditation and prayer have a calming effect on the nervous system, but having a sense of spirituality is equally powerful. In an impressive study at the University of Colorado Department of Medicine, doctors looked at the effects of spiritual well-being in patients with heart failure. They found that greater spiritual well-being, and in particular *having a sense of meaning and peace*, was strongly associated with less depression. The study suggests that enhancing spiritual well-being may be a potential therapy to reduce or prevent depression and thus improve outcomes in people with heart failure. I have to applaud this study. For doctors to suggest in a peer-reviewed medical journal that spiritual well-being might be a beneficial therapy for heart patients is quite brave and an extremely important step in bringing humanity back to medicine.

A further connection between spirituality, depression and energy is beginning to surface as researchers are refining ways to study spirit. At Johns Hopkins School of Medicine in the US doctors found that daily spiritual experiences in older adults with arthritis were strongly associated with less depression and increased energy. This

'Having a sense of meaning and peace is the most powerful factor of all, associated with significant improvement in overall physical functioning, general physical health, mental health, social functioning, pain and vitality. I cannot name any other single lifestyle factor that would cover so many bases.'

would not surprise a Rinpoche because, according to Buddhist doctrine, meditation produces energy. For example, meditation produces mindfulness, which is considered a source of energy that powers awareness of what is happening in the present moment. With daily spiritual exercises, the Johns Hopkins arthritis patients were tapping a source of energy, and they were able to report back to researchers that they felt more energetic.

One of the most powerful studies of spirituality comes from Dr Harold Koenig, co-director of the Center for Spirituality, Theology and Health at Duke University Medical Center in the US, and one of the giants in the field of research on spirituality and health. Over a 21-month period he and his team examined 811 people, 50 years or older, who had been admitted to Duke's Medical Center. Participating in organized religious activity resulted in fewer hospitalizations and shorter acute hospital stays. And when the researchers looked at people who needed to go from the hospital for longer-term care at a nursing home or care facility, those who had religious activities and professed a sense of spirituality had significantly reduced long-term care days. (The effect was strongest for African-Americans and women.) In this study, spirituality was a simple, side-effect-free, feel-good way to reduce long-term care hospital stays.

Spirituality is a powerful healing tool, but it is underutilized. The same people who tell me that they see themselves as spiritual, routinely admit in the next breath that they do *not* have a regular contemplative practice to cultivate that spirituality. My response is to encourage them to engage in daily practice – even if it's simply the two-minute meditation or prayer that I prescribe for them first thing in the morning (see the 21-Day Plan, Day One). You – and everyone – should cultivate your inner life by following the spiritual connection that is meaningful for you. Ultimately, I want you to go beyond a two-minute practice once a day to cultivate a spiritual attitude. Try it: you'll feel protected and connected.

'Spirituality would be a pharmaceutical gold mine if it could be bottled and sold.'

Prayer

By one estimate, 42 per cent of all adults in the UK pray regularly, with about 26 per cent praying at least once a week. And despite most doctors' reluctance to broach the topic it appears that many people know instinctively that prayer belongs in healthcare. In a study published in the venerable *Archives of Internal Medicine* and conducted at the University of Pennsylvania in the US, researchers found a strong natural bias toward the power of prayer to heal: of 177 people visiting an outpatient lung specialist, 51 per cent described themselves as religious and yet a full 90 per cent of the patients believed that praying can influence recovery from an illness.

'Some intriguing studies strongly suggest that prayer works even if you *don't know* you're being prayed for, and even if you are not a follower of the religion of the person who's praying for you.'

I once broached the topic of prayer with a patient who was having a very difficult time in her life; her child had been diagnosed with diabetes just after she'd completed treatment for breast cancer. In my office, she looked depleted and miserable, having come to ask for treatment for a sinus infection. When I turned the topic to spiritual resources, and asked if she ever prayed, she replied, 'Oh, yeah, you mean like for the placebo effect?' From her point of view, and for many people, prayer is a sort of turbo-charged version of the power of positive thinking.

This is not to say you've got to enlist a prayer group to maintain your health. Praying clearly also has physiological benefits for the person doing the praying. I'm fascinated by the studies that show that there are changes in the brain during prayer.

Brain activity measured with functional MRIs and PET scans indicate that different levels of brain functioning may be attained as a person gets 'better' at praying. Herbert Benson established that brainwave activity commonly shifts toward calming alpha waves during a relaxation exercise such as conscious breathing. But when people with advanced praying skills, like Buddhist monks or

The Power of Prayer

One of the most widely acclaimed prayer studies was conducted several years ago at CalPacific Medical Center by doctor Elizabeth Targ and her group. What was so unique about this study is it was double-blinded – meaning the patients didn't know they were being prayed for – and it utilized prayers by people from eight different spiritual traditions including Christians, Jews, Buddhists and Native Americans. Advanced-stage AIDS patients (who at the time they volunteered for the study all had the same degree of illness [including similar T-cell counts]) were assigned on a rotating basis to the prayer givers, each one receiving prayer from a different healer each week. The results were nothing short of astonishing. When compared to the people who didn't receive prayers, the prayed-for patients had seven times fewer days spent in the hospital, and four times fewer new hospitalizations, a sixfold reduction in new AIDS-related illnesses, two thirds fewer severe illnesses, one-third fewer doctors' visits, and significantly less psychological distress. What I like about this study is it managed to isolate the effects of prayer from the effects of believing in prayer, which removes the placebo effect from the equation.

The first major rigorous double-blind study of prayer, published in a peer-reviewed medical journal in 1988, was conducted by Randolph Byrd, staff cardiologist at the University of California, San Francisco School of Medicine. In Byrd's study, 393 patients in the coronary care unit were prayed for by Christian groups. During their hospital stay the prayed-for patients had significantly fewer cases of congestive heart failure, cardiopulmonary arrest and pneumonia; and they required less medication and fewer intubations (insertion of a breathing tube). This was a real shot in the arm for those of us who felt frustrated in our efforts to have spirituality's positive role in healthcare acknowledged more.

In a follow-up study, published in the Archives of Internal Medicine in 2001, researchers examined the effect of prayer on 990 patients in the Coronary Care Unit of St Luke's Hospital in the US state of Missouri. This study was triple-blinded; neither the doctors nor data analysts knew which patients had been prayed for; and the patients didn't know they were being prayed for. The prayers were given by a diverse group of people trained to pray for better recovery. The patients did not have the dramatic outcomes of the Byrd study, but improved in every measurement compared to the group who were not prayed for.

evangelical Christians, are at prayer, their brainwaves shift toward a frontal midline theta rhythm, which reflects intense mental concentration as well as a meditative state characterized by relief of anxiety – it's what people often call a flow state, when you're concentrating so hard on something that you think only a few minutes has passed when it's actually been a half-hour. Other studies suggest prayer has immune-boosting, anti-inflammatory properties due to the relaxation response's effect on the vagus nerve, which regulates feedback between the automatic nervous system and the immune system. Again, few drugs come close to having such sophisticated and highly desired effects.

> 'Electro-encephalograms (EEGs) show shifts in the brain's energy during prayer.'

Prayer and Medicine

As tantalizing as prayer studies are, I agree with visionary doctor and philosopher Dr Larry Dossey that evidence-based research is not the *only* avenue for bringing prayer and spiritual intention to medicine. In his book *Healing Beyond the Body*, Dossey writes, 'Unable to see how prayer could work, too many people insist that it *cannot* work.' It's possible that studies of prayer by their very design interfere with the effects. When I was scientific advisor to the first conference on Native American medicine to be held in North America, we encountered resistance from the leaders of several nations who felt that to take their prayer practices out of context would destroy their efficacy. One tribal elder explained to me that healing prayer is part of a holistic system, which includes community and social support, and sometimes involves specific dietary restrictions and herbs, sweat lodges and movement exercises. To some, taking out one element and subjecting it to some sort of scientific scrutiny was unthinkable.

Regardless of what tradition prayers come from, I think most rational people will agree that science will never 'prove' *how* prayer works. Some scientists have attempted to measure the energy that people emanate while praying. Philosophies that believe in the efficacy of prayer, from Larry Dossey's theory of non-local mind to the Buddhist concept of collective consciousness, more or less boil down to the idea that when you pray you connect to the absolute – a larger energetic reality that is within you and also surrounding you, throughout the universe. This connection of personal to universal energy or consciousness is what allows your intention to effect change across space and time.

For me in my practice, and for my patients who pray, it's enough to know that prayer *does* work. We can cite research as well as evidence from thousands of years of practice by spiritual leaders and their religious communities, but we frankly just know it in our hearts. I see no reason for the medical establishment to continue to keep people's spiritual lives out of the consulting room. The most rational reason to encourage a contemplative practice is that prayer is one more powerful tool in your healing armamentarium to increase energy and promote total well-being.

Religion

When I was growing up in a conservative town in northern California, my mother was consistently religious and had us attend services regularly at the local Episcopal Church. The leader of our church was an extremely charismatic priest, L. Douglas Gottschall, who had been canonized (an elite designation) by the archdiocese for his work in trying to uncover the location of King Solomon's mine and other sacred treasures in Africa and the Middle East. Canon Gottschall wore a ring on his left hand that he said he found during his religious treasure hunts. Every Wednesday evening, he used this ring as part of weekly faith-healing services. As an acolyte, I often assisted him while infirm parishioners came to be healed. I grew accustomed to seeing very smart, respectable people from our community come in to be touched by the ring and healed. I actually saw someone come in barely able to walk with assistance and walk out with a nearly perfect gait. I was pretty mystified by this as a youth, but from what I now know about religion I am no longer surprised. Combine that

'Religion can combine almost all of the connectivity factors:
social support, belief in a higher power, cultivating a
spiritual practice, music, art and community service are all
wound up in one big powerful package.'

with the force of a spiritually powerful person like Canon Gottschall,
and you've got a major healing centre.

Some of the benefits of religious involvement can be explained
by healthier lifestyle habits. For example, Seventh Day Adventists
and Mormons have been shown to have lesser cancer incidence and
increased longevity linked to moderate lifestyles shaped by their re-
ligions. But some studies factor out healthy lifestyle habits and still
show beneficial results from religious practices. Let's take a look at a
few of the studies that argue in favour of following a religious tradition's centuries-old blueprint for getting connected.

What the Research Says

In medicine, when we want the big picture we turn to epidemiology, which tells us the common tendencies in groups of a whole lot
of people. A number of such studies have established the protective effects of religious involvement. One study of 6,545 residents of
California that went on for 31 years likened the general protective
benefits of religion to the known benefits of high socio-economic
status; non-church attenders had significantly higher rates of death
from cancer and circulatory, digestive and respiratory diseases. More
recently, Duke University's Harold Koenig and colleagues examined
records of a nationwide cohort of 8,450 men and women aged 40
years and older from 1988 to 1994, seeking associations between
religious service attendance and mortality. Incredibly, the statistics
yielded up a dose-response relationship. At each level of increased
attendance the risk of dying decreased – from no attendance, to less
than weekly, to the lowest risk of dying for people who attended religious services more than once a week.

In a 1997 study showing a beneficial dose-response relationship

'Religion appeared to reduce inflammation and strengthen the immune system independent of mood.'

between religion and health, Koenig and his team enlisted 1,718 elderly people and looked for a correlation between religious attendance and immune system strength. More non-church attenders had elevated levels of harmful inflammatory molecules than occasional attenders. People who attended religious services once a week or more were 49 per cent *less likely* to have elevated levels of harmful molecules than were non-attenders.

In study after study the message is clear: having a religious practice is good for you. In one compelling study, elderly surgical patients who were both socially active and found strength and comfort in their religious faith were *14 times* less likely to die during the six months following surgery than their less religiously connected counterparts. Those who reported attending religious services at least every few months had about half the death rate of those who never or rarely attended services. Once again, greater frequency conferred stronger results.

Hundreds of published studies provide so much evidence supporting the power of religious practice to improve health and well-being that noted epidemiologist Jeffrey Levin – who has reviewed most of the research connecting religion and health – is an advocate of a new approach to medicine called *theosomatic* medicine. In his book *God, Faith and Healing*, Levin defines this approach to medicine as 'a view of the determinants of health based on the apparent connections between god or spirit or faith in god – and the well-being of the body'. The studies have shown religion to be as powerful and in many cases more powerful at extending longevity than some of our most powerful medications. If you are at all inclined to attend religious services regularly, I highly recommend that you do so.

Community

I live in New York City – a giant metropolis of more than 8 million inhabitants; you'd think it might be a lonely place with such high potential for anonymity, but I am constantly amazed at how people manage to create their own special, meaningful communities. There are communities based on shared nationality and shared love of the arts; dog lovers find each other; fashion followers find each other; musicians, punk-rockers, artists, architects, furniture buffs, comic book buffs, philanthropists . . . you name the group, there's a tight-knit community of them in New York. Each of these microcommunities is a centre of collective energy, and their ranks are continuously energized by including others.

The human instinct to gather together has powerful benefits. Pioneering cardiologist and bestselling author, Dean Ornish, has elegantly explained feelings of isolation can have significant adverse effects on health and energy. One simple but illustrative study showed that people with the fewest social ties (3 or less) had 4.2 times greater risk of catching a cold than those with the most (6 or more) social ties. You might think: OK, big deal, so you've got a cold. But many other studies have shown that loneliness and isolation can significantly depress the immune system as well. One fascinating study compared the immune systems in people who simply had the belief that there was available social support for them to those who felt they had no support. Those who had the perception of social support had a stronger response to a hepatitis B vaccination, producing more antibodies than those who felt they had poor social support.

A Health Phenomenon

Researchers may have hit on an explanation for this phenomenon. Investigators at UCLA's David Geffen School of Medicine in the US found that feelings of isolation are linked to alterations in the activity of genes that drive inflammation, the body's first immune response. This hard scientific link between isolation and inflammation helps explain why loneliness has been associated with inflammatory conditions such as heart disease.

We are hardwired to be social animals. Highly sophisticated neural circuitry that connects your brain structures makes it possible to process others' verbal and non-verbal cues (and intentions). This is what author Daniel Goleman calls 'neural WiFi'. In his book *Social Intelligence*, Goleman writes, 'The most telling news here may be that the social brain represents the only biological system in our bodies that continually attunes us to, and in turn becomes influenced by, the internal state of people we're with.' When you have a positive supportive community, the good vibes, so to speak, resonate in your body.

The meaning of a supportive community can be extremely diverse. It can be a church or parenting group, a choir or crossword puzzlers, quilters, readers or knitters, cake bakers or community gardeners. I was once visiting friends in a tiny town in Colorado and a vintage car show came to town. Being an admirer of custom cars I wandered over and found a vibrant community in action of individuals who had come together over a mutual love of old cars. They sat all day in the blinding August sun talking about their cars and their respect for what each had accomplished with his or her car. They have a tremendous love for the skill, patience, time and effort it takes to lovingly restore these cars. After eight hours, they hopped in their cars and drove to another town to do it all over again. They felt fulfilled.

'Too many people expend way too much energy negotiating energy-draining interpersonal relationships at work, and spend zero time cultivating supportive community relationships.'

A common problem for people today is that they have many daily interactions that don't add up to a community. Some companies have tried to improve the current situation in the workplace by having a company outing or other system-wide social event to shift the energy of a working community to become more nurturing. These give employees a chance to interact on a more human level – to engender a closer sense of community to help change what is all too often a stressful, competitive, energy-draining workplace environment. Because most people have to spend the majority of their time in the workplace, we need to strive to create a sense of community at work.

Impersonal Interaction

With the rise of the internet, some people feel as if they have forged new communities while sitting alone in the comfort of their living rooms. In some ways the benefits of web activities are similar to keeping a diary – greater self-understanding, a raising of consciousness about issues on a personal and international level, a gaining of insights into events – with an interactive audience. My only concern is whether these relationships are authentic. You may be talking to someone impersonating the friend you want. It's hard for anyone over the age of 30 to understand, but people who spend an inordinate amount of time in internet communities lose important interpersonal skills and the scope of energy that comes with interacting face to face. I feel that people are spending too much time shut up in their energy-draining, blue-light dominated computer world: I'd rather see you get out and enjoy the natural world and interact with real people whom you enjoy so that you experience the vital source of connecting with others' direct energy.

Intimate Relationships

Intimate relationships are based on love and we find them within the nuclear family, with a spouse or significant other, in extended families of close relationships, and with one or two close friends and confidantes. These are the people you can go to when the chips are down. In today's society the definition of family has shifted considerably from the nuclear family of fifty years ago.

Many characteristics of families have changed. There are now fewer with children under the age of 18 (our population is getting older because the baby boom is over). The average age at marriage has increased, and the number of babies born in the UK to women over thirty-five has more than doubled during the past decade. In fact, the pregnancy rate in women over forty is rising faster than in any other age group. In the UK, more than 25,000 women each year become mothers in their fifth decade. What's more, single-parent families have increased from 1 per cent of families with children in 1971, to some 25 per cent in 2008. More parents are devoting less time to their own children and more to their own parents. This 'sandwich generation' is pulled in multiple directions with longer average workdays and commute times, and the intrusion of television and computers into family life eroding time spent together. The role of family life has shifted dramatically. But intimate relationships still play a central role in people's lives and health.

Intimate relationships should be a source of healing energy, but too often can be one of energy-draining negativity. For example, having caring parents is a good predictor of health in later life. A Harvard study that looked at 35 years of people's lives found the vast majority (91 per cent) of people who *did not* perceive themselves to have had a warm relationship with their mothers had diagnosed diseases by midlife including coronary artery disease, hypertension, ulcers and alcoholism. Only 45 per cent of participants who *did* perceive themselves to have had a warm relationship with their mothers had these same health problems. A similar association between perceived warmth and closeness with fathers predicted future illness. Other research has established that hostility in the marital relationship lowers immunity.

'As you change the energy you bring to relationships, the energy you receive will begin to shift. Your intimate connections should be a source of positive energy.'

I strongly recommend that you cultivate mindfulness in your intimate relationships regardless of your family structure – whether you're part of a home that some would see as fractured or you're trying to recreate a *Waltons*-style traditional family. This means that you bring a freshness to every encounter. Many people are locked into habitual knee-jerk responses to their loved ones that ultimately drain the energy out of the relationship. Think about the attitude – the energy you are projecting to your loved ones. You cannot change your teenagers' pubescent moods, but you can shift the energy that you bring to the relationship with your teenager or your spouse, sibling, life partner or the people who you count among your intimate acquaintances.

I often recommend that my patients reach out for help in repairing their intimate relationships. Couples and families can find help in couples or family counselling. The goal is for each person to understand the other and to feel understood, and to reach a point in which behavioural and attitudinal changes stop the habitual negativity in a relationship. Compromise is seen not as a giving in, but as a positive step to satisfying the needs of each person. The improvement comes not just from valuing all that has been, and all that can be, but in the sheer good fortune you have to be in a loving supportive relationship. The improvement that comes from changing attitudes, expectations and behaviours within the relationship is most often a noticeable increase in positive energy, joy and health.

Giving Back

A patient and friend of mine, a corporate executive, spends one night a month supervising the men's ward of a homeless shelter. I asked him: isn't this a stressful, energy-draining activity? His answer was, 'It's the opposite, it's uplifting.' He's deeply moved by the stories he hears. He says there are so many good people there whom fate just seemed not to shine on. That night at the shelter is one of the most satisfying things he does with his life and in many ways it seems more important to him than his regular job. He doesn't sleep much on those nights, but he comes away more energized than if he had spent a weekend at a spa.

You don't have to do something quite as dramatic as spending the night in a homeless shelter, but there are simple things you can do that can help you give energy to others. You can help your neighbour move boxes or organize a cake sale to raise funds for your local animal shelter or volunteer your time to any charitable organization – there are as many ways to give back as there are people in need. The passion that comes from compassion is a potent form of vital energy.

Music and Art

The creative arts have restorative powers and some are formal healing therapies: music and art therapy, dance therapy and expressive writing or keeping a diary are increasingly recognized as powerful therapeutic tools. In a study in the venerable *Journal of the American Medical Association*, expressive writing was shown to significantly improve asthma and rheumatoid arthritis. The benefits of music therapy in particular have been well established with hundreds of published studies.

Listening to music has also been shown to improve biochemical parameters such as the production of substances that improve brain functioning, reduction of inflammatory chemicals and adrenalin. Neuroscientist Daniel J. Levitin puts his finger on the beauty of music in his book *This Is Your Brain On Music:* 'When we love a piece of music, it reminds us of other music we have heard, and it activates memory traces of emotional times in our lives. Your brain on music is all about . . . connections.' Quite simply, the creative arts take us out of ourselves and help us share the energy of the universe.

Nature

I was visiting a dear friend in a coronary intensive care unit, one of the *least* natural places on the planet, and I saw an extraordinary example of the power of nature. I was his last visitor of the day, it was late, and visitors were no longer allowed in the unit. He'd just had a small heart attack and emergency coronary angioplasty, a proce-

'Listening to music has been shown to improve fatigue, stress, pain, anxiety, depression, sleep, hypertension, exercise performance and recovery.'

dure that requires manipulating the vital coronary artery. He was feeling pretty delicate. I really didn't feel like leaving him and I felt he didn't want me to go. A nurse came in and asked, 'Would you like to be visited by a vol-

'Therapy with animals such as dogs, cats and horses has been shown to promote healing.'

unteer?' Seeing the expectant look on the nurse's face my friend gave a polite OK. With a huge smile she said, 'His name is Red.' In walked a volunteer with an officially trained, hospital-credentialled therapeutic dog! My friend's face lit up. And I left knowing that his heart was a bit lighter, simply because of the unexpected canine visitor.

If dogs are allowed in an ICU, you can bet there's been a good deal of research into canine therapy. Visits by dogs have been shown to decrease postoperative pain in children, to reduce depression and increase oxygen saturation in patients undergoing chemotherapy, and to decrease blood pressure and depression in nursing home patients.

Horses are playing a greater role in both physical and psychological rehabilitation medicine. Studies have shown that equine therapy benefits people with multiple sclerosis, cerebral palsy and spinal cord injury. Animals provide a wonderfully healing interface with nature.

In one fascinating study, researchers told a group of residents in a nursing home to take more responsibility for themselves, including caring for an inexpensive plant. The control group was given a plant and told the nurses would take care of it. The group given responsibility for the plant was dramatically more engaged in activities in the community, they were more alert and had better moods. (A full 93 per cent of the plant-caretaking group showed improvement, versus an actual decline in overall well-being of the control group.) I'm not suggesting you force yourself to start gardening, but there are many ways to get connected to nature, and the important thing is to start now, today, reaching out beyond yourself and interacting with the energy that's all around you.

Energy Medicine

As a doctor I sometimes recommend that my patients see energy healers, which most doctors do not do. Over the years I have seen some remarkable turnarounds in people working with practitioners of Qi gong, Reiki and therapeutic (healing) touch in particular. All of these involve the transfer of beneficial healing energy from one person to another. Early on in my career I was sceptical of these practices, but my eyes were opened about fifteen years ago when a patient of mine with chronic Lyme disease – which caused her partial blindness, impaired balance, difficulty walking and problems with concentration and memory – was healed by an energy practitioner. This woman struggled for four years with the disease, had seen a dozen specialists but had had no significant improvement in her condition for over two years. Out of desperation she turned to a Qi gong practitioner she'd heard about through friends. Incredibly, after a one-and-a-half-hour session her eyesight dramatically improved, she was able to walk unassisted and had more mental energy than she'd had since the disease began. While the results did not produce complete reversal, the improvement was dramatic and far better than anything conventional medicine had provided. When I last saw her, she felt emboldened to discuss beginning to taper off her medication with her neurologist.

'The point is to remind yourself that you're part of something beautiful and much bigger than yourself, whether nature for you means interacting with your pet, visiting your favourite beach or taking a walk in your local park.'

What happened here? Well, no one really knows. There have been attempts to measure energy emanating from renowned healers; from the cruder early days using photography to wonderfully inspired recent research from psychologist Dr Gary Schwartz at the University of Arizona in the US using highly sophisticated bio-photon imaging to measure energetic emissions from healers' hands. In one study examining the effects of Reiki for cancer patients undergoing conventional therapy, there was a significant decrease in fatigue, pain and anxiety after seven Reiki sessions over two weeks. Another randomized, controlled study showed decrease in heart rate and blood pressure in patients after three Reiki treatments compared to control groups.

Probably the best studied energy practice is therapeutic (healing) touch, which for thirty years has been part of the nursing curriculum at many top nursing schools. Therapeutic touch doesn't actually involve touching; it's achieved by a transfer of energy from the practitioner's hands to the receiver. In one powerful study therapeutic touch decreased pain, anxiety and suppressor T lymphocytes (which help regulate a balanced immune response) in burn patients. Another study published in *The Journal of Holistic Nursing* showed an increase in haemoglobin (red blood cell) levels in healthy students compared to controls. Numerous other studies, particularly in nursing journals, show benefits from the use of therapeutic touch in the hospital, particularly with pain and mood states.

My colleague Dr Dolores Krieger introduced therapeutic touch to nursing schools. I couldn't agree more with her belief that the ability to engage energy in the healing process should be at the core of healthcare. I would only caution you to find the best practitioner. One study showed that Reiki practitioners had poor results on days they weren't feeling well. This is definitely an area in which having a referral from a trusted source is key. If you are in a hospital where therapeutic (healing) touch is offered I highly recommend you take advantage, as nurses are the standard bearers of these traditions.

The Interconnected Web

I was fortunate enough recently to meet Edgar Mitchell, a visionary scientist, the sixth astronaut to walk on the moon (he shares with Alan Shephard the record for longest moonwalk) and founder of the Institute of Noetic Sciences. He is one of the few human beings who experienced a greater spiritual connectedness while hurtling through space. Looking at the beautiful blue Earth from his spaceship on the return flight, Edgar was overwhelmed with the intimate knowledge that he was connected to his home planet. In a moment of deep insight, he realized that he was also connected with everything – his energy was entangled with that of everything and everyone – through time and space. That experience led eventually to his founding of the Institute of Noetic Sciences, which conducts research into the healing power and the energetic nature of consciousness.

In Chapter 1 you learned about a neuropeptide web that interconnects parts of your body separated by space – it allows your thoughts to send chemical messengers that affect your digestive tract, your emotions to affect your cardiovascular system, your hormones to affect your moods – and vice versa. Researchers are beginning to redefine their view of all matter in terms of this underlying energetic web. While the neuropeptide web communicates by chemical reactions, physicists have been able to demonstrate that instantaneous communication between subatomic particles occurs on an energetic level at speeds faster than the speed of light.

Working on an infinitesimally minute level of the smallest known subatomic particles and the forces that bind them together, physicists performing experiments with particle accelerators (the massive tools they've designed to split atoms) have demonstrated that the objects we perceive as matter – from your loved ones to this book you're reading – are actually made of collections or patterns of energy. Quantum physicists have further established that this energetic matter seems to be infinitely mutable (it can be in two places at once and move backwards in time, which is termed *non-locality*) and it is continuously interacting with other matter that enters its energetic field, becoming perpetually entangled with it even across vast expanses of space.

'Where most of us see empty space separating one living thing from another, physicists have shown all these empty spaces to be filled with energy that allows for continuous sharing of energy and information across space.'

Energy in Action

You and I have no problem understanding that energy can transcend space in nearly instantaneous time: when someone plays a violin, you can hear the music a hundred metres away – travelling over invisible waves at the relatively slow speed of sound. When you turn on a light bulb you accept with little fanfare that the light fills the room in an instant, but it did in fact have to travel at the speed of light, transmitting the energy of the light's photons from the bulb to your dinner table. One of my favourite examples of invisible, energetic information transfer in everyday life is of a remote-control garage-door opener: when you press the button, an electromagnetic signal travels seemingly instantaneously to a receiver that opens the door. I'd like you to accept this image of energy just as you accept that a violin string transmits sound energy. Your thoughts can conceivably emanate like the energy of the door-opener to be received by others and vice versa.

This new science of energy has enormous implications for healing, and at the same time explains many of the healing phenomena I have witnessed over years of practising medicine. The energetic web that underlies all matter helps explain the beneficial power of belief in any cure to heal illness and also informs us how the destructive power of negative thoughts can do us harm on a physical level. The existence of this web also helps explain how my patient was healed by Qi gong, why being in a supportive community can be so powerful, and why helping others can be so energizing. The discoveries of quantum physics strongly suggest that all of us have the power to affect not only our own health, but also each other through the interaction of energy – including the energy of thought and emotion.

This very real energetic web tying together all matter allows for a cause and effect relationship between consciousness (the energy of thought) and healing (the returning of physical processes to normal). The transformative power of our own thoughts and intentions and of the thoughts and intentions of others involves an energetic process that transcends space, in what Larry Dossey has described as 'non-local mind'. As a doctor I have witnessed the benefits of *non-locality*; I have come to see the value of tuning in to our energetic selves. I've come to think of this process as plugging into an *inter-connected web* – the source – of energy that ties us all together and makes us part and parcel of the universe, of each other, and, perhaps, of the absolute.

Part two

21 Days to Optimal Energy

Power up, Cleanse, Maximize

The Source Day-by-Day

WELCOME TO THE SOURCE DAY-BY-DAY. My 21-Day Plan for Increasing Your Energy and Feeling 10 Years Younger consists of three vital phases that will purify and maximize your body's energy-generating capacity. For each day you will find a one-page summary of the plan for that day, followed by more detailed discussions of various aspects of the day that may contain new or unfamiliar concepts. Here, a quick overview of the three weeks:

- **Week One: The first step is to increase, or *power up*, your energy-generating capacity. This requires reducing stress and gradually eliminating alcohol, red meat, wheat, sugar and processed and chemically treated foods – all of which cause inflammation. You will eat nutrient-dense (primarily whole) foods every three to four hours to stabilize your blood sugar and provide blocks of energy. You will begin regular guided relaxation. You will breathe more (using breath work every day), and drink more water and other healthy fluids (350ml every two hours), rest more (closing in on the desired eight hours' sleep a day), move more (20 to 30 minutes a day), and remove toxins, including negative thoughts (with a daily stress log).**

- **Week Two: The second step is to reset your metabolism by *cleaning out* the toxins. During this recharge phase, I will guide you through a one-day juice cleanse that will dramatically reduce inflammation and enhance detoxification. You'll follow that with a gentle recovery day. You will eliminate foods that may bring your energy down via allergic or other adverse food reactions. You will regularly consume power foods** such as greens, green tea, mushrooms, non-wheat whole grains, flax, berries and fish. You will practise powerful yogic breathing exercises and incorporate massage and other body work designed to help flush out toxins and increase vitality. You will continue to sleep more, exercise moderately, maintain hydration and manage stress better.

- **Week Three:** The third step is to move beyond lifestyle changes to more advanced energy-generating techniques to *maximize* your energy. Inflammation, glycation (sugar ageing) and the level of toxins in your body will have all decreased dramatically. With your new habits, you will be extracting more energy from food, coping with stress rather than letting it undermine you, raising your pulse rate daily to use energy more efficiently, and getting superior sleep. You will be ready for deeper body work such as Reiki or acupuncture. If, despite introducing all of the above, your energy is still not optimum, I will add powerful supplements to further maximize your energy supply.

Negotiating Change

Bad news up front: in order to restore your energy over the next 21 days I will ask you to eliminate red meat, sugar, alcohol, coffee, wheat and processed foods. Why should you do this? Because these foods tend to cause allergic, inflammatory, insulin-related and other reactions that put a strain on your natural energy supply. For some people, this is a welcome challenge and change (the plan offers many enticing substitutes for all of the above) as they have been wanting a reason to cut out these foods that they've guessed are not doing them any good. For others, the elimination of these long-time gustatory companions will seem impossible. Do you *have* to get rid of all of them? Not exactly. I'm willing to negotiate with you rather than lose the chance to bring your energy back because you're worried you won't be able to get off and stay off them. I will offer you a way to work the plan in increments.

> **Check for Illness First**
> *It's essential that you be screened by your doctor for an underlying cause of your fatigue before starting the plan. Certain parts of the plan – including the cleanse and the sauna – may not be suitable for people with certain conditions. See page 16 for a discussion of what to look for with your doctor.*

One Step at a Time

My first recommendation for you if you can't go 'cold turkey' on what I call energy-negative foods is that you eliminate only one or two target offenders at a time. There are two ways to choose the first to go: you can eliminate the items you consume the least of, which is the easiest (but less effective) route; or you can follow a classic allergy-elimination paradigm and stop eating the offenders that you consume most often. What you flood your system with on a consistent basis is likely to do the most harm and cause the most potent cravings. Removing that offender will yield the greatest results. Removing your most energy-negative food will likely provide you with the best motivation to continue to comply.

The biggest impediment is fear of crashing, particularly from sugar and coffee withdrawal. Some people really do feel their lives and personal energy will come to a screeching halt, or at least be terribly disrupted, if they don't get their accustomed stimulants. This brings me to my second negotiating tactic. If you can't go off your energy-negative foods cold turkey, try gradual withdrawal. In the 21-Day programme, for instance, you gradually reduce coffee, and substitute green tea, which gives you a more gentle lift. You don't have to give up the taste of sweetness altogether, as you will have plenty of fruits and natural sugars in the plan, but refined (white) sugar is off the list. The upside is that, once white sugar is gone, the compulsion for sweetness often goes away.

I'll take a small change in habit over no change any day. One patient began the programme as she was moving to a vineyard in Italy! Drinking no alcohol was out of the question so I suggested she take one glass of wine with dinner every other day rather than her accustomed two or three glasses every night. She reported developing a more discerning palate by drinking less. She also found it easier to get out of bed in the morning and had fewer headaches.

Focus on the Positive

The simplest way to negotiate change is to focus on the positive. Rather than think of the plan as some sort of Spartan regimen, think of it as a new experience. My patients often report that the plan expanded their horizons. Some patients have even planned ahead trips to Asia at the end of 21 days, after having been introduced to its multitude of flavours and energy practices.

I'll offer one more incentive; you do not have to be on the plan for a lifetime, and you do not need to cut out these foods forever. Cutting out wheat, for example, doesn't always make a difference. Go ahead, try it again after abstaining for three weeks and see how you feel. Moderation is your mantra . . . everything in moderation.

WEEK ONE: POWER UP!

'Reduced to our own body, our first instrument, we learn to play it, drawing from it maximum resonance and harmony.'

YEHUDI MENUHIN

Day 1

- **Power Mind: Learn the early morning wake-up call**
  - **Establish an Evening Stress Log**
  - **Take the Energy Quiz (see page 13)**
- **Power Food: Organic menu**
  - **Eat every 3 to 4 hours: Avoid blood-sugar swings**

- – A Quick Look at Inflammatory Foods
- – Increase water: Drink 5 to 6 glasses per day
- • Power Exercise: Baby steps
- • Power Rest: 8 hours
  - – Meet the Sleep Plan: 8 hours' sleep 4 nights per week; asleep by 11pm 2 to 3 nights per week

Early Morning Wake-Up Call

On the first morning of the plan when you wake up I want you to be aware that you are in the midst of a critical transition from sleep to waking – your hormones, neurotransmitters, muscle fibres and blood cells are ramping up in preparation for meeting the challenges of the day. Awakening can be a stressful time, but you are going to transform this stressful moment of the day into an energy-generating opportunity. You will dissolve negative or worrying thoughts that can sap your energy and wreak havoc on your body throughout the day.

Before bounding up, sit on the edge of your bed, spine straight, hands relaxed on the thighs. Take three deep breaths – drawing from your abdomen to the count of 4, hold for one count and exhale from

The Remedy

The following conditions are significantly improved by regular elicitation of the relaxation response with controlled breathing, meditation and other methods.

- • Anxiety
- • Asthma
- • Cardiac arrhythmias
- • Chronic pain
- • Headaches
- • Hot flushes

- • Hypertension
- • Insomnia
- • Irritable bowel
- • Lower back pain
- • Mild/moderate depression
- • PMS

From Herbert Benson, *The Relaxation Response*

your abdomen to the count of 6. Now sit quietly focusing only on your breath. When thoughts of your day come into your consciousness, allow them to leave. Focus on your breathing. If thoughts persist try repeating a mantra to calm your frantic mind (love, energy and peace are a few to try) – or use images (clouds, ocean, loved ones). Stay this way for at least 2 minutes, which is long enough to begin to elicit the relaxation response. See Chapter 1 for more on how this relaxation exercise benefits your health.

Do not fear that if you relax in the morning you won't perform as well at work. You will soon find out what neuroscientists know about meditation and breath work – it stimulates portions of the brain involved in mental focus. You'll find you have better energy and more laser-like focus with the Early Morning Wake-Up Call.

Eat Every 3 to 4 Hours to Avoid Blood-Sugar Swings

For the 21-Day Plan you will eat every 3 to 4 hours to avoid a drop in blood sugar. Low blood sugar produces an immediate energy drain; not only does your body have insufficient sugar to manufacture energy, but the hormone changes required to compensate for lack of blood sugar cause energy expenditure.

A Quick Look at Inflammatory Foods

The organic menus of the 21-Day Plan eliminate all major inflammatory foods. When digested, certain foods – like alcohol, red meat, sugar and artificial ingredients – turn into substances that promote the creation of inflammatory molecules. These molecules, consisting mainly of a class called cytokines, are part of the immune system and are beneficial to the body in the short term (for example, they help in attacking infections). But a steady diet of foods that promote inflammatory substances can worsen or even cause inflammatory conditions such as arthritis, asthma, heart disease and chronic pain. Inflammation drains energy and can even cause weight gain. By following the menus of the 21-Day Plan you will significantly reduce inflammation. (See Chapter 2 for a more complete list of inflammatory foods.)

Increase water

During the 21-Day Plan you will drink between 250 and 360ml of water every two to three hours. (Non-caffeinated, minimally sweetened beverages like herbal tea count towards this.) Inadequate hydration causes the body to extract water from non-vital tissues in order to shunt water to key organs (heart, brain and kidneys). Such stop-gap water management can produce a significant drop in overall energy. Scientists have even shown that insufficient hydration can have a negative effect on memory.

What's in your water?

Every drinking water supply is different. Here are examples of contaminants repeatedly detected in the water supply, and the best type of filter to eliminate the problem. You can obtain a report on your own water supply by contacting your local water supplier.

Contaminant	Common Source	Potential Health Effects	Best Filter
Chlorination by-products	Water chlorination practices	Potential carcinogen	Carbon (filters particles down to a fraction of a strand of hair)
Lead	Plumbing, brass alloy faucets	Kidney, nervous system damage	Carbon
Mercury	Crop run-off, battery disposal	Kidney, nervous system disorders	Reverse osmosis (filters particles down to a single atom)
Microbes	Animal or human waste	Gastrointestinal illness	Reverse osmosis
Atrazine	Run-off from use as herbicide	Promotes breast tumour growth	Reverse osmosis

Source: www.nsf.org

Finding clean water: You're going to be drinking a lot of water over the next 21 days, so let's make sure it's healthy. Tap water has become suspect in many areas. Out-of-date water treatment facilities do not adequately remove many 21st century industrial chemicals that can contaminate ground water, streams and reservoirs. Well water has no oversight whatsoever, and can easily be contaminated from local run-off, for example from lawn chemicals. Old pipes that carry water to you can leach contaminants and breed bacteria. Home filtration is by far the best, least expensive and most ecologically prudent way to ensure your water is clean. Your second-best bet is high-quality bottled (preferably in glass) water, which is fairly well regulated in the UK and Europe.

Shopping for a water filter: Water filters can be placed where the water enters the house or underneath the kitchen sink. Carbon filters are sufficient for removing most contaminants, but reverse osmosis is considered to be the best filtration technology, though it requires a small water tank under the sink. One of my favourite filter manufacturers is Culligan, but there are many quality brands: look for NSF International certification on the package label of whichever filter you choose. Although this is an American standard for drinking water products, it's now internationally recognized.

Power Exercise: Baby Steps

If you don't already have an exercise routine, start powering up your metabolism simply by walking for 20 minutes, but keep in mind that you are working towards the Power Up Workout (Day Three). You may already have a regular exercise routine, in which case keep it up! If you don't exercise (like approximately 65 per cent of the population), I'm going to make it simple for you. Begin by taking a 20-minute walk each day. Studies show that walking is sufficient exercise to give life-extending benefits, whether it's on your way to the bus, at lunch time, on the way home, or an evening stroll. Begin to make it part of your life.

Establish an Evening Stress Log

My goal is for you to begin to pinpoint the stressful moments in your day. With that in mind, I'd like you to get a notebook and keep a stress log that will help you recognize the stressors in your life. On almost a daily basis people tell me they are fine when I ask about stress, and then wind up near tears later in the conversation when they start to talk about (and actually recognize) the difficulties in their lives. Stress is cumulative, which is to say that relatively small stresses can have great impact when stress is loaded upon stress on a chronic daily basis. With this log you will begin to see patterns of stress that you can address. Once you've identified and named the stressful moments in your day, I hope you can begin to let them go each evening and, eventually, address them in order to reduce them.

Write down the three most stressful moments of your day. These can include an encounter with a difficult person, upsetting thoughts or horrendous traffic on your morning commute. The point is to note where and when your blood starts to boil. Note the time and place and nature of the stress. Rate on a scale of 1–6 the level of stress, and give yourself a grade for how you coped with it. Once you've put it down in print, that's where it should stay. Now let it go.

Meet the Sleep Plan
8 hours of sleep 4 nights a week
Asleep by 11pm 2 or 3 nights per week

During the 21-Day Plan you will develop regular, healthy sleep patterns, which means that most nights you'll get to bed around the same reasonable time and clock 8 hours of sleep. Tonight, you're going to try for 8 hours. You've got nothing to lose and everything to gain. When it comes to sleep your body is just like your mobile phone battery: if you don't charge it long enough, it runs out faster. The same goes for your body: inadequate sleep = inadequate energy. As folksy as this wisdom sounds, we now have solid scientific evidence about what the body actually needs to do while you sleep. It takes 8 hours for the body to optimally repair and regenerate cells, lower blood pressure (by as much as 10 per cent), and manufacture protective and functional hormones as well as other key chemicals you need for energy generation. If you don't sleep long enough and deeply enough, your body will be inadequately recharged.

Scientists have pinpointed 8 hours as the ideal amount of sleep. Considering that the majority of us get less than 7 hours of sleep, I'm going to be realistic and ask that you shoot for 8 hours at least 4 nights a week. I've added in bed by 11pm 2 or 3 nights a week because I know many people try to make up for sleep shortages on the weekends, but if that means sleeping from 1am to 9am I'm still not happy. Research shows that the hours of sleep before midnight are more productive in their repair and regeneration of cells than the hours of sleep after midnight. In Chinese medical terms, it's best to be sound asleep between 11pm and 1am, when the body's Qi energy replenishes itself.

Day 2

- **Power Mind: Early morning wake-up call**
  - *Establish Breath Breaks**
  - *Evening Stress Log*
- **Power Food: Organic menus**
  - *Eliminate Chemical Toxins with Organics*
  - *Increase Chewing*
  - *Juice Cocktails vs Dessert*
- **Power Detox:** *Identify environmental energy drains at home*
- **Power Exercise:** *The Power of Walking*
- **Power Rest: Asleep by 11pm**
  - *Calming Bedtime Routine*

  *Note: New concepts for you are *italic*.

Early Morning Wake-Up Call

This morning as you transit from sleep to waking, I want you to feel the energy in your body as it moves from its dormant state to its active state. Highly trained Buddhist monks can control the energy in their bodies to such a degree that they can raise their body temperatures even while sitting outside in the winter. I'm not suggesting you aspire to monk-like power, though anything is possible! My goal is to make you aware of the energy you possess.

This morning as you practise the Early Morning Wake-Up Call, become aware of sensations of energy in your body – move your fingertips together and feel a tingling or vibration, or look for a release of tension from your spine or facial muscles. Take just two minutes, or as long as you'd like, to begin to feel relaxed and energized.

As you make your way through the Power Up! plan, I want you to practise the Early Morning Wake-Up Call every day. You can keep it simple, as I've set it out for the first two days, or you can try different focuses for your meditative time. For instance, try the focus of the Connectedness exercises – mindfulness, forgiveness, letting go of grudges. If you already have a contemplative or spiritual practice, take this morning time to deepen it. Simply using a mantra that evokes a higher power can magnify the benefits of the relaxation response. As you work with this exercise, find ways of making it your own and of making it meaningful.

Establish Breath Breaks

During the 21-Day Plan I want you to reap the benefits of the relaxation response that you elicit with the Early Morning Wake-Up Call throughout the day by taking Breath Breaks. The breath is the best means you have for directly changing aspects of your autonomic nervous system, which functions without conscious intervention to regulate the activities of the heart, muscles and glands. By simply breathing deeply and rhythmically, with intention, you can slow your heart rate, lower your blood pressure, improve your digestion, strengthen your immune system and calm your nervous system.

Take a Breath Break every time you are aware that you are breathing. Do this frequently – sitting, walking, eating, while in a tense meeting. You will immediately feel the tension in your body release. You will be less tight, less hunched in the neck and shoulders. You will have a calmer mind, slower pulse – and a slower life and greater energy. Here's how:

- **Inhale with a slow, deep abdominal breath (allowing your breath to expand your abdomen) to the count of 4.**
- **Pause, holding in this fresh oxygen, for one count.**
- **Exhale slowly (allow your abdomen to contract) to the count of 6.**
- **Pause for one count. (Repeat two more times.)**

Eliminate Chemical Toxins with Organics

Eating organic fruits and vegetables is the best way to begin eliminating toxins from your body and get cleaner energy from your food. A growing number of scientists and doctors, myself included, harbour deep concerns about the wide array of pesticides, herbicides and other chemicals used to grow foods. Apples and strawberries, for example, carry an average of five different pesticides per piece of fruit and can be sprayed up to 25 times during the growing cycle. While the chemical industry conducts some research on the individual effects of pesticides, scant research exists on the effects of continuous exposure to numerous pesticides on a daily basis, which is the average exposure for people eating non-organic, conventional foods. I want you to reduce this cumulative load of industrial chemicals by buying as much organic food as you possibly can.

If you want to prioritize your organic purchases, a quick rule of thumb is that produce and dairy come first, followed by meats and then all other foods. It's more important to purchase organic thin-skinned fruits and vegetables such as berries, peaches, apples, tomatoes and almost all vegetables. (Onions are about the only vegetable that I don't insist on being organic because they rarely carry pesticides) Thick-skinned fruits such as oranges, bananas, melons and avocados offer less exposure to pesticides because their edible insides are more protected from chemical contamination by the thick peel. (For more on organics, see Chapter 3.)

Increase Chewing

During the 21-Day Plan I want you to practise chewing more, at least 12 times per mouthful. Chewing is the first step in the process of transforming your food into energy. Unfortunately, few people chew enough. Most of us inhale our food, which increases the amount of energy needed to digest it and reduces the amount of nutrients and energy you extract from it.

Here's how it works. Many of the enzymes in your pancreas are also present in your mouth. When you chew well, your food is predigested by the time it hits your stomach. With improper chewing, you throw large chunks of whole food into the stomach, which churns and acidifies the partially chewed food, but cannot finish the job. This leads to indigestion and chronic poor absorption of nutrients, especially when your stomach doesn't have much acid (as can happen most notably when taking acid-suppressing drugs). The undigested food is difficult for the chemicals from the gall bladder and pancreas to break down fully. The remainder of the digestion then falls to the intestinal bacteria, which are not entirely cut out for the work, and in the process create gas, bloating and cramping.

Just like mum told you, wolfing your food is bad – it leads to low energy. Chewing more is an easy way to reduce digestive problems and receive more energy from your food. Another key benefit of chewing more is eating less: when you eat slowly and chew well, you absorb your food more efficiently and get the 'all-full' signal faster.

Juice Drink vs Dessert

Your dinner menu today includes a juice cocktail, Papaya Fizz, and no dessert. The drink has healthy antioxidants and enzymes in the papaya, but it also contains a fair amount of natural fruit sugar – enough to give up eating dessert as well. Throughout the 21 days the dinner menus alternate between juice cocktails and dessert. Feel free to substitute either one, if you prefer a special drink with dinner each night, then skip dessert or have a small bowl of berries. If you prefer dessert, go for any one of the desserts and skip the cocktail.

Identify Environmental Energy Drains at Home

For the 21-Day Plan I want you to identify and eliminate major sources of chemical toxins in your home that may very well be draining your energy. I think the best approach is to evaluate the pollutants in your home that might target your physical vulnerabilities – do you have asthma, eczema, a family history of cancer, recurring bronchitis or headaches every time you shower? Or do you wake up with a stuffy nose every morning, which goes away by lunch? Are you exposing yourself to respiratory, hormonal, skin or immune system disruptors? You can make quick changes that will stop your home from sapping your energy.

Take an inventory of possible environmental sources of toxicity listed in 'Home Sweet Toxin', below, and seek out healthier alternatives. The amount of exposure you have to any given toxin is the key to your evaluation. Items you are widely exposed to are more important than those you are minimally exposed to. For example, when evaluating your personal-care products, those that come in contact with large amounts of skin (i.e. moisturizers or bath products) should be more carefully scrutinized than those that come in contact with only a small portion of skin. You are likely to spend more continuous time in your bedroom than any other room in the house, so first evaluate your bedroom for possible offenders. One exception to the dose-exposure rule: I have zero tolerance for plastic shower curtains, Teflon pans and microwaving in plastic containers – get rid of them, now! (See Chapter 3 for more on environmental toxins.)

The Power of Walking

During the 21-Day Plan I want you to derive maximum benefit from 20 to 30 minutes of walking. First I suggest you make peace with the concept of walking. Take a moment to recognize how lucky you are to be freely mobile. Walking is a privilege and a joy and a way of knowing the world that many of us forego for convenience. Many of us don't walk well and, rather than holding our bodies erect when

Home Sweet Toxin

Your domestic haven could be making you sick and tired. Below are some of the biggest offenders. In the US, I subscribe to The Green Guide (greenguide.com) and greenerchoices.org for useful information on making a healthy household. In the UK, try Environment and Greener Living advice centre at www.direct.gov.uk. See also www.ectopia.co.uk

Products	Toxic Chemicals	Potential Health Risks	Healthier Alternatives
Mattresses	Polyurethane, formaldehyde, toluene, PBDE (flame retardants)	Respiratory disruptor, carcinogen, neurotoxin	Natural-fill (wool or cotton), untreated mattress or pillow topper
Fitted carpets	Adhesives and stain-proofing agents can outgas formaldehyde	Carcinogen, skin irritant	Jute, wool, hemp, or sea grass area rugs installed with VOC* -free adhesives
Paints	Benzene, formaldehyde, toluene, xylene	Carcinogen, neurotoxin	Look on labels for no -VOC or low-VOC paints, and let dry ventilated for 72 hours. Pregnant women should not paint
Cosmetics	Phthalates, parabens, preservatives, coal tar, triclosan, DEA, heavy metals, sodium lauryl sulphate	Endocrine (hormone) disruptor, carcinogen, antibiotic resistance, neurotoxin, skin toxin	Look for these worst offenders on labels and try to avoid them. For cosmetics the organic claim is not heavily regulated
Cleaning products	Chlorine bleach, ammonia, acids, fragrance, DEA and TEA	Respiratory, eye, skin irritants, carcinogens, endocrine disruptors	Soap, water, baking soda, vinegar, lemon juice and borax. Be mindful of ventilation
Plastic and vinyl shower curtains	Off-gasses plasticizers for as many as 5 years	Endocrine (hormone) disruptor	Go for washable cotton, canvas, silk or rayon
Kitchenware	Teflon, PVC (plastic)	Carcinogens, endocrine disruptor	Cook with enamelled cast-iron or seasoned stainless steel; microwave and store in Pyrex, not plastic

* Volatile organic compounds (VOCs) are noxious gases emitted from certain compounds that can be inhaled or absorbed by the skin over time.

we walk (which we're designed to do), we simply allow our bodies to slump down upon our legs and feet, which are forced to drag around dead weight all day long. Let's wipe the slate clean and start over.

Think of these as the first steps of your new life. Imagine you're walking on sand, with your toes lightly pressing on the ground (this is why doctors have always recommended soft shoes for toddlers – humans should engage their toes when they walk). Set down your heel gently (there should be very little sound, and certainly no elephantine thumping). Feel the toes activated and the ball of your foot pushing off as your foot prepares to leave the ground. Keep your length of stride reasonable: don't reach with your legs. Slightly rotate your pelvis under while tightening your bottom and abs (this will eliminate swayback and flaccid bottom muscles). Spine position is erect, with your abdominals lightly contracted, chest expanded, shoulders back and down (not up). Your head should feel as though there is a string gently pulling you up from the crown, the muscles under your chin slightly tight, and your head positioned to balance a book.

Feel the elongation of your spine. Feel the effortlessness of your body as it moves through space. Feel blessed that you have the ability to walk freely. Use this time to move and to relax your mind. And breathe as though you need the oxygen, which you do!

Calming Bedtime Routine

From a very young age, bedtime rituals are the first step towards getting a proper night's sleep. You need a calming ritual that begins to organize your nervous system, not stimulate it. Bedtime laggards, who stay up later than planned, are about twice as likely as early-to-bed types to be on the internet or doing work related to their jobs during the hour before going to bed. And 87 per cent of the population reports watching television before bed. Be mindful of how a programme will affect your stress levels. TV and most other electronic devices overstimulate the brain and make it harder to move into a sleep zone, which requires a lot of soothing alpha brainwaves. Go for soothing evening activities that make your brain sleep-prone.

It's important to fall asleep relatively quickly, not tossing and turning when the lights go out, which is a sure sign you haven't prepared yourself properly for sleep. People who take 30 minutes or more to fall asleep are more likely to sleep less than six hours on weekdays; they experience at least one symptom of insomnia and report that they get less sleep than the minimum they say they need to function at their best. On average, it takes 23 minutes to fall asleep, which means ideally you should have lights out by 9:35pm, and begin calming activities by 8:30pm!

The best activities for the hour before bed are: practise relaxation exercises (see Days 3, 4, 5, 8 and 15), calm reading (no page turners), take a hot bath with lavender oil, listen to soothing music or drink calming tea with chamomile and valerian.

Day 3

- **Power Mind: Early morning wake-up call** *with Sun Salutation*
  - **Daytime: Breath Breaks**
  - *The Two-Minute Energy Boost*
  - **Evening Stress Log**
- **Power Food: Organic menus**
  - *Eliminate Wheat*
  - *Why Drink Green Tea?*
- **Power Exercise:** *The Power Up! Workout in a nutshell*
  20 to 30 Minutes' Walking
  30 Crunches, 20 Push-ups (bent-knee OK)
- *Power of Connection: Establish positive emotional actions*
  - *Letting Go of Grudges*
- **Power Rest: 8 hours' sleep**
  - *Tips for Falling Asleep: Progressive Relaxation*

Sun Salutation

If you can add the incredibly powerful yogic asana (position) Sun Salutation to your Early Morning Wake-Up Call every day or every other day or once a week, you will start the game on a better energetic plane. I'd like you to get instruction on Sun Salutations from an expert, but overleaf is a detailed illustration of how to complete the posture once. Classically, Sun Salutations are done in pairs, starting first with one foot, then the other. Most importantly: don't rush; feel the energy moving through your body.

The Two-Minute Energy Boost

During the 21-Day Plan you will give up your accustomed pick-me-ups – the cup of coffee or the bar of chocolate – and learn to generate quick energy in much healthier, longer-lasting ways, through breath work and relaxation exercises. Your Two-Minute Energy Boost can be any movement – from a yoga posture to hopping up and down – that gets your blood moving. The key is to use exercises that you can do anywhere anytime, with minimal space and no equipment. You can even do them where others can watch you because they are unobtrusive; you may even give others the idea to do the same. Here is a list of the energy-generating exercises that I explained in detail at the end of Chapter 4.

- Abdominal breathing
- Seated warrior
- Downward facing dog
- Qi gong energy ball
- Hopping
- Rock out with your iPod

Eliminate Wheat

As you go through the 21 days I am going to have you eliminate certain foods that could be either directly toxic to your health and energy, or produce an energy drag via allergies and other processes. In my experience, wheat is the most sensitizing food – nearly 50 per cent of my patients become sensitive to wheat by the age of 40. This

Sun Salutation

Sun Salutation is an energizing combination of seven yoga postures, always performed in this order. You begin by placing one foot back, complete the series, then start again with the other foot. Before attempting this, spend time with an instructor or an instructional video to learn and perform it with good alignment.

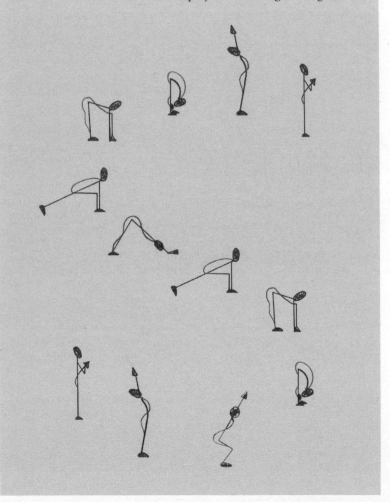

means that even though their allergy testing may be non-reactive, wheat produces subtle health problems – most commonly fatigue, but also other physical problems such as headaches indigestion, and joint aches. Additionally many more people have subtle allergies to wheat, measurable either by skin tests or through blood tests – the latter creating a reaction that can occur up to three days after consumption. And the 5 per cent of people with actual gluten-intolerant coeliac disease can become quite ill after the tiniest bit of wheat. (See Chapter 2 for more information on allergy testing.)

The main trouble-maker is the New World wheat hybrid that is most commonly used in North America for 'wheat' in breads, pasta and almost all baked goods (even commercial oat bread routinely contains wheat as the main grain). This grain has had limited commercial success in the UK and Europe; however, modern refining techniques do strip most of the nutrients from European wheats, and there is no question that wheat is over-eaten in the UK. In the menu plan, for the few times we include bread, we ask that you try one of the delicious Old World varieties such as kamut or spelt, to which most people are not sensitive. (And for coeliac substitute with non-gluten flours such as quinoa, rice, potato or corn.) Your body will tell you if cutting out wheat is the right thing for you. Either you will notice much more energy when you eliminate wheat, or you will feel immediately bad again when you reintroduce it after three weeks of clearing it out.

Why Drink Green Tea?

Health benefits: Green tea is one of the most powerful healing foods on the planet. All green and black teas come from the same plant worldwide, *camellia sinensis*, but they are prepared with different processes that affect the healthful compounds in the leaves. Green tea is dried while black tea is fermented (oolong is partially fermented), and the fermentation process reduces some of the most important health-giving substances present in *camellia sinensis*.

Green tea has catechins – some of nature's most potent antioxidants, which also may help keep your metabolism working at a higher level (potentially releasing more calories from fat). A cup of regular green tea does have some caffeine – 10–30mg, versus 100–150mg for coffee – but the lift you get from green tea tends to be less of the roller-coaster ride you get from coffee, largely due to the amino acid theanine present in green tea, which counteracts the effects of caffeine by promoting production of calming brain neurotransmitters. If you find that you are sensitive to the caffeine in green tea you can clear 80 per cent of the caffeine while retaining most of the other beneficial ingredients by steeping your tea bag for one minute, then pouring out that tea and making a second cup of tea from the same bag.

Shopping: Green tea aficionados know the best quality leaves are harvested in the spring. Tea lovers wait all year for the *first picking* of the spring teas as the ultimate prize. But you do not need to go to these lengths to find green tea that is both delicious and health- and energy-promoting. Fortunately, there has been an explosive growth in quality teas available at your local supermarket (loose or packaged individually in tea bags) from companies like Tazo, Traditional Medicinals and Jing. Loose, good-quality green teas are available from most healthfood shops and larger supermarkets. Once you make a cup of green tea, colour is a sure sign of freshness. Sounds obvious, but it really should be green. Poorer quality teas have been oxidized (made stale by exposure to air), which lends a pale brown colour indicating loss of the beneficial substances. When buying green, look for green in your cup!

The Power Up! Workout in a Nutshell
20 to 30 minutes walking
30 crunches, 20 push-ups (bent-knee OK)
Studies have shown that a brisk 30-minute walk three days per week gives you the cardiovascular benefits of more strenuous running or other more intense aerobic exercise. For example, it lowers blood pressure, helps repair the inside of the blood vessels, and reduces the

inflammatory marker, CRP, the most powerful predictor of the risk of heart disease. Make sure to set three days a week aside to engage in aerobic walking. This is what is called *conversational aerobics* – your heart rate is raised, your metabolism increased, but you are still able to have a conversation while doing it, rather than feeling intensely winded. We will go into how you can maximize the aerobic benefits of simple walking in Day 5.

Crunch, Crunch, Crunch

To jump-start your core you need to strengthen it; and the best way to accomplish this on your own, without the need for an instructor, is the core crunch – an improvement on the old-fashioned sit-up. Lie on your back; bend your knees so that your lower back presses against the floor. Rest your hands loosely against the back of your neck. Do not pull your neck up with your hands! Engage your abdominal muscles, and slowly roll your upper body off the floor, keeping your neck in a straight line with your spine. Stop just after your shoulders leave the mat. The secret to doing this most efficiently and safely is to treat your abdominal muscles and your ribcage as a single unit – and to breathe throughout the exercise. After you have elevated about 7 or 8cm, slowly roll back down – without rounding your shoulders – then repeat. The motion should be smooth and slow, no jerking up and down, and no holding your breath. Do this until your muscles are just beginning to ache (for some people early on, just two or three proper core crunches can be excruciating!). Rest for a minute or two and do two more sets.

Work your way into proper push-ups

As we discussed earlier, research shows that strength builds quicker when you increase load rather than repetition. If you have never been able to do more than a couple of push-ups at a time, here's how to get stronger. Increase the challenge throughout the session, with your last push being hardest. For beginners, start your push-ups from a standing position, place your toes about 60cm from a wall, place your hands flat against it with arms stretched straight out, and slowly bring your nose to the wall by bending your arms, keeping your core engaged, body in a straight line like a plank. Do this a dozen times, rest, then move onto the floor for two rounds of bent-knee push-ups – straight spine, core engaged. Finally, do one perfect all-out push-up, on your toes, body straight as a board. Next time, end with two perfect push-ups, and soon you'll be up to six ... then on to 30!

Power of Connection: Establishing Positive Emotional Actions and Letting Go of Grudges

I want you to keep your daily stress log so that you can focus on particular patterns of behaviour that are counterproductive to you; holding grudges is a biggie. You need to be able to receive the positive energy of others in your community. What you project out is so often what comes back to you; ruminating on those who've wronged you is a sure to draw more negativity. Today I would like you to focus on how much and how often you hold grudges against others. Rather than thinking of the wrongs others have done to you, try thinking of what you can do to help others – it's a wonderful way to take your mind off yourself. Holding onto negative thought patterns will eat you up inside. I'm not suggesting you should become best friends with your nemesis, but let the negativity go.

Tips for Falling Asleep: Progressive Relaxation

This is a simple and effective way to release tension that's keeping you awake, shift the focus of your thoughts away from nagging worries, and at the same time say thank you to your body for all of the hard work of the day. Start with your toes: inhale deeply and squeeze and scrunch your toes as hard as you can. Now exhale completely while releasing your toes, and say a small thank-you to them for walking you through your day. Progress upwards through the major muscles of your body, contracting and releasing – thighs, buttocks, abdomen, then hands, arms and shoulders, and finally the face. As you move through your body, feel your limbs relax and begin to get heavier, and continue quiet deep breathing afterwards as you drift off to sleep.

Day 4

- **Power Mind: Early morning wake-up call**
  - Daytime: Breath breaks
  - Two-Minute Energy Boost
  - Evening Stress Log
- **Power Food: Organic menus**
  - *Still No Alcohol...Why?*
  - *Cutting Back on Coffee*
- **Power Detox:** *Identify environmental energy drains at work*
- **Power Exercise: Power-Up! Workout**
- **Power Rest: Asleep by 11pm**
  - *Tips for Nighttime Awakening: Dream remembrance*

Still No Alcohol...Why?

I am asking you to avoid alcohol for these three weeks principally to let your body's detox machinery rest. As discussed in detail in Chapter 3, people are highly variable in their abilities to detoxify alcohol – and other drugs. For some, the build-up of toxic by-products (such as acetaldehyde) can produce considerable lasting fatigue. Some are very sensitive to the yeast and fermentation by-products contained in alcoholic beverages. But for everyone, abstention from alcohol and other drugs gives the detox systems (especially enzymes in the liver) the chance to rejuvenate and work on clearing out some of the many other energy-draining toxic substances present in your body, such as pesticides, preservatives and other pollutants. In addition, alcohol can affect sleep patterns, and sleeping for three weeks without any alcohol in your system should help give you more restful, energy-generating sleep. You will find a half-dozen non-alcoholic cocktails included in the menu plan. I recommend serving them in fun glasses, and fulfilling the need to quaff without the alcohol.

Cutting Back on Coffee

For the rest of the 21 days I'd like you to eliminate coffee (or at least significantly cut back on it). Too many people use coffee as their energy drug – drinking it throughout the day to keep their energy up. The problem is that each time you drink coffee or high-caffeine beverages, you get a lift for a couple of hours, but then are susceptible to a follow-up energy crash – leading you to drink more. Caffeine is a drug that can cause withdrawal symptoms, which means that the nervous system becomes dependent on it. That dependence produces a yo-yo effect with energy going up and down. Cutting back on coffee will break the cycle of the yo-yo effect. Once you get past the withdrawal you can expect to have more consistent energy throughout the day. And, like alcohol, caffeine can affect sleep patterns, so getting it out of your system will give you a chance at a better night's sleep. I'm not recommending that you go cold turkey because I know this can be disruptive. If you know that you get severe withdrawal symptoms, taper your consumption by 50 per cent each day and substitute regular green tea for the coffee you give up. By the fifth day of the plan shoot for cutting out caffeine altogether. Just give yourself three weeks to try it.

Identify Environmental Energy Drains at Work

Work can drain your energy, but usually we think this is due to difficulties with co-workers, or work that is too much or too stressful. All too often, however, the physical environment itself is an unrecognized work energy drain. Consider making the following changes.

- **Get a HEPA air filter.**
- **Get an air-filtering plant such as a fern or large palm.**
- **Ask for any copy machine or inkjet printer to be removed from**

your immediate area (both can emit micronized particles of toner, considered air pollutants).

- Turn off overhead fluorescent lighting if you can, which is draining to the eyes. A better light source is natural light from a nearby window and a desk lamp that sheds light on your work without excessive glare.
- Get a glare screen for your computer.
- Consider using amber glasses that block the blue light from computers which can throw off your biological clock, disrupting your sleep cycle (see page 198).
- If you're constantly on the telephone, use a headset to minimize nerve and muscle strain.
- If you're on your mobile frequently, use an earpiece.
- Keep an emergency vitamin packet in your desk drawer for the times that you're exposed to sick co-workers or clients.
- Wash hands frequently, specially during cold and flu season.

Tips for Nighttime Awakening: Dream Remembrance

In my practice, waking up in the middle of the night is a far more prevalent problem than having trouble falling asleep initially. If you awaken in the wee hours, say, 4am, dream remembrance may be a big help. At that hour, your brainwaves shift towards the vivid dreaming rapid eye movement (REM) phase. It's often at this time that people spring up to consciousness where stressful thoughts – that you haven't brought under control during the day – quickly commandeer attention and keep you awake. (For more on sleep phases see Chapter 5.)

As you get a glimmer that you are coming out of a dream and beginning to wake up, latch onto that dream, hold onto it and try to conjure every detail. Allow your mind to drift fully into the dream. In sleep medicine this is called rebound sleep, which is the natural tendency to go back into the stage you were in before waking up. By training your mind, you can take advantage of what your body really wants to do – sleep. If you lose the dream, use your morning meditation exercise to lock onto a state of mental relaxation that will keep conscious thoughts at bay. This is a mind game – your mind will try to bring in conscious thoughts (almost always incessant worries), but you have to keep them from entering centre stage. By using your dream to distract from your worries, you keep yourself in sleep mode, which is where you need to be in the middle of the night.

Day 5

- **Power Mind: Early morning wake-up call**
  - *Why Massage Matters*
  - Daytime: Breath breaks
  - Two-Minute Energy Boost
  - Evening Stress Log
- **Power Food: Organic menus**
  - *Shopping for Fish*
  - *A Word on Calories*
- **Power Exercise: Power Up! Workout**
  - *The Power of Walking – Find Your Target*
- **Power of Connection: Positive emotional action**
  - *Cultivating Forgiveness*
- **Power Rest: 8 hours' sleep**
  - Tips for Falling Asleep: *10-minute meditative breath work*

Why Massage Matters

I'd like you to have a couple of massages during the 21-Day Plan. Many people think of massage as a luxury, but it has powerful health benefits that put it closer to the necessity category. Massage therapists use hands, fingers, elbows and forearms to manipulate soft tissue, targetting muscles, tendons, ligaments, joints and connective tissue as well as lymphatic vessels. Studies show numerous positive effects of massage include relaxation, improved sleep and strengthened immune system along with relief of fatigue, pain, anxiety and nausea. Massage is terrific for the circulatory system; it's been shown to lower blood pressure and heart rate. In one study at Massachusetts General Hospital in the US, massage reduced diastolic blood pressure, calmed breathing and reduced psychological distress and pain in patients undergoing cardiac catheterization. In another study, a back massage for spouses of patients with cancer resulted in improved mood, reduced stress and increased the activity of natural killer cells (powerful immune defenders).

Massage can also be energizing. For fatigue, the deeper the massage the better. Shiatsu (deep-tissue massage based on acupressure points that releases muscle tension) has been shown to significantly reduce fatigue after chemotherapy. And people with advanced kidney disease experienced a dramatic improvement in fatigue and depression after receiving acupressure massage (using strong finger pressure to target and release acupuncture points). Athletes have known for centuries that sports massage (a general muscle rubdown) relieves soreness and fatigue. The type of massage you get is less important than the often nearly intuitive ability of the massage therapist to locate and effectively release tension points (also known as trigger points) in your body. If you've never had bodywork you will be amazed at how energizing it can be, or if you're familiar with massage, think of this as permission to spend the time and money on your well-being. There are massage therapists who specialize in pregnancy massage, which is a wonderful idea, especially in the last trimester when muscles and connective tissue are under such stress. (Note: If you are being treated for a medical condition, especially if you're taking blood thinners, have significant musculoskeletal injuries, or vascular problems like tendency to clots, get permission from your doctor before having a massage.)

A Word on Weight

If you follow the 21-Day Menu plan you will be well within a healthy calorie range *and* composition. The increase in obesity in the last 20 years has been blamed on the quantity of what you eat – too many calories in the super-size-me era. But it's also a matter of the quality of what you eat. Refined carbohydrates significantly change the relationships between insulin, leptin and many other hormones that control your weight and satiety. Recent research shows that eating fats that increase inflammation keeps you from losing weight. In my plan you won't go hungry, but you *will* eat a balance of complex carbohydrates, healthy fats and lean protein, with an abundance of plant foods that will make the kilos fall off, even while you feel satisfied.

Shopping for Fish

Over the course of 21 days you will eat fish four separate times, reaping the benefits of this source of rich anti-inflammatory omega-3 fatty acids. For each recipe we have selected species of fish that are nearly free of mercury and other chemical toxins, and that are classified by multiple regulatory agencies as safe to eat four or more times a month (see Chapter 3). You'll see that each recipe works with more than one kind of fish, so that you can be flexible and select whichever safe fish is fresh and available on the particular day you shop. As I discuss in Chapter 3, wild fish is preferable to farmed fish because fish farming is a largely unregulated industry that can produce fish lower in healthy fats and higher in chemicals and additives (there are some exceptions; see page 118). For updates on the safety of wild fish stocks, I recommend you check one of my favourite online resources – www.edf.org or the Monterey Bay Aquarium's Seafood Watch (www.mbayaq.org/cr/seafoodwatch.asp), both of which list fish caught and farmed internationally. If you frequent a good fish market, you will find your local fishmonger is an excellent source of information on what is fresh and healthy in your area, though sometimes even the most responsible fishmongers can't verify where the fish they sell comes from.

When it comes to being choosy at the fish counter I would follow Julia Child's lead, as she wrote in *The Way to Cook*: 'When you buy fish, open the package just outside the checkout counter (they rarely let you sniff before you choose it) and take a very careful, unhurried whiff. If it smells fishy or chemical or not right in any way, take it immediately to the store manager, give him a whiff, and get your money back.' She also recommends placing fish on ice in the fridge (double-bagged in Ziploc freezer bags to keep water out). This is timeless advice from a master. In my recipes, culinary nutritionist Stefanie Sacks further recommends that before you cook it, you first wash your fish with lemon and salt, then rinse with water and pat dry with a paper towel. Following all of the above, you should have a non-fishy, delicious fish-eating experience.

The Power of Walking – Find Your Target

For the first couple of days I had you out taking a brisk walk, but now I'd like to get a little more scientific about exactly how brisk – and how aerobic – that walk is going to be. After many years of working with patients to get them into shape and increase their energy,

220 – Your Age = Your Maximum Heart Rate

Now to find your target heart rate, you simply go back to secondary school mathematics and calculate 70 per cent of your maximum.

(220 – Your Age) x .70 = Target Heart Rate

For example, if you are 40 years old:

220 – 40 = 180 (that's the max)
180 x .70 = 126 (that's the target)

A 40-year-old's Target Heart Rate *is 126 beats per minute. Finally, in order to know you're hitting your target, you need to monitor your pulse during exercise. You can buy a heart-rate monitor, or you can simply monitor yourself by pausing briefly to measure your pulse for 15 seconds (sorry, this requires one final maths problem).*

Target Heart Rate ÷ 4 = 32
(your 15-second Target Pulse Rate)

To find your pulse, pause your exercise, place your index and middle fingers lightly on the thumping artery in your neck or inner wrist. Don't use your thumb – it has a pulse of its own.

and after extensive reviews of the literature over the years, it's clear the best possible prescription for exercise is 90 minutes a week of movement that raises your heart rate to 70 per cent of its maximum capacity (60 per cent if you're unfit). The box on the previous page shows how you calculate your target and hit your exercise bulls-eye.

Cultivating Forgiveness

Yesterday I talked about releasing grudges from your thought processes. Try taking the next step – forgiving the person who wronged you. Not paying lip service to forgiving, but really letting go of the wrong, and forgiving the offender. It is amazing how many people in the world do things – unintentionally or purposefully – that harm others. But holding an inner resentment creates a negative energy cycle within you; it reduces your energy. Forgiving does not mean that you have to seek to spend time with the person, though you may have to spend time with him or her at work or socially. Feel compassion toward the other. The act of forgiving, either silently or openly with a direct communication, is incredibly liberating and energizing. If you have been harbouring painful feelings for many years, you may have difficulty resetting them on your own. If you have a hard time with this exercise or feel you're thinking negatively all the time, you may benefit from working with a therapist to get past this draining emotional carousel.

10-Minute Meditative Breath Work

Throughout the 21 days I am offering a variety of tips for falling asleep; what works for you will be highly individual. But one thing that is nearly universal to people who have trouble falling asleep is the inability to deal properly with stress (although sometimes it's simply that too much stress overwhelms normally adequate coping skills). To help turn off the thought processes at bedtime, try invoking the morning relaxation exercise, only take it further – try it for 10 minutes. Let your thoughts dissipate and stay focused only on your breathing or your mantra for 10 minutes. You can work on your problems tomorrow. Do this sitting up, then get into bed and try to stay focused in the same neutral mental place. Incorporating this 10-minute meditative breath work into your bedtime routine – and consciously banishing worrying thoughts – can make it much easier to drift off to sleep.

Day 6

- Power Mind: *Lounge in bed upon awakening and daydream*
  - Early Morning Wake-Up Call
  - *Potter in the Morning*
  - Get a Massage
  - *Read Your Stress Log: Identify triggers of negative emotion*
  - *Start Making an Action Plan*
- Power Food: Organic menus
  - *The Perils of Red Meat*
  - *Cooking with Spices*
- Power Exercise: Power Up! Workout
- Power of Connection: *The Communal Meal*
- Power Rest: *Power nap*
  - 8 hours' sleep
  - Practise the Sleep Tips that Work for You
  - *Sleep Cycles: What are they?*

Lounge in Bed upon Awakening and Daydream

Take time for yourself today; you've earned it. Instead of jumping out of bed (or crawling if your energy is not yet optimal), lounge and relax before getting up. Let your mind drift to pleasant thoughts or back to your dreams. Reflect back on all you accomplished in the first phase of this plan, and the fresh energy you can look forward to having as you enter the *Cleanse* phase of the plan. Society makes us too goal-oriented, so this will be a day to relax and connect with a sense of inner peace. When you get up, practise your Early Morning Wake-Up Call to allow peacefulness to fill you.

Potter in the Morning

Let there be no hurry – that's today's mantra. If you have chores, stay mindful as you go about them; don't allow yourself to feel dragged down by the weight of all that is expected of you. Know that you will get to what needs to be done.

Read Your Stress Log
Identify Triggers of Negative Emotion and Start Making an Action Plan

Up to this point I've had you focus on what causes stress during your day: home, work, relationships, tasks, past issues, anticipation of difficult times ahead … you name it. I also encouraged you to let go of some of your more destructive thoughts – to release grudges, to feel more compassionate and to be forgiving. Think about the week to come. Are there easy or practical ways to eliminate stresses? Can you adjust your schedule so you are not so pressed for time during your commute? What may give you similar – or new – stress, which you can minimize with prior planning? With whom can you make peace? How can you better generate the positive energy that you feel within, and give it out to others? Are there any coping strategies that you can adopt for next time? Perhaps you can take a breath break before you encounter a difficult co-worker to help you maintain control. Make reducing stress a priority; you'll be amazed at how much you gain.

The Perils of Red Meat

Here I am telling you to relax, and then I bring up the somewhat troubling concept of eliminating a food you may love to eat. But you need to hear this if you are like the majority of my patients who really don't understand why I want them to eliminate, or at least cut back on, eating red meat. Most people who don't have a cholesterol problem think they're fine eating meat. Cholesterol and saturated fat are particularly dangerous for people with cardiovascular disease, but they are not the only problem with red meat. Animal fat, particularly from red meat (beef, pork, lamb and veal), can cause overproduction of inflammation-promoting molecules called cytokines, which are implicated in numerous health problems including cancer, heart disease and arthritis. Some people are more susceptible than others to developing inflammation. (See Chapter 2 for more on inflammation.) In addition, conventional, non-organic meat can carry antibiotics and pesticide residues, all of which I want you to avoid. Let's see how you feel after three weeks off red meat. Some people feel so wonderful, they never go back to eating meat. Others find they crave it, or actually get energy from it, and in that case there are healthier meats you can eat (see Day 14); but after your 21 days of not eating meat, consume all meat in moderation.

Cooking with Spices

Classic Western cooking imparts flavour by incorporating salt and saturated fat (cream and butter). These two standards both hold and enhance flavours, but they are substances I am encouraging you to leave behind for three weeks – and I want you to use dramatically less of them forever. With the 21 days of menus you will replace salt and fats with spices, herbs and oils that not only impart fantastic flavour, they are some of the most powerful healing substances on the planet. Tonight you will have curry-roasted chicken for dinner. Curry contains turmeric as well as other beneficial spices. Studies have shown that turmeric works on every mechanism involved in reducing inflammation in the body; there is extensive literature about its use as a therapy for inflammatory diseases including cardiovascular disease and some cancers. How wonderful to eat your chicken with a substance that has the potential to prevent a heart attack and cancer! Rosemary, oregano, cinnamon and garlic all have copious research studies attesting to their ability to help the body detoxify, resist infection, regulate blood sugar and reduce inflammation. Leave the salt and fat behind – switch to healthy herbs and spices to energize your food, and import it with exotic new flavours that will satisfy your palate.

The Communal Meal

Today, consider hosting a meal with friends or family. There is little that is as effective for feeling connected to others as a shared meal – with people you enjoy. I'm not suggesting inviting all the folks who grate on your nerves at obligatory holiday meals. The curry-roasted chicken is a perfect, exotic dish to serve as a conversation piece. And you'll note the menu includes a non-alcoholic cocktail to kick off the meal. Invite a group you meet with regularly – surprising them by hosting an event at your place. Or do one of my favourite things – bring people together from different walks of life who will stimulate and be stimulated by each other. Rotate the places at the table throughout the meal so everyone gets to talk with everyone else. Put your positive energy into making others feel part of a greater collective energy.

Sleep Cycles: What Are They?

You should move between the two types of sleep – non-rapid eye movement and REM – about every 90 minutes throughout the night, with the first four stages being more dominant in the first half of your sleep and the fifth vivid dreaming stage being more dominant in the wee hours of the morning. Today, just keep in mind that getting 8 hours of uninterrupted sleep allows adequate time to cycle through all of the stages of sleep. For a full understanding of sleep cycles, check out Chapter 5.

Day 7

- **Power Mind: Early morning wake-up call**
  - **Take the Energy Quiz**
- **Power Food: Organic menus**
  - *Dr Merrell's Morning Shake*
  - *Indulge in a Treat: Dark chocolate*
- **Power Exercise: Take a day off**

- **Power of Connection:** *Establish your local spot to connect with nature*
- **Power Rest: Power nap**
  – 8 hours' sleep

Dr Merrell's Morning Shake

Tomorrow you will enter the *Cleanse* phase of this plan, during which you will begin each day with my breakfast shake (see recipe, page 309). This shake gives a marvellous head start on nutrition for the day. It supplies enough calories to be in line with weight maintenance: a great balance of lean protein, health-promoting fats, complex carbohydrates and fibre, and powerful healing nutrients. This shake incorporates in your breakfast many of the key Power Foods discussed in Chapter 2. It is antioxidant, anti-inflammatory, nutritious and energy-generating. This is a whole meal – you can use it for the rest of your life as breakfast, or a meal replacement, or an energy snack during the day. It is very satisfying – the good fats, protein, complex carbohydrates and fibre leave you feeling satisfied easily until lunch. (Though I recommend a mid-morning snack each of the 21 days just to prevent you from going famished into lunch.)

Indulge in a Treat: Dark Chocolate

Quick quiz: What is one of nature's most powerful antioxidant foods – four times more powerful than green tea? It's chocolate, scientific name *theobroma coca* (theobroma translated literally means food of the gods). It has many health-giving nutrients, powerful antioxidants and chemicals (including phenylethanolamine) that actually improve mood. Recent studies show it lowers blood pressure, and I'm sure more good news is to come. So why is there any controversy about it? Because the chocolate most of us grew up on – and which is still the most widely consumed – is mainly sugar, often with dairy added. Studies that show chocolate's benefits were done on chocolate with at least 80 per cent cocoa mass and very little sugar. Regular commercial chocolate is closer to 10 per cent cocoa, with most milk chocolate at between 10 and 15 per cent. Even many traditional darker chocolates max out at 30 per cent cocoa. The caveat here: for chocolate to work best for health and energy, it needs to be at least 75 per cent cocoa, though I'll settle for 70 per cent. If not, the rest is mostly sugar and dairy products. People accustomed to high sugar and dairy chocolate may gag on 80 per cent-plus. I must say, 90 per cent and over is too bitter even for me, a cocoa lover. But the sweet spot should be 75 to 85 per cent. In this zone, the bitterness of pure cocoa has been softened with some sugar and cocoa butter, and the natural flavonoids that are so healthy are still abundant. You don't need to eat the whole bar: a few squares should do it. A good organic bar is probably your best bet; try Green & Blacks's, which uses the finest ingredients and a wallop of pure cocoa. Go ahead: indulge and enjoy in moderation one of nature's great energy foods.

Establish Your Local Spot to Connect with Nature

Today I want you to take the time to get out into nature. Remembering you are part of something beautiful and much larger than yourself and experiencing awe at that beauty are an essential part of connectivity and of tapping the energy of the universe. While it would be wonderful if you could take a walk in the cathedral of a redwood forest or along the edge of the Grand Canyon or the White Cliffs of Dover, today's exercise can be something as simple as sitting under your favourite tree and truly feeling the energy and wisdom of the tree that's been around for a long time ... perhaps longer than any human. Think of the tree's connectedness to all living things, many of which have come before you. Even inanimate objects like beautiful rock outcroppings can be equally inspiring. My daughters and I like to skip rocks at a local beach. This is a very mindful time when we're just present with each other and with nature. Wherever it is you love to spend time in nature, make it a regular habit.

Power Nap

I am definitely a fan of short naps, and suggest taking them at least once a week during the 21-Day Plan. The ideal nap is 15 to 20 minutes long, which allows just enough time to catch the first two stages of non-rapid eye movement sleep that leave you feeling refreshed and, studies show, better able to perform tasks that require thinking and memory. A nap that lasts from 20 minutes to an hour may be too long; it's very likely to leave you feeling groggy as it takes you to a deeper stage without completing a full cycle. While a 90-minute daytime nap will probably take you through an entire sleep cycle and give you energy, it is likely to throw off your body clock and make it harder to fall asleep at bedtime. Take a 20-minute power nap today, then get up and do a two-minute energy boost. You'll feel like a new person.

WEEK TWO: CLEANSE

'Matter in its subtlest form is prana, a vital energy which is inseparable from consciousness.'

HIS HOLINESS THE DALAI LAMA, from *The Universe in a Single Atom*

Day 8

- Power Mind: Early morning wake-up call
  - Daytime: Breath breaks
  - Two-Minute Energy Boost
  - *Book a Massage for Today*
  - *Evening Laugh Log*
- Power Food: Organic menus
  - *Essential Nutrients: Probiotics*
- Power Detox: *Foods that detox*
- Power Exercise: Power Up! Workout
  - *Investigate Local Yoga Classes*
- Power Rest: Asleep by 11pm
  - *Sleep Tip: Squeezing lemons*
  - *Evaluate your Mattress and Pillow*

Book a Massage

I've told you why I want you to have a massage, but the question is, where to get one? As is the case with all healthcare practitioners, word of mouth trumps almost all other recommendations. If you don't know where to go, local spas are usually a good bet. Some gyms have good masseurs or masseuses, but spas, which usually cater to a different crowd, are often able to attract more experienced masseurs. Many masseuses with private massage practices or who make home visits are more experienced – they have enough referrals to support a private practice. On the other hand, private masseuses are more likely to have developed their own eclectic style, so make sure to find out exactly what the massage technique is before booking. Local massage schools can give referrals to less expensive massages from students or recent graduates.

Evening Laugh Log

Last week I had you keep track of things that added stress to your life, and some things you could do to lessen the burdens. This week, I want you to keep track of those things that make you feel good. I call it a laugh log – but the log is not limited to things you find hilarious. Note what makes you smile, feel warm-hearted, fulfilled and hopeful. Accentuate the positives in your life – in preparation for cultivating them more each day.

Essential Nutrients: Probiotics

I've asked you to add probiotic (helpful bacteria) powder to your shake every morning as part of the cleanse in order to repair and restore your gut, which also strengthens your immune system. There is no supplement class as powerful as probiotics to help digestive function, which is the foundation of a healthy internal detox system (see Chapter 3). In fact, I think of probiotics (including acidophilus and bifidophilus) as the Mr Fix-Its of digestive health. When the many different types of bacteria get out of balance, however, they can throw your digestion and immune system out of whack. Recent research even suggests that obesity is partly due to improper bacterial colonization of the gut – a person can have too much of certain types of bacteria that extract calories from food! You will improve your health and energy when you set your gut on the right track with probiotics.

It's good if you regularly eat yogurt, which is milk fermented with acidophilus. But you'd have to eat about 10 yogurts to get the amount of probiotics contained in a good supplement. Try to find a higher potency (one billion or greater organisms per capsule) in a refrigerated liquid form or powder concentrate. (There is evidence that the 'GG' or 'VSL' strains are most effective.) Use quality freeze-dried capsules when you travel. Unlike some of our natural intestinal bacteria, probiotics do not colonize (set up house and multiply) in the intestines – they are mostly eliminated within five days after you ingest them – so to maintain their presence you have to consume probiotics regularly. Buy the powder or liquid, put it in your shake, and let Mr Fix-It take care of things.

Investigate Local Yoga Classes

The key to starting a yoga practice is going slow and finding a small class. Such classes are tough to find today with so many people getting into yoga, and getting competitive about it! Before you put yourself in someone's hands, check out his or her credentials. Your best bet is to go to a well-known, long-standing yoga studio, preferably one that employs instructors with certification from recognized schools (such as Iyengar, Integral, Sivananda, Kripalu, the British Yoga Teachers' Association or the International Yoga Therapy Association). Working one on one with an instructor produces dramatically better results than group work, but many people choose the more economical option of classes where the group dynamics can also help provide a real energy lift. In my experience, classes tend to move quickly, but beginners need to go slowly. Hurrying through postures you're just learning can render them useless and also cause injury. If you can't procure a private session, invest in a video series from a top yogi such as beginner DVDs from Jivamukti or Shiva Rea. For most people learning yoga is extremely visual, so the ideal would be to slowly go through a beginner video with a mirror close at hand to match your movements to those of the yogis on the video. For more on getting started with a yoga practice, see Chapter 4.

Sleep Tip: Squeezing Lemons

This short form of muscle relaxation utilizes the image of squeezing lemons. As you lie in bed, pick up two imaginary lemons, hold them straight out in front of you, making a fist. Inhale deeply as you squeeze as hard as you can until all of the 'juice' is out of the lemons. Now toss them away as you exhale completely and let your hands go limp. Try this three times.

Evaluate your Mattress and Pillow

Is your pillow making you tired? A pillow is supposed to support your head so that your neck, airways and spine remain in a natural position with good alignment throughout the night. Bottom line: a pillow should support your head and take pressure off your neck.

Pillows frequently contribute to allergies, which prevent a good night's sleep. If you are chronically congested, try a hypoallergenic foam pillow and place it inside a dust-mite blocking pillow protector that goes under the pillow case (www.greenguide.com and www.allergyuk.org are both great resources for information on pillow allergies). (Mattress quality is also critical for proper sleep: for details on this, refer to Chapter 5.)

Day 9

- **Power Mind: Early morning wake-up call**
  - **Two-Minute Energy Break**

- Breath Breaks
- Evening: Laugh log
- Power Food: Organic menus
  - *Preparing for the Juice Cleanse*
- Power Exercise: Power Up! Workout
  - *Heart Monitor vs Pedometer*
- Power of Connection
  - *Contemplative Time*
- Power Rest: Asleep by 11pm
  - *Light and Your Sleep Hormones*

Preparing for the Juice Cleanse

One of the most powerful tools I have to help jump-start my patients' health is a juice cleanse. Tomorrow, it's your turn; you will ingest only fresh vegetable and fruit juices every three to four hours, maintaining your nutrient and calorie intake while giving your digestive tract and natural detox system a rest (see Chapter 3 for more on this). In order to prepare for the cleanse, please read the juice recipes in the recipe section and collect all of the ingredients today. It's essential that you drink fresh juice that you make yourself at home or that is made for you, to your specifications, at a reliable restaurant or healthfood shop. Fresh juice lasts for up to three to four hours before enzymes begin to degrade, so you can only make or buy what you will consume within that period of time. If you are going to purchase a juicer, look for one that includes the fruit or vegetable fibre in the juice. At lunch and dinner you can have a cup of shiitake-miso broth (leftover from tonight's soup). On the cleanse day *especially* you should not drink caffeine or alcohol. A note on store-bought bottled juices: they can be used as a stop-gap when you can't get fresh juice. Make sure to buy organic. Also make sure there is less than 100mg of sodium per serving: many conventional vegetable juices contain high levels of sodium. (For more on the health benefits of the cleanse, please see Chapter 3.) The other essential element of tomorrow's cleanse is drinking plenty of fresh water.

Heart Monitor vs Pedometer

Several years ago the American Heart Association announced that taking 10,000 steps a day reduces the risk of heart disease, which caused a mini-bubble in the market for pedometers that count your steps. This guidance was immediately echoed by the British Heart Foundation. But if you want to more effectively increase your energy you have to take a *brisk* walk that raises your heart rate to 70 per cent of its maximum capacity, which makes a heart rate monitor the key gadget to employ. A heart rate monitor takes your pulse with a sensor strapped around your chest and transmits the data to a digital read-out on a special wristwatch so that you can make sure your heart rate increases gradually to 60 or 70 per cent of its maximum for your age. Keep your heart revved for a total of 90 minutes a week and your energy will also rise.

Light and Your Sleep Hormones

Light has a significant effect on your sleep. The primary sleep hormone, melatonin, is produced in darkness, with the peak time being the early hours of the morning. Keep your room very dark when you sleep. Darken your bedroom at night, and throw open the curtains and start moving outside in the morning. (For more on light therapy and sleep hormones, see Chapter 5.)

Day 10

- **Power Mind: Early morning wake-up call**
  - Two-Minute Breath Work
  - Evening: Laugh log
- **Power Food: Organic menus**
  - Juice Cleanse (see menus and recipes)
- **Power Exercise: Gentle yoga or 20-minute walk or both**
- **Power Rest: 8 hours' sleep**

The Juice Cleanse

This is an exciting day, one you've been preparing for. A juice cleanse is one of the most effective means to repair and rejuvenate; it protects your DNA and improves your ability to create energy. The Juice Cleanse is laid out in detail in Part III, Menus and Recipes. It's critically important that you carefully follow the menu for the day and drink all of the liquids as recommended so that you can maximally repair and restore. The key to this cleanse is that it provides essential nutrients to support your body's detox abilities, and drinking copious amounts of water helps flush out toxins as well as prevent dehydration.

I want you to consider this a tranquil day. Gentle yoga or a 20-minute walk is fine, but no exertion. Continue your breath breaks. This sort of cleanse is known to help cultivate mindfulness. With less energy spent on digestion, you are likely to feel more alert throughout the day. Have a quiet evening and take time to reflect on the positives in your life. Finishing with a good 8 hours' sleep is essential.

Day 11

- Power Mind: Early morning wake-up call
  - Daytime: Two-minute energy break
  - Breath Breaks
  - Evening: Laugh log
- Power Food: Organic menus
- Power Detox: *Foods that detox*
- Power Exercise: Power walk 30 minutes
- Power of Connection: Positive emotional action
  - *Get Inspired! Buy Tickets to an Upcoming Show or Event*
- Power Rest: Asleep by 11pm

Foods That Detox

In this phase of the plan, you focus on cleaning out your body in order to free up energy. Many of the foods you will eat this week and throughout the plan help boost your body's detox capacity. Here is a quick list of some of the best foods to help your body detoxify; for more complete information about these foods' amazing properties, see Chapter 3.

- **The brassica family (cruciferous vegetables): broccoli, cauliflower, kale and Brussels sprouts**
- **The allium family (sulphurous vegetables): onions, leeks, chives, garlic and shallots**
- **The thistle family: artichokes, dandelions and burdock**
- **Green tea**
- **Nuts and seeds**
- **Seaweed: arame, hijiki, kombu and wakame**
- **Spices: turmeric and ginger**
- **Red berries**

Walking Clubs

If you find it difficult to take up walking on your own, try to do it with a friend. Equally satisfying is finding a walking club in your local area and doing it with a group. The sense of community that comes from this shared desire to be healthier can be wonderful. For details of local walking clubs, visit www.walking-uk.com; both short- and long-distance walking and rambling clubs are listed by county. The British Walking Federation (www.bwf-ivv.org.uk) also provides information about local walking clubs and events. The WHI (www.whi.org.uk) is a joint initiative of the British Heart Foundation and Natural England, and is focused on promoting 'health walks' as a means of improving fitness.

Get Inspired! Buy Tickets to an Upcoming Show or Event
The power of art and entertainment can sweep you out of your everyday rut. Today, plan to treat yourself to an uplifting event. If you're like me, you will have been looking at the newspapers saying: I wish I could see this or go to that. Take yourself up on that challenge. A musical, concert or play not only transports you away from daily concerns, it also plugs you into the energy of others. Try to maintain the good feelings generated during the event.

Day 12

- **Power Mind: Early morning wake-up call**
  - **Daytime: Two-minute breath work**
  - **Evening: Laugh log**
- **Power Food: Organic menus**
  - *Healthy Fats*
- **Power Exercise: Power Up! Workout**
- *Power of the Playground*
- **Power of Connection:** *Say You're Sorry*
- **Power Rest: 8 hours'sleep**
  - *Have a TV-free Night*

Healthy Fats

If you've been following the menus – and I sincerely hope that you have – then you know I am not the sort of doctor who is completely against having fat in your diet. The 21-Day food plan has a healthy balance of monounsaturated and omega-3 fats from olive oil; nuts, seeds and nut butters; avocados and fish. The key is that my menus have no transfats and almost no saturated fat from animal foods. Shifting from saturated to healthy fats changes the way your body responds to inflammation: producing anti-inflammatory rather than pro-inflammatory immune messengers. Your body also needs sufficient healthy plant and fish oil fats to dissolve the fat-soluble vitamins. Your body also utilizes essential fatty acids from healthy oils to build beautiful cell walls that have integrity and can protect your DNA and the many other structures, including the energy-generating mitochondria, that reside inside every one of your cells. A moderate amount of fat in the diet promotes satiety; you may have noticed that, as public health policy shifted toward non-fat foods, our waist-bands have expanded. You will also find your skin is more supple with eating healthy fats. Bottom line: you will have more energy and, yes, feel and look younger, as you replace bad fats with good.

Power of the Playground

OK, kids, weather's great, it's time to get out and play. After 12 days on the plan you should begin to feel the urge to get outside and move after you've been cooped up inside all day. This is part of the process of re-energizing your body. Today, as you get ready to work out I want you to try to remember the days of your youth when you couldn't wait to get out and run around. When you go outside, embrace the day, breathe deeply as you warm up and feel your body coming alive. You might even hop on your bike today instead of walking, or grab a skipping rope and try to get all the way through 'Teddy Bear, Teddy Bear'. Reflect on the joy of going out to play, and then have a go at it!

Say You're Sorry

I've talked about the energetic lift of letting go of grudges and forgiv-ing others. Today, I want to turn that 180 degrees and have *you* ask someone for forgiveness. This is hard. Asking for forgiveness means swallowing your pride and saying you're sorry; it means admitting you were wrong and that you've hurt someone else. You cannot be sure of the reaction that your apology will bring, but you will have to let go of expectations. If you feel it's appropriate, ask this person what you can do to make it right – or just express that the apology comes from your heart. It is the energy you project that will sig-nificantly affect the result. Think about it carefully and rehearse the script if necessary. In my experience, saying, 'I'm sorry if I hurt you' is less effective than saying, 'I'm sorry for what I did'. This exercise will help reduce a lot of stress-filled negative emotional energy in your life. It will not necessarily bring back a relationship. But it is part of moving on and cleaning up your emotional baggage. Even if the object of your apology doesn't express open appreciation and forgiveness, your act of giving of yourself will cause a positive energetic shift that will reverberate for quite some time.

Have a TV-free Night

Breaking a bad habit can be incredibly energizing. Nighttime television watching is a habit that's been clearly linked in studies to getting less sleep. Tonight, turn off the TV, and pursue other, more relaxing activities. Take a walk after dinner, listen to your favourite CDs (remember the days when you could just sit and go through the sleeve notes?), read a book, meditate, take a long hot bath. Get out of your habitual, evening couch-potato mode, and you will find that you have better sleep and perhaps even more interesting dreams.

Day 13

- **Power Mind: Lounge in bed**
  - Early Morning Wake-Up Call
  - Potter in the Morning
  - *Review What Made You Laugh This Week*
- **Power Food: Organic menus**
  - *Big 12 Trouble-Makers*
- **Power Detox:** *Supplements for detox*
- **Power Exercise:** *40 minutes of movement*
- **Power of Connection: Concert or event**
- **Power Rest: 8 hours' sleep or asleep by 11pm**
  - *Sleep Tips: Apnoea, snoring and other impediments*

Review what made you laugh this week

Last week you kept your stress log, and at the end of the week, reviewed it for patterns. I'd like you to review it again this week, but with the goal of getting more of the joy and laughter into your life. My feeling is that as you fill your life with more joy, you'll have less room for stress. When you keep track, you may see that things aren't as bad as they seem. As you're relaxing and pottering about today take the time to reflect on what you love about your life.

The Big 12 Trouble-Makers

As you get ready for your final week of the plan and begin to think of life after the plan, I want you to consider your relationship to the 12 most highly reactive foods. Ask yourself, 'Might I have a food sensitivity or allergy?' Over the past 13 days, if you've been following the plan, you haven't had most of these foods. Do you feel better? As you add them back, do you notice any reaction? If you think you may have a food allergy, a trip to an allergy specialist for testing can be well worth the time and effort. Identifying chronic energy-draining food sensitivities and allergies – and eliminating those foods for good – is one of the easiest ways to increase energy. (For more on allergies, see Chapter 2.)

- Wheat
- Milk
- Corn
- Sugar
- Soya
- Peanuts
- Coffee
- Alcohol
- Yeast (fermented) foods
- Citrus fruit
- Shellfish
- Eggs

Supplements for Detox

You are at the end of a week of cleansing your system. You should be feeling more energetic at this point, but if you're still not as full of vigour as you want to be, it may be you have a history of being exposed to many toxins. Maybe you were a smoker once, or ate a diet loaded with preservatives or poor-quality meats and produce. Maybe you worked in a factory, or in a 'sick building'. Take a look at the supplements for increasing your detox capacity in Chapter 3.

40 Minutes of Movement

OK, I know I've been telling you that 30 minutes of exercise is sufficient, and it is. But I don't want you to think that's the maximum amount. On the weekend, when you have more time, consider adding more exercise to your routine. Adding more movement to your day (gentle movement so that you're not sore on Monday like a weekend warrior) is one of the most energizing, life-affirming things you can do with your time.

Apnoea, Snoring and Other Impediments to Sleep

Nothing interferes with restorative sleep more than an abnormal breathing pattern – caused by apnoea, heavy snoring, or even chronic sinus congestion – that reduces the oxygen supply to your bloodstream and to the rest of your body. What used to be considered just plain old snoring has been increasingly identified by researchers as a cause of significant health problems. For example, sleep apnoea (when breathing is frequently obstructed for at least 10 seconds throughout the night) has been associated with numerous health problems including hypertension (high blood pressure), heart disease and heart attack. And only recently chronic sinus has been recognized congestion as a factor in poor sleep. Amazingly, Breathe Right Nasal Strips that hold your nostrils open to allow in more air can be a quick fix for minor problems. In Chapter 5, I cover a number of possible solutions to sleep-breathing problems. Furthermore, if you or your spouse or partner suspects you might have altered breathing or severe snoring (and if you constantly wake up exhausted), self-help measures may not be enough: please make an appointment with your doctor to get a referral to a sleep specialist.

Day 14

- **Power Mind: Early morning wake-up call and Congratulate yourself!**
  - Take the Energy Quiz
  - *Get Ready to Maximize*
- **Power Food: Organic menus**
  - *Life After the Plan: Healthier meats*
- **Power Exercise: Take a day off**
- **Power of Connection: An e-mail-free day and Write a letter to someone who's always on your mind**
- **Power Rest: 8 hours' sleep**
  - *Bedroom Feng Shui*

Get Ready to Maximize

By now you should have made major changes to your energy on many fronts. Congratulations for staying with the plan! You are about to move into Week Three when the changes will be consolidated and made part of your ongoing lifestyle. Remember there's absolutely no reason that you can't increase your energy throughout your life. Whether you continue to find more vitality and energy through a more varied and plant-based diet, more regular exercise, a cleaner environment and more restorative sleep – or by extending your connections with others or deepening your spiritual or contemplative practice ... never say never!

Life after the Plan: Healthier Meats

I have had you eliminating red meat during the plan, and limiting poultry. You will most likely feel better energy as a result. If you have no medical conditions that warrant avoiding meat (heart disease, history of colon cancer or autoimmune disorders) and want to resume meat consumption after the plan, limit how often you do so and consider healthier options. Commercially raised red meats and poultry have much higher saturated fat content than wild animals and game. Instead of commercial meat, try venison or rabbit, which have about the same saturated fat as chicken – much less than beef. The lowest fat in a land animal is ostrich, which may sound weird, but there are commercial ostrich farms and many butchers now carry ostrich meat (which tastes like a cross between chicken and veal, and can be used in chicken and beef recipes). Also consider wild poultry – heritage species, or birds such as quail, pheasant and partridge, which have less fat than chicken. At the very least, try to find organic (or natural and chemical-free), free-range meats that will contain minimal additives and chemicals.

How you cook your meat and what you eat it with also makes a difference to how healthy it is. Charred meat is high in carcinogens called heterocyclic amines. Brown your meat as you cook it through; don't burn it. Research published in the journal *Carcinogenesis* demonstrated that eating broccoli along with meat increases the liver enzyme system's removal of heterocyclic amines. Further, eating a diet rich in essential fatty acids (from olive oil, nuts and fish) counteracts the build-up of cholesterol from saturated fat. In one study conducted by nutrition scientists in Spain, volunteers who ate a mixture of minced beef and ground walnuts had more antioxidants in their bloodstreams that helped to counteract the harmful inflammatory effects of red meats. Next time you make a burger, mix it with some ground walnuts, don't burn the meat and have a large helping of broccoli on the side. But you'll be even healthier if you eat a veggie burger.

An E-Mail-Free Day and Write a Letter to Someone Who's Always on Your Mind

As you know by now I'm a true believer in reaching out to the energy of others, and making amends with those who have left negative energetic footprints in your life. Along with that comes the need for reflection on how you are communicating with people on a daily basis. I am a fan of e-mail as a work tool, and as a way of keeping in touch with far-flung relatives, but I find that it gets in the way of maintaining real connections with the people in your daily life and even interferes with the need to make deeper connections with your inner life. Today, leave the e-mail alone. Sit down and revisit the art of letter writing. You might even want to get some new stationery to energize your writing further.

Bedroom Feng Shui

Feng shui is a Chinese art of aligning energy within a space to create harmony and health. The physical placement of objects is important, as is colour, the orientation of objects and the relation of the space to nature. Naturally, in the bedroom the goal is to create a harmonious, calm, peaceful and healthy environment. The placement of your bed is of the utmost importance; feng shui principles in general require the head of the bed to be against a solid wall with no windows, your head should not be in line with the exit door, nor should you be able to see yourself in a mirror from the bed. Equally important is minimizing clutter in the bedroom – absolutely no piles of books or papers collecting dust. Your belongings, from the contents of your pockets to your shoes and ties to your magazines and perfume bottles, are best kept behind doors in the bedroom to keep the energy flowing and not caught up in a bunch of material objects. Matching bedside tables are thought to promote harmony for couples. And it's considered a good idea to have a comfortable, relaxing chair in the bedroom (placed so the back does not face the door) to promote the tranquil feelings you want to engender at bedtime. Feng shui is as much science as art. I'm certainly no feng shui expert, but I have seen remarkable transformations in people's lives as a result of working with feng shui practitioners. If you're interested in pursuing the topic further, you can consult good books on feng shui or a feng shui school that can provide references to practitioners. The Feng Shui Society (www.fengshuisociety.org.uk) is a good web resource that lists consultants and teachers in the UK, and Feng Shui Tips (www. fengshuitips.co.uk) provides lots of helpful ideas to transform your home or office.

WEEK THREE: MAXIMIZE

'If you miss the present moment, you miss your appointment with life.'
THICH NHAT HANH, from *The Art of Power*

Day 15

- Power Mind: Early morning wake-up call
  - *Start Planning Your Holiday*
  - *10-Minute Evening Unwind*
- Power Food: Organic menus
  - *Essential Fatty Acids*
- Power Exercise: Power Up! Workout
- Power Rest: Asleep by 11pm
  - *Life After the Plan: Consistency is key for restorative rest*

Start Planning Your Holiday

Over the years I have become emphatic about people taking holidays. I don't mean extravagant breaks that cost an arm and a leg. I mean getting away from your everyday existence, preferably communing with nature and taking the time to unwind. I recently came across a sad study that found that fewer Brits are taking holidays for fear of reprisals at their jobs. One study found that 72 per cent of British workers don't use their full holiday entitlement, and 7 per cent *never* take a holiday. I cannot imagine a worse scenario for creating stress than one in which you can't take time off from work for fear of losing your job. Everyone needs time off at least twice a year (Christmas and New Year don't count because those can actually be stressful or exhausting holidays). Ideally one of these should be for two weeks. The real holiday, when you begin to feel unplugged and recharged, usually starts in the second week. Start planning now, and keep in mind that a good break leaves you energized, not needing a holiday from the holiday!

10-Minute Evening Unwind

During the first two weeks of the plan, I had you keep stress and laugh logs, the purpose of which was to review your day in the context of your coping skills. Rather than worrying about how your day went, you identified the important emotional moments from your day, then took a step back and reviewed how you managed to cope with them. Then you put any ruminations on your day behind you. If keeping a log particularly resonated with you, please continue to keep it up for 10 minutes in the evening. If writing is not your thing, I'd like you to set aside 10 minutes a day to mentally review and detach from the events of your day. I call this the 10-Minute Unwind – the key is to keep the events of the day in the context of your coping skills. If you could have done better, make a note of that and work out how to get it right the next time. If you had a wonderfully joyous moment, lock that into the treasury and feed off it when the going gets rough. Then let it go, and move onto the tranquillity of your evening routine.

Essential Fatty Acids

I've talked about the healthy plant and fish fats you're eating in the menu plan, but I want to zero in briefly on the important component of those fats, essential fatty acids (EFAs). Your body can't make EFAs – they have to come from the diet, and most people don't get enough. When your diet is low in EFAs (as is the average Western diet), your body's ability to fight hundreds of energy-draining inflammatory processes is reduced. You need some source of EFAs every day. If after the 21-Day Plan you find yourself slipping back into old eating habits, take an omega-3 supplement.

Life After the Plan: Consistency is Key to Restorative Rest

If I can have you remember one tip on maximizing your sleep, it would be for you to go to bed at approximately the same time every night. Maintaining a consistent bedtime and bedtime routine has been shown to be a crucial part of maintaining healthy sleep cycles.

Day 16

- **Power Mind: Early morning wake-up call**
  - Two-Minute Energy Boost
  - 10-Minute Evening Unwind
- **Power Food: Organic menus**
  - *What's the Best Multivitamin?*
- **Power Exercise: Power walk 30 minutes**
- **Power of Connection:** *Investigate energy practitioners in your area*
- **Power Rest: 8 hours' sleep**
  - *Gentle Sleep Aids*

What's the Best Multivitamin?

By following the 21-Day Menu Plan with its highly diverse foods and wealth of nutrients, most people won't need a multivitamin. When you eat a rainbow diet, packed with vegetables, fruit and lean protein, food alone does have all the nutrients you need. But eating a well-rounded diet is most people's Achilles heel, so, during times of high stress or travel, when eating becomes erratic, or if you have a medical condition, you may need to take a daily multivitamin. In that case, look for a food-based (as opposed to synthetic) multivitamin, which will come as close as scientifically possible to mimicking the nutrient value of food, which has numerous beneficial compounds we have yet to even identify. Vitamin E is a good example. Most supplements only contain one form of E, alpha tocopherol. But in nature (for example, in wheat germ) – and in more sophisticated multivitamins – the whole family of vitamin E is used, including alpha and gamma tocopherols and tocotrieniols. Vitamin C is another good example. A good multivitamin should include the bioflavonoids that always accompany vitamin C in nature. Same for the A vitamins, the carotenoids; beta carotene should come with its whole family (including lycopene, lutein and zeaxanthin). For a more complete discussion of multi-vitamins, see Chapter 2.

Gentle Sleep Aids

If you now have a better diet, increased exercise, you've curtailed alcohol and coffee, and are practising relaxation exercises, but you are still having trouble falling asleep or staying asleep, there are some gentle sleep aids you can take at bedtime. I reviewed these in detail in Chapter 5, but please reserve these for use on an occasional basis. Using them chronically means you may need to do more work with your sleep habits or seek the help of a sleep specialist to solve your sleep problems.

Investigate Energy Practitioners in Your Area

I can't imagine a more appropriate topic for the week of maximizing energy than locating and having a session with an energy practitioner trained in the art of working with energy fields. I say art because Reiki, therapeutic touch, healing touch, energy healing, Johrei or any of the dozens of other energy medicine practices are not fully – or even partially – understood by science. However, a number of excellent nursing journals have demonstrated very positive results with energy healing, particularly with the use of Reiki and therapeutic touch in healthcare settings. Finding a good practitioner requires some perseverance and luck. The interaction is highly personal, and each practitioner brings his or her own background, energy and training to the experience. Some specific courses confer a certificate; Reiki, for instance, offers standardized mastery levels from 1 through 5. There is no regulatory body for these practices (although there is a voluntary self-regulation group set up for each discipline under the auspices of the General Regulatory Council for Complementary Therapies), however, so finding the right person to work with you and your energy is usually best done by getting a referral from someone you trust who has had a positive experience. I have witnessed some remarkable results with my patients so I know it's worth giving it a try. For more detail on energy medicine, see Chapter 6.

Day 17

- **Power Mind: Early morning wake-up call**
  - Five-Minute Breath Work
  - Book a Massage for Day 20
  - 10-Minute Evening Unwind
- **Power Food: Organic menus**
  - *Do You Need an Energy Supplement?*
- **Power Exercise: Power Up! Workout**
  - *Maximizing the Routine: Innovative movement*
- **Power of Connection:** *Random acts of kindness*
- **Power Rest: Asleep by 11pm**

Do You Need an Energy Supplement?

If you feel your energy is still substandard, now may be the time to try supplements that have been used to help increase energy, mood and vitality. These are described in detail in Chapter 2 and include Russian rhodiola, Ayurvedic ashwaganda, Chinese cordyceps and Chinese and American ginseng. Specific energy-supporting and energy-generating vitamins, minerals and other nutrients can also be helpful. There is an abundance of energy formulas for sale from supplement manufacturers, but you should exercise extreme caution, as some of these formulas can have unpredictable effects and side-effects. Choosing the right supplement is very important. This almost always requires the input of a knowledgeable medical professional working with you, especially if you have medical problems or are taking medication.

Maximizing the Routine: Innovative Movement

At this point in the plan you are advancing your fitness level to a point where you can begin to branch out. I highly recommend exploring the world of martial arts (such as tai chi, karate and aikido) and martial arts hybrids (like tae bo, jujitsu or capoeira) – exercise systems designed to work specifically with your energy. Start with a local martial arts school. Many gyms, particularly in urban settings, are beginning to offer classes that are strictly martial arts or that incorporate aspects of martial arts. Make sure to ask if beginners are welcome.

Random Acts of Kindness

One of the most powerful ways you can generate energy is to give of yourself to others. From random acts of kindness to working with a community group, by giving to others you connect with a larger energy source that enhances your own. As discussed in Chapter 6, community service and helping others is one of the most rewarding, energy-producing activities you can do, and it's been shown to reduce depression. You receive back many-fold times more energy than you give when you give selflessly, out of love and compassion for humankind – both giver and recipient are enveloped in a more healing energy environment. Today, do something that helps. I'm not asking you to sign on for hundreds of hours of obligations to a charitable organization if you don't have the time or inclination. Try some random acts of kindness. All too often ambitious intentions fall by the wayside, but it's the little things – like brightening someone else's day with a positive comment – that most frequently add up to big changes.

Day 18

- **Power Mind: Early morning wake-up call**
  - **– Breath breaks**
  - **– 10-Minute Evening Unwind**
- **Power Food: Organic menus**
  - **– *A Note on Bitters***
- **Power Detox: *Antioxidants – to have or have not***
- **Power Exercise: Power walk 30 minutes**
- **Power Rest: 8 hours' sleep**

A Note on Bitters

Quaffing a teaspoon of bitters is a great way to assist digestion occasionally and stop the energy drain of slow or poor digestion. Made from bitter herbs such as gentian and thistle, many digestive bitters were originally manufactured as patent medicines. All bitters – whether alcohol-based Angostura, alcohol-free Swedish Bitters, or bitter aperitifs (Campari, Cinzano and Fernet Branca) – stimulate the flow of all of your body's natural digestive chemicals. Only a teaspoonful is needed, and only on occasion. (Enzymes sold in health-food shops as digestive aids can work sometimes, but then only supply one part of the digestive picture, the pancreas's enzymes.)

Antioxidants – To Have or Have Not

The majority of people who come to me taking more than one vitamin supplement per day use some form of antioxidant. For most, the old-fashioned vitamins E-C-beta carotene has given way to newer antioxidant tablets containing more exotic ingredients such as quercetin, pycnogenol, grapeseed and resveratrol. Do you need these? Rarely. With the menus in the 21-Day Plan, you are eating many foods that are anti-inflammatory and antioxidant. And your lifestyle these three weeks produces dramatically fewer free radicals in the first place. Food can be your medicine here. Fruits, vegetables, herbs and spices should be doing most of the work for you, so that you don't need supplements. Tablet forms should be reserved for the handful of people whose lifestyle and health risk factors predispose them to heavier free radical burdens (such as heart disease, chronic arthritis, inflammatory bowel disease and recent smokers). In these instances, taking a tablet may be useful: the caveat is that you should take one that has ingredients containing as much of the whole food as possible, rather than only one extracted molecule from a food. This is best done in consultation with a knowledgeable integrative medical professional, such as a dietitian or nutritionist, or another experienced practitioner.

Day 19

- **Power Mind: Early morning wake-up call**
  - *Mindfulness Meditation*
  - **Breath breaks**
  - **10-Minute Unwind**
- **Power Food: Organic menus**
  - *Other Supplement Options*
- **Power Detox: *How green is your grass?***
- **Power Exercise: Power Up! Workout or class**
- **Power Rest: 8 hours' sleep**

Mindfulness Meditation

I want you to begin to cultivate what the great healer/philosophers Jon Kabat-Zinn and Thich Nhat Hanh teach us – be mindful all day. In his book *True Love*, Nhat Hanh explains mindfulness as: 'Mindfulness is like a light, enabling concentration to really be there, and that also makes it possible for us to look deeply into the heart of things.' Mindfulness is the opposite of multi-tasking. It's about being in the moment – not thinking of 20 other things you want to do – especially the things that worry you most; and in that moment absolutely feeling love and compassion towards yourself, the task you are engaged in, or the person you are with. Whether you are washing dishes, driving the car, practising breath breaks or sitting in a meeting, be mindful.

Mindfulness meditation is rather like filling your cup of consciousness with positive energy. Again, I like Thich Nhat Hanh's explanation in *True Love*: 'Our immediate awareness is something like our living room. The task of the meditator is not to chase away or suppress the energy of anger that is there but rather to invite another energy that will be able to care for the anger.' It's quite extraordinary that it's possible to effect such a transformation with your thoughts.

I recommend you explore the books and tapes published by Kabat-Zinn and Thich Nhat Hanh. For today, you can try one of the mindfulness meditations in Chapter 1. Or, as you do your breath work today, try the following healing meditation from Thich Nhat Hanh, *The Energy of Prayer*:

> *Breathing in, I see myself as a five-year-old child.*
> *Breathing out, I smile to the five-year-old child.*
> *Breathing in, I see the five-year-old child, who is myself, as very*
> *fragile and vulnerable.*
> *Breathing out, I smile to the five-year-old child in myself, with*
> *understanding and compassion.*

There are infinite varieties of mindfulness meditations you can use to transform your energy. Try a few. Occasionally, I encounter patients who simply can't get the hang of it on their own, but there are excellent meditation teachers and coaches who can help. Your stress will be reduced, you will make more meaningful connections with those around you, and you will feel an energy surge as you begin to banish the many negative thoughts that interfere all day in coping with life's challenges.

How Green Is Your Grass?

Yes, I'm talking about your lawn. The suburbs may be blanketed with grass as green as the hills of Ireland, but they are also awash with chemicals that achieve the green. Over 5400 tonnes of herbicides and pesticides are applied around UK residences each year. Over 175 pesticide products, containing over 14 active ingredients, are specifically produced to control lawn problems in the UK. Most of us know to stay off the lawn after a treatment until the grass has had a good soaking. But few people think to have their well water checked for the presence of chemicals like atrazine, a weed-killer that has now been banned on non-cropped land, but still appears in products for home and garden use. In the UK atrazine is the pesticide most frequently found contaminating groundwater. Think about the chemicals you're putting on your grass. Investigate integrative pest management lawn services that use organic methods to control the lawn, and in this case, perhaps try to think *less* green. The good news for your own drinking water is that a simple activated carbon-based water filter like the ones commonly available in supermarkets can filter out atrazine and other chemicals. Reduce and remove ... that's your mantra.

Day 20

- **Power Mind: Lounge in bed**
  - **Potter in the Morning**
  - **Get a Massage**
  - *Crisis Management*
- **Power Food: Organic menus**
- **Power Exercise:** *Get a game*
- **Power of Connection: Positive emotional action**
  - **Reach Out – Make plans with friends for the weekend**
- **Power Rest: Afternoon nap**
  - **8 hours' sleep**

Crisis Management

Unfortunately, many people use food as crisis-management medicine. Comfort foods – rich in refined carbohydrates and fats – provide instant emotional rewards: they raise blood sugar, giving an immediate energy boost, and briefly elevate neurotransmitters, counteracting the effects of stress hormones. But this short-lived fix causes all manner of destructive inflammation, glycation and oxidation. An abrupt elevation of your happy molecules – blood sugar and neurotransmitters – is always followed by a crash in the same, leaving you much worse off than when you began, suffering from low blood sugar levels and the roller-coaster ride down. Don't medicate yourself with junk food; support yourself with nature and natural nurture.

> ### My Crisis Management First Aid Kit
> - **Lean protein and whole grains** *(for sustained energy).*
> - **A cup of green tea** *contains L-Theanine for a gentle lift.*
> - **Licorice (sweetened with molasses) or licorice root** *to support the adrenals (chew every couple of hours).*
> - **Protein shake** *made with fruit and veggie juices (once a day).*
> - **A square of 70 percent or greater dark chocolate** *(1–2 times per day).*
> - **Tonic herbal tea,** *such as chamomile (as often as needed).*
> - **Antianxiety tincture,** *Bach Flower "Rescue Remedy."*
> - **Calming essential oils** *like lavender (dab on the wrist daily).*
> - **Adaptogenic herbs,** *ashwaganda or cordyceps (twice daily).*
> - **Multivitamin** *to support increased energy demands (daily).*
> - **Relaxation exercises,** *morning meditation, yoga stretches, and frequent breath breaks (daily).*

Get a Game

Game-playing is a bit of a lost art, and I'd encourage you to consider reviving it. I grew up watching my parents play bridge monthly and my father play his weekly golf game (even through the frigid winter months). I came to appreciate the value these games had in keeping them connected with friends and in truly energizing their lives even at times when the going was rough for my father at work or my mother was besieged by having four teenaged boys in the house. One of my patients who was going through a very rough time in her life joined a volleyball team (a game she'd not played since high school), which became a real anchor for her during turbulent times. She'd go out and forget about her troubles during the training sessions and matches and get a bit of a workout to boot. Computer games don't count in my book – they cause you to lose sleep and can be addictive. Keep the level of competition healthy. One of my patients felt little stress at home or work, but became highly anxious in his ultra competitive weekly golf outings. If you're consumed by winning, then game playing may have moved out of the health-promoting category for you. In that case, perhaps taking up a new sport would be a better idea.

Day 21

- **Power Mind: Early morning wake-up call and Congratulate yourself – Take the Energy Quiz – You are graduating today**
- **Power Food: Organic menus**
- **Power Exercise: A day off or Your favourite new workout**
- **Power of Connection:** *Connecting to a greater energy*
- **Power Rest: 8 hours' sleep**

Connecting to a Greater Energy

You've been through a transformative journey these past 21 days. You've fixed a lot of mechanical energy problems and healed emotional energy drains. I'd like you to finish this journey with the intention to connect to a greater energy beyond yourself – through family, community, religion, nature or spirituality. Your vital spirit touches others; it energizes them and is magnified back to you in a reverberating circuit. Beyond your ability to see or even comprehend fully, the universe exists as a limitless energy field that you can tap for greater personal energy. Today, take some contemplative time to commune with this energy of the cosmos, with a higher power, that which is the absolute. You are a vital part of it. You can sense it within you and around you. Breathe, relax and feel joy.

Part three

Menus and Recipes

with Stefanle Bryn Sacks, MS

Culinary nutritionist Stefanie Bryn Sacks contributed the menus and recipes for the 21-Day Plan. Stefanie has helped many of my patients transform their eating lives and I think you will find that her menus and recipes presented here will do the same for you.

Pantry Notes

A food processor is required for some of the recipes. You don't need to get a huge expensive piece of equipment; many good small models can be found for under £40.

Agave syrup (nectar) is a sweetener derived from the leaves of a plant native to Mexico, and is a good alternative to table sugar as it has a low glycaemic index.

Certified organic is the best choice when choosing animal foods such as eggs, dairy or meats, meaning the animal has been raised without hormones or antibiotics, given organic feed and treated humanely.

Curry powder can be found at all supermarkets. Make sure the one you choose does not contain monosodium glutamate (MSG) or artificial ingredients.

Gomasio is an Asian seasoning made from sea salt, sesame seeds and seaweed. One teaspoon has 80mg of sodium while one teaspoon of table salt has 2,360mg sodium.

Juices, which are naturally sweet, are typically high in natural fruit sugar (fructose). Many juices on the market today contain added sugar whether in the form of high fructose corn syrup, glycose syrup, cane sugar or even other juices and juice extracts. When buying juices, try to choose those that are 100 per cent juice (preferably 100 per cent single fruit juice).

Mirin is a seasoned, rice-based wine often used in Japanese cuisine. It is similar to sake but has a lower alcohol content. Mirin can be found in shops where soy sauce and tamari are displayed. Make sure to buy real mirin versus those products that call themselves mirin but are only corn or glucose syrup, water and flavourings.

Quinoa (pronounced keen-wah) is a whole grain native to South America. It can be substituted for rice in most recipes. It has one of the highest protein contents of any grain.

Rapeseed oil mayo is rich in heart healthy monounsaturated fats, giving it a healthier fat profile than traditional mayonnaise. Rapeseed mayonnaise can be found at some shops or you can order it on the internet.

Red curry paste is made with red chillies and is commonly found in the Thai or international food sections of supermarkets.

White miso is a Japanese seasoning paste made from soya that can be found refrigerated in the produce or dairy sections of many Asian supermarkets. Don't substitute sweet white miso, which can change the taste of the recipe.

Whole cardamom pods encase the tiny brown seeds that are ground to make the powdered spice. Cardamom has a peppery floral essence. The pods can be found in most spice departments. Look for unbleached, green varieties.

Stefanie Bryn Sacks, MS

A note for vegetarians and vegans: this plan is designed to help everyone transition towards a plant-based diet. If you are already there, you can substitute the poultry or fish dishes with any one of the many vegetarian dishes in the menus and recipes.

DAY 1

Breakfast
- Plain low-fat Greek yogurt topped with honey, wheat germ and walnuts
- Blueberries
- 350ml (12 fl oz) filtered water
- Green tea (decaf or regular) or herbal tea

Snack
- Burst of Energy Trail Mix (page 338)
- 350ml (12 fl oz) filtered water

Lunch
- Lemon Parsley Hummus Wrap (page 334)
- 350 ml (12 fl oz) filtered water or decaffeinated, unsweetened drink
- Herbal tea

Snack
- Rice cake with almond butter (1 tbsp)
- 240ml (8 fl oz) filtered water or decaffeinated, unsweetened drink

Dinner
- Garlic Roasted Asparagus (page 323)
- Walnut-Pesto Wild Salmon (page 331)
- Harvest Wild Rice (page 324)
- Citrus Mint Mixed Berries (page 340)
- 240ml (8 fl oz) filtered water

DAY 2

Breakfast
- Almond butter (1 tbsp) and strawberries on wheat-free toast
- 350ml (12 fl oz) filtered water
- Green tea (decaf or regular) or herbal tea

Snack
- Rice crackers with Lemon Parsley Hummus (leftover)
- 350ml (12 fl oz) filtered water or decaffeinated, unsweetened drink

Lunch
- Watercress Rocket Salad (page 321)
- Rye crispbread
- 350ml (12 fl oz) filtered water
- Herbal tea

Snack
- 2 dark (70+%) chocolate squares
- 240ml (8 fl oz) filtered water or decaffeinated, unsweetened drink

Dinner
- Papaya Fizz (page 344)
- Mixed Salad Leaves with Balsamic Vinaigrette (page 318)
- Vegetarian Chilli (page 337)
- Brown rice (follow directions on package)
- 240ml (8 fl oz) filtered water

DAY 3

Breakfast
- Vegetable Goat's Cheese Egg-White Omelette (page 311)
- 350ml (12 fl oz) filtered water
- Green tea (decaf or regular) or herbal tea

Snack
- Red grapes
- 350 ml (12 fl oz) filtered water or decaffeinated, unsweetened drink

Lunch
- Vegetarian Chilli (leftover)
- 350ml (12 fl oz) filtered water
- Herbal tea

Snack
- Rice crackers with Walnut Pesto (leftover)
- 240ml (8 fl oz) filtered water or decaffeinated, unsweetened drink

Dinner
- Juicy, Sweet Roasted Broccoli (no kidding!) (page 324)
- Tofu Vegetable Stir-Fry (page 335)
- Rice noodles or 100% buckwheat soba noodles (follow directions on package)
- Coco-nutty Banana (page 341)
- 240ml (8 fl oz) filtered water

DAY 4

Breakfast
- Power Up Granola (page 310) with soya or rice milk and mixed berries
- 350ml (12 fl oz) filtered water
- Green tea (decaf or regular) or herbal tea

Snack
- Rice cake with hard-boiled egg
- 350ml (12 fl oz) filtered water or decaffeinated, unsweetened drink

Lunch
- Mediterranean Tuna Salad (page 318)
- 350ml (12 fl oz) filtered water
- Herbal tea

Snack
- Freshly cut veggies with Guacamole (page 339)
- 240ml (8 fl oz) filtered water or decaffeinated, unsweetened drink

Dinner
- Cool Mint Lemonade (page 343)
- Rocket Salad with Crushed Walnuts and Goat's Cheese (page 316)
- Warm Puy Lentils (page 329)
- Herb-Marinated Chicken (page 333)
- 240ml (8 fl oz) filtered water

DAY 5

Breakfast
- Wheat-free toast topped with goat's cheese and chopped watercress
- 350ml (12 fl oz) filtered water
- Green tea (decaf or regular) or herbal tea

Snack
- Small apple
- 350ml (12 fl oz) filtered water or decaffeinated, unsweetened drink

Lunch
- Herby Chicken Salad (page 319)
- 350ml (12 fl oz) filtered water
- Herbal tea

Snack
- Celery with almond butter (1 tbsp)
- 240ml (8 fl oz) filtered water or decaffeinated, unsweetened drink

Dinner
- Sweet Spinach Salad (page 320)
- Quinoa with Spring Onions and Toasted Sesame Oil (page 325)
- Miso-Baked Cod (page 330)
- Dark Chocolate Dairy-Free Mousse (page 342)
- 240ml (8 fl oz) filtered water

DAY 6

Breakfast
- Plain low-fat Greek yogurt topped with honey, wheat germ and walnuts
- 350ml (12 fl oz) filtered water
- Green tea (decaf or regular) or herbal tea

Snack
- Antioxidant Fruit Salad (page 315)
- 350ml (12 fl oz) filtered water or decaffeinated, unsweetened drink

Lunch
- Nitrate-free sliced turkey with avocado in a wheat-free wrap
- 350ml (12 fl oz) filtered water
- Herbal tea

Snack
- 2 dark (70+%) chocolate squares
- 240ml (8 fl oz) filtered water or decaffeinated, unsweetened drink

Dinner
- Cranberry Tea Infusion (page 343)
- Sautéed Kale with Garlic (page 326)
- Cinnamon Roasted Acorn Squash (page 323)
- Curry Roasted Chicken (page 332)
- 240ml (8 fl oz) filtered water

DAY 7

Breakfast
- Scrambled Tofu with Vegetables (page 312)
- Wheat-free toast
- Blueberries
- 350ml (12 fl oz) filtered water

Snack
- Half grapefruit
- 350ml (12 fl oz) filtered water or decaffeinated, unsweetened drink

Lunch
- Vegetarian Cobb Salad (page 320)
- 350ml (12 fl oz) filtered water
- Herbal tea

Snack
- Burst of Energy Trail Mix (page 338)
- 240ml (8 fl oz) filtered water or decaffeinated, unsweetened drink

Dinner
- Mango-Peach Freeze (page 344)
- Watercress Rocket Salad (page 321)
- Red Lentil Soup (page 313)
- 240ml (8 fl oz) filtered water

DAY 8

Breakfast
- Dr Merrell's Morning Shake (page 309)
- 350ml (12 fl oz) filtered water
- Green tea (decaf or regular) or herbal tea

Snack
- Burst of Energy Trail Mix (page 338)
- 350ml (12 fl oz) filtered water or decaffeinated, unsweetened drink

Lunch
- Red Lentil Soup (leftover)
- Rye Crispbread
- 350ml (12 fl oz) filtered water
- Herbal tea

Snack
- Freshly cut veggies with Guacamole (page 339)
- 240ml (8 fl oz) filtered water or decaffeinated, unsweetened drink

Dinner
- Warm Hijiki Salad (page 321)
- Tofu Vegetable Stir-Fry (page 335)
- Brown rice (follow directions on package)
- Fresh berries
- 240ml (8 fl oz) filtered water

DAY 9

Breakfast
- Dr Merrell's Morning Shake (page 309)
- 350ml (12 fl oz) filtered water
- Green tea (decaf or regular) or herbal tea

Snack
- Rice Crackers with Lemon Parsley Hummus (page 339)
- 350ml (12 fl oz) filtered water or decaffeinated, unsweetened drink

Lunch
- Leafy Greens and Chickpea Salad (page 317)
- 350ml (12 fl oz) filtered water
- Herbal tea

Snack
- Apple half with almond butter (1 tbsp)
- 240ml (8 fl oz) filtered water or decaffeinated, unsweetened drink

Dinner
- Shiitake Miso Soup (page 314)
- Quinoa with Sliced Avocado (page 325)
- Fresh berries
- 240ml (8 fl oz) filtered water

DAY 10 – JUICE CLEANSE

7:30am
- Dr Merrell's Morning Shake (page 309)
- Green tea (decaf or regular) or herbal tea

9:00am
- 240ml (8 fl oz) filtered water or decaffeinated, unsweetened drink

10:30am
- 240ml (8 fl oz) Dr Merrell's Veggie Juice (page 343)

12:00pm
- 240ml (8 fl oz) Shiitake Miso Broth (leftover)
- 240ml (8 fl oz) filtered water
- 240ml (8 fl oz) decaffeinated, unsweetened herbal tea

1:30pm
- 240ml (8 fl oz) Dr Merrell's Veggie Juice

3:00pm
- 240ml (8 fl oz) herbal decaffeinated, unsweetened drink
- 240ml (8 fl oz) filtered water

JUICE CLEANSE continued...

4:30pm
- 350ml (12 fl oz) Dr Merrell's Fruit Juice (page 344)

6:00pm
- 240ml (8 fl oz) Dr Merrell's Veggie Juice
- 240ml (8 fl oz) Shiitake Miso Broth (leftover)
- 240ml (8 fl oz) filtered water

7:30pm
- 240ml (8 fl oz) decaffeinated, unsweetened beverage

9:00pm
- 240ml (8 fl oz) Dr Merrell's Veggie Juice

10:30pm
- 240ml (8 fl oz) decaffeinated, unsweetened herbal tea

DAY 11

Breakfast
- Dr Merrell's Morning Shake (page 309)
- 350ml (12 fl oz) filtered water
- Green tea (decaf or regular) or herbal tea

Snack
- 1 small apple
- 350ml (12 fl oz) filtered water or decaffeinated, unsweetened drink

Lunch
- Leafy Greens and Chickpea Salad (page 317)
- 350ml (12 fl oz) filtered water
- Herbal tea

Snack
- Freshly cut veggies with Guacamole (page 339)
- 240ml (8 fl oz) filtered water or decaffeinated, unsweetened drink

Dinner
- Cucumber Wakame Salad (page 317)
- White Bean Kale Soup (page 315)
- Brown rice (follow directions on package)
- Fresh berries
- 240ml (8 fl oz) filtered water

DAY 12

Breakfast
- Dr Merrell's Morning Shake (page 309)
- 350ml (12 fl oz) filtered water
- Green tea (decaf or regular)
  or herbal tea

Snack
- Celery sticks with almond butter
  (1 tbsp)
- 350ml (12 fl oz) filtered water or
  decaffeinated, unsweetened drink

Lunch
- Power Protein Mixed Green Salad (page
  318)
- Half grapefruit
- 350ml (12 fl oz) filtered water
- Herbal tea

Snack
- Power Up! Granola (page 310)
- 240ml (8 fl oz) filtered water or
  decaffeinated, unsweetened drink

Dinner
- Sweet and Spicy Kale (page 328)
- Red Curry Tofu with Basil (page 335)
- Quinoa (follow directions on package)
- Fresh berries
- 240ml (8 fl oz) filtered water

DAY 13

Breakfast
- Dr Merrell's Morning Shake (page 309)
- 350ml (12 fl oz) filtered water
- Green tea (decaf or regular)
  or herbal tea

Snack
- Burst of Energy Trail Mix (page 338)
- 350ml (12 fl oz) filtered water or
  decaffeinated, unsweetened drink

Lunch
- Immune-Boost Soup (page 311)
- Wheat-free bread drizzled with extra-
  virgin olive oil
- 350ml (12 fl oz) filtered water
- Herbal tea

Snack
- Orange wedges
- 240ml (8 fl oz) filtered water or
  decaffeinated, unsweetened drink

Dinner
- Tangerine Spritzer with Papaya Ice
  (page 344)
- Braised Chard (page 322)
- Vegetable Biryani (page 336)
- 240ml (8 fl oz) filtered water

DAY 14

Breakfast
- Dr Merrell's Morning Shake (page 309)
- 350ml (12 fl oz) filtered water
- Green tea (decaf or regular)
  or herbal tea

Snack
- Power Up! Granola (page 310)
- 350ml (12 fl oz) filtered water or
  decaffeinated, unsweetened drink

Lunch
- Rosemary Butternut Squash Soup
  (page 313)
- Black Bean Salad (page 316)
- 350ml (12 fl oz) filtered water
- Herbal tea

Snack
- Half grapefruit
- 240ml (8 fl oz) filtered water or
  decaffeinated, unsweetened drink

Dinner
- Scrumptious Brussels Sprouts (page
  327)
- Trout with Lemon and Herbs (page 330)
- Brown rice (follow directions on
  package)
- Berry Parfait (page 340)
- 240ml (8 fl oz) filtered water

DAY 15

Breakfast
- Plain low-fat Greek yogurt topped with
  honey, wheat germ and walnuts
- 350ml (12 fl oz) filtered water
- Green tea (decaf or regular)
  or herbal tea

Snack
- Burst of Energy Trail Mix (page 338)
- 350ml (12 fl oz) filtered water or
  decaffeinated, unsweetened drink

Lunch
- Rosemary Butternut Squash Soup
  (page 313)
- Watercress Rocket Salad (page 321)
- 350ml (12 fl oz) filtered water
- Herbal tea

Snack
- Rice cake with hard-boiled egg
- 240ml (8 fl oz) filtered water or
  decaffeinated, unsweetened drink

Dinner
- Mango-Peach Freeze (page 344)
- Sweet and Spicy Kale (page 328)
- Vegetarian Chilli Burritos (page 338)
- 240ml (8 fl oz) filtered water

DAY 16

Breakfast
- Dr Merrell's Morning Shake (page 309)
- Wheat-free toast drizzled with extra-virgin olive oil
- 350ml (12 fl oz) filtered water
- Green tea (decaf or regular) or herbal tea

Snack
- Antioxidant Fruit Salad (page 315)
- 350ml (12 fl oz) filtered water or decaffeinated, unsweetened drink

Lunch
- White Bean Kale Soup (page 315)
- Ryvita with goat's cheese
- 350ml (12 fl oz) filtered water
- Herbal tea

Snack
- Power Up! Granola (page 310)
- 240ml (8 fl oz) filtered water or decaffeinated, unsweetened drink

Dinner
- Juicy Sweet Roasted Broccoli (no kidding!) (page 324)
- Halibut Puttanesca (page 329)
- Brown rice (follow directions on package)
- Dark Chocolate Dairy-Free Mousse (page 342)
- 240ml (8 fl oz) filtered water

DAY 17

Breakfast
- Vegetable Goat's Cheese Egg-White Omelette (page 311)
- 350ml (12 fl oz) filtered water
- Green tea (decaf or regular) or herbal tea

Snack
- Red grapes
- 350ml (12 fl oz) filtered water or decaffeinated, unsweetened drink

Lunch
- Nitrate-free sliced turkey with avocado in a wheat-free wrap
- 350ml (12 fl oz) filtered water
- Herbal tea

Snack
- Half apple with almond butter (1 tbsp)
- 240ml (8 fl oz) filtered water or decaffeinated, unsweetened drink

Dinner
- Peach Spritzer with Cranberry Ice (page 344)
- Crunchy Pak Choi with Tangy Chilli Vinaigrette (page 323)
- Red Curry Tofu with Basil (page 335)
- Quinoa with Spring Onions and Toasted Sesame Oil (page 325)
- 240ml (8 fl oz) filtered water

DAY 18

Breakfast
- Power Up! Granola (page 310) with soya or rice milk and mixed berries
- 350ml (12 fl oz) filtered water
- Green tea (decaf or regular) or herbal tea

Snack
- Grapefruit wedges
- 350ml (12 fl oz) filtered water or decaffeinated, unsweetened drink

Lunch
- Vegetarian Cobb Salad (page 320)
- 350ml (12 fl oz) filtered water
- Herbal tea

Snack
- Celery and carrot with Lemon Parsley Hummus (page 339)
- 240ml (8 fl oz) filtered water or decaffeinated, unsweetened drink

Dinner
- Rocket Salad with Crushed Walnuts and Goat's Cheese (page 316)
- Turkey Bolognese over Spaghetti Squash (page 333)
- Berry Parfait (page 340)
- 240ml (8 fl oz) filtered water

DAY 19

Breakfast
- Plain low-fat Greek yogurt topped with honey, wheat germ and walnuts
- 350ml (12 fl oz) filtered water
- Green tea (decaf or regular) or herbal tea

Snack
- Freshly cut veggies with Guacamole (page 339)
- 350ml (12 fl oz) filtered water or decaffeinated, unsweetened drink

Lunch
- Power Protein Mixed Green Salad (page 318)
- 350ml (12 fl oz) filtered water
- Herbal tea

Snack
- Power Up! Granola (page 310)
- 240ml (8 fl oz) filtered water or decaffeinated, unsweetened drink

Dinner
- Cranberry Tea Infusion (page 343)
- Quick Italian Vegetable Soup (page 312)
- Warm Puy Lentils (page 329)
- Brown rice (follow directions on package)
- 240ml (8 fl oz) filtered water

DAY 20

Breakfast
- Wheat-free toast drizzled with extra-virgin olive oil and sliced hard-boiled egg
- 350ml (12 fl oz) filtered water
- Green tea (decaf or regular) or herbal tea

Snack
- Rice crackers with Walnut Pesto (page 332)
- 350ml (12 fl oz) filtered water or decaffeinated, unsweetened drink

Lunch
- Quick Italian Vegetable Soup (leftover)
- Black Bean Salad (page 316)
- 350ml (12 fl oz) filtered water
- Herbal tea

Snack
- Fresh berries
- 240ml (8 fl oz) filtered water or decaffeinated, unsweetened drink

Dinner
- Spiced Coconut Cauliflower (page 327)
- Curry Roasted Chicken (page 332)
- Harvest Wild Rice (page 324)
- Dark Chocolate Chunk Almond Biscuits (page 341)
- 240ml (8 fl oz) filtered water

DAY 21

Breakfast
- French Toast (page 309)
- Blueberries
- 350ml (12 fl oz) filtered water
- Green tea (decaf or regular) or herbal tea

Snack
- Burst of Energy Trail Mix (page 338)
- 350ml (12 fl oz) filtered water or decaffeinated, unsweetened drink

Lunch
- Mixed Salad Leaves with Balsamic Vinaigrette (page 318)
- Red Lentil Soup (page 313)
- Wheat-free bread drizzled with extra-virgin olive oil
- 350ml (12 fl oz) filtered water
- Herbal tea

Snack
- Half grapefruit
- 240ml (8 fl oz) filtered water or decaffeinated, unsweetened drink

Dinner
- Steamed Artichokes with Lemon Aioli (page 328)
- Walnut-Pesto Wild Salmon (page 331)
- Quinoa Tabbouleh (page 326)
- Spiced Apples with Pecan Crumble (page 342)
- 240ml (8 fl oz) filtered water

Breakfast Recipes

Dr Merrell's Morning Shake

As well as containing many antioxidant flavonoids, blueberries, raspberries and blackberries also contain ellagic acid, which block the harmful effects of many pollutants, including cigarette smoke. Flaxseed (linseed) meal and flaxseed oil are one of the best non-fish sources of omega-3 fatty acids, which help decrease the likelihood of developing inflammatory and chronic diseases like heart disease and cancer.

SERVES 2

200g (7oz) mixed frozen berries
  (or chopped fresh pineapple or papaya*)
240ml (8 fl oz) pineapple juice
  (or pomegranate or cherry juice)
120ml (4 fl oz) water
180ml (6 fl oz) unsweetened soya milk
  or rice milk (for soya allergies use whey
  protein powder**)
1½ tsp fresh ginger root, peeled and finely
  chopped (or ½ tsp ground cinnamon or
  turmeric)
1 heaped tbsp ground flax (linseed) meal
1 tsp flaxseed (linseed) oil
1 tbsp probiotic powder or liquid***

Combine all ingredients in a blender and purée until smooth.

*Can chop pineapple or papaya ahead of time and store in airtight container or bag in fridge for up to 3 days. **Combine 2 heaped tbsp of powder with 120ml (4 fl oz) water (use instead of soya milk). ***Make sure contains, at least, acidophilus and bifidophilus.

French Toast

Cinnamon appears to have a unique ability to help the body metabolize sugar. The essential oils found in the bark that's ground to make the spice contain three known active compounds that may account for this effect, and a wide range of other potentially beneficial phytochemicals.

SERVES 2

2 medium eggs
60ml (2 fl oz) unsweetened soya milk
1½ tsp pure vanilla extract
¼ tsp ground cinnamon
½ tbsp rapeseed oil*
1 tbsp butter, unsalted
4 slices bread, wheat-free
2 tbsp maple syrup or agave syrup (nectar)

1. In a medium bowl, combine eggs, soya milk, vanilla and cinnamon; mix well with fork.
2. Heat oil and butter in large sauté pan on medium.
3. Soak bread in egg mixture. Then gently place bread in pan and cook until browned on each side (about 3 minutes per side). Repeat with remaining bread slices.
4. Serve with maple syrup or agave syrup.

* If using a non-stick pan, use 1 tbsp oil instead of oil and butter.

Power Up! Granola*

Nuts are packed with nutrients, including high-quality protein and minerals like calcium and iron. The monounsaturated and polyunsaturated fats in nuts help lower LDL or bad cholesterol. Wheat germ contains plenty of the nutritional building blocks of energy, especially vitamins B and E.

SERVES 8

- 65g (2¼oz) whole raw almonds, coarsely chopped
- 50g (1¾oz) pecans, coarsely chopped
- 50g (1¾oz) walnuts, coarsely chopped
- 50g (1¾oz) rolled oats
- 30g (1oz) wheat germ
- 15g (½oz) unsweetened coconut flakes
- ¼ tsp ground cinnamon
- 1 tbsp maple syrup
- 60ml (2 fl oz) brown rice syrup
- ½ tbsp rapeseed oil

1. Preheat oven to 180°C/350°F/gas 4.
2. Cover baking tray with greaseproof paper; set aside.
3. Place chopped nuts in a bowl with remaining ingredients and mix well.
4. Spread mixture onto baking tray; bake for 10 minutes.
5. Remove from oven (it will look like a big biscuit), allow granola to cool for 10 minutes and break into chunks.
6. Once thoroughly cooled, store in airtight container in cool, dry place for up to three weeks. Can measure individual servings into small plastic bags for on-the-go eating.

* Make once for entire 21-Day Plan.

Scrambled Tofu and Vegetables

Tofu contains isoflavones, which have a beneficial effect on hormone-sensitive tissues such as the breast and prostate. Curry powder contains numerous phytochemicals including the curcumin in turmeric, which has demonstrated significant anti-inflammatory activity helpful for preventing heart attacks and strokes.

SERVES 2

- 1 tbsp rapeseed oil
- 1 small onion, diced
- 1 small courgette, diced
- ½ block extra firm tofu, crumbled
- 2 tsp low-salt tamari soy sauce
- ½ tsp curry powder
- ⅛ tsp salt

1. In a medium frying pan, heat oil on medium and fry onion until translucent. Add courgette and fry for another 3 minutes.
2. Drain tofu well. Crumble tofu into pan and mix well. Add tamari, curry powder and salt, mix well and cook for another 3 minutes.

Vegetable Goat's Cheese Egg-White Omelette

Egg whites carry half the calories and almost all of the protein of whole eggs; and they deliver the antioxidant mineral selenium (useful for heart muscle maintenance) as well as magnesium, which is beneficial for nerve and muscle function.

SERVES 2

6 egg whites, separated from yolks
½ tbsp extra-virgin olive oil*
1 tbsp butter, unsalted
15g (½oz) spring onions, thinly sliced
15g (½oz) broccoli florets, finely chopped**
60g (2oz) goat's cheese
freshly ground pepper, to taste

1. Using two bowls, separate whites from yolks (discard yolks). Add spring onions and broccoli to whites and mix well.
2. In a medium frying pan, heat olive oil and butter on medium.
3. When pan is hot, pour in egg. As edges start to set, gently lift edges, tilting pan slightly to allow uncooked egg to flow underneath cooked parts.
4. When most of the egg is set, spread goat's cheese over top of the omelette. Cook for another minute, until cooked entirely through.
5. Fold omelette in half over itself and slide onto plate.

* If using a non-stick pan, use 1 tbsp oil instead of oil and butter. ** Fresh or frozen. If frozen, run package under hot water for 30 seconds to defrost before chopping.

Soup

Immune-Boost Soup

Broccoli and garlic are a powerful combination, providing plenty of vitamins A and C, which boost immune function; sulphurophanes that aid in cancer prevention; and allicin, a sulphur-containing compound in garlic that has antibacterial properties shown to be effective against colds and stomach viruses. Coriander has anti-inflammatory and anti-microbial activity, and aids in processing of fats and cholesterol.

SERVES 4 (includes leftovers)*

1 tbsp extra-virgin olive oil
1 clove garlic, coarsely chopped
½ small onion, diced
1 small carrot, cut into rounds
½ tsp paprika**
¼ tsp ground coriander
1 small head broccoli, trimmed and coarsely chopped
1 litre (1¾ pints) water
pinch of salt
freshly ground pepper, to taste

1. In a medium pan, heat oil on medium. Fry garlic, onion, carrot and spices for 3 to 5 minutes, until soft.

2. Trim and coarsely chop broccoli. Add broccoli and water to pot and simmer, covered, on low for 15 minutes (until broccoli is soft).

3. Uncover and cool for 5 to 10 minutes. Place in blender and purée until creamy.***

4. Season with salt and pepper.

* Store leftovers in airtight container in fridge for up to 3 days or immediately freeze for up to 3 months. ** Preferably smoked Spanish paprika, but regular will do. *** Be cautious when puréeing warm/hot items in blender. Hold top down firmly with hand. Otherwise, top could easily pop off while puréeing, creating a mess.

Quick Italian Vegetable Soup

Garlic and onion are rich in sulphur, which the body uses as part of the liver's detoxifying mechanism. Onions also have quercetin, one of the most powerful antioxidants that acts as a natural antihistamine. Oregano is both anti-microbial (inhibits the growth of bacteria) and antioxidant (studies suggest it carries four times as much antioxidant activity as blueberries).

SERVES 4 (includes leftovers)*

2 tbsp extra-virgin olive oil
1 clove garlic, finely chopped
1 small onion, thinly sliced
2 tsp dried oregano
1 tsp dried thyme
1 medium yellow squash, sliced lengthwise and cut into half moons
1 medium courgette, sliced lengthwise and cut into half moons
75g (2½oz) red pepper, thinly sliced
285g (10oz) bag mixed frozen vegetables (whichever are your favourites)
2 tbsp balsamic vinegar
1 litre (1¾ pints) water
1 handful parsley, stems tied with string
½ tsp salt
freshly ground pepper, to taste
4 tsp Parmesan cheese

1. In a large pan, heat oil on medium. Add garlic, onion and dried herbs and fry until onion is translucent (about 3 minutes).

2. Add remaining vegetables (including frozen), balsamic vinegar, water and parsley. Cover, bring to the boil, then reduce heat and simmer for 20 minutes.

3. Discard parsley and season with salt and pepper. Serve with a sprinkling of Parmesan.

* Store leftovers in airtight container in fridge for up to 3 days or immediately freeze for up to 3 months.

Red Lentil Soup

Lentils are a good source of minerals and lignans, fibre compounds that can bind to oestrogen receptors and interfere with the cancer-promoting effects of oestrogen on breast and prostate tissue. Celery delivers phytochemical compounds known as coumarins, which are associated with cancer prevention and are capable of lowering blood pressure.

SERVES 4 (includes leftovers)*

1 tbsp extra-virgin olive oil
1 small onion, thinly sliced
2 stalks celery, diced
250g (9oz) red lentils
700ml (1¼ pints) water
480ml (16 fl oz) low-salt vegetable stock
pinch of salt
freshly ground pepper, to taste

In medium pan, heat olive oil on medium, add vegetables and fry until soft (about 3 minutes). Add lentils, water and stock. Simmer, uncovered, for about 30 minutes. Season with salt and pepper.

* Store leftovers in airtight container in fridge for up to 3 days or immediately freeze for up to 3 months.

Rosemary Butternut Squash Soup

Butternut squash delivers more than twice the recommended daily intake of vitamin A, making it a truly immune enhancing food. Rosemary contains rosmarinic acid, a powerful anti-inflammatory compound.

SERVES 4 (includes leftovers)*

1 medium (900g/2 lb) butternut squash
700ml (1¼ pints) water
1 large sprig fresh rosemary
pinch of salt

1. Peel squash, cut lengthwise and remove seeds; cut into large cubes.
2. Combine squash, water and rosemary in medium pan. Cover and cook on medium to low until squash is soft (about 20 minutes).
3. Cool for 5 to 10 minutes. Remove sprig of rosemary and discard. Add squash to blender with half the cooking liquid and purée. Add more cooking liquid as needed to achieve thick, creamy consistency.**
4. Season with salt.

* Store leftovers in airtight container in fridge for up to 3 days or immediately freeze for up to 3 months. ** Be cautious when puréeing warm/hot items in blender. Hold top down firmly with hand. Otherwise, top could easily pop off while puréeing, creating a mess.

Shiitake-Miso Soup

Research is currently underway into the many complex beneficial compounds in shiitakes including lentinan, which has been shown to strengthen the immune system, and eritadenine, shown to lower cholesterol levels. Miso is a fermented soya-bean paste that is a good source of minerals and the B vitamins useful for making energy.

SERVES 4 (includes leftover broth for cleanse)*

6 medium dry shiitake mushrooms
240ml (8 fl oz) warm water (to soak
   mushrooms)
1.75 litres (3 pints) water
1 small onion, thinly sliced
1 large carrot, thinly sliced into rounds
10 medium fresh shiitake mushrooms,
   stems removed and thinly sliced
2 slices fresh ginger root, unpeeled, 5mm
   (¼ inch) thick
1½ tbsp white miso
3 stalks pak choi, thinly sliced
Low-salt tamari soy sauce, wheat-free,
   to taste
gomasio, to taste

1. In bowl, soak dry mushrooms in 240ml (8 fl oz) warm water.
2. Prepare vegetables.
3. Place water plus all vegetables (including ginger) except for pak choi in a large pan. Cover and bring to boil. Turn down heat and simmer, covered, for 20 to 40 minutes.
4. Meanwhile, when soaking mushrooms are soft, remove from water, slice thinly (you may need to remove tough stems) and add to simmering soup with soaking liquid.
5. When soup is finished, turn off heat, remove and discard ginger. Add miso, mixing thoroughly. Add pak choi.
6. Season with tamari and gomasio.

* With whatever is leftover, strain the broth, discard vegetables and save in the fridge for the Cleanse day.

White Bean Kale Soup

Beans are a superb source of cholesterol-lowering fibre as well as antioxidants. They also deliver folic acid and vitamin B6, which help lower levels of homocysteine, the amino acid that causes plaque to stick to arteries. Kale delivers a host of cancer-preventing phytochemicals as well as more than 70 per cent of the RDI of vitamin C in a single serving.

SERVES 4 (includes leftovers)*

1 tin (425g/15oz) white (cannellini) beans, drained and rinsed
1 tbsp extra-virgin olive oil
1 small onion, thinly sliced
1 clove garlic, finely chopped
2 vine-ripened tomatoes, diced
700ml (1¼ pints) water
700ml (1¼ pints) low-salt vegetable stock
1 sprig fresh thyme
1 sprig fresh oregano
1 small bunch kale, ripped from stem or cut into small pieces
pinch of salt
freshly ground pepper, to taste

1. In a large pan, heat olive oil on medium. Fry onion and garlic until lightly golden. Add beans, tomatoes, water, stock and herbs. Simmer, covered, for 15 minutes.
2. Remove and discard herb stems. Add kale and continue to simmer, covered, for 20 minutes more.
3. Season to taste.

* Store leftovers in airtight container in fridge for up to 3 days or immediately freeze for up to 3 months.

Salad Recipes

Antioxidant Fruit Salad*

Papaya delivers several antioxidant carotenes along with Papain, an enzyme that helps to digest proteins. Kiwi fruit is high in vitamin C and the antioxidant lycopene, and is associated with promoting respiratory tract health. The pigments in blueberries carry powerful antioxidant flavonoids. Mint contains the antioxidant rosmarinic acid, which blocks the production of hay fever-producing leukotrienes.

SERVES 2

170g (6oz) papaya, peeled, halved, seeds removed and cubed
1 kiwi, peeled and sliced into rounds
60g (2oz) blueberries
1 tbsp fresh mint leaves, coarsely chopped

In a bowl combine all ingredients and mix gently.

* Can be made the night before if desired. You can also buy ready-made fresh fruit salad if easier (make sure it is fresh fruit and not a fruit cocktail with added sugar).

Rocket Salad with Crushed Walnuts and Goat's Cheese

One of the only cruciferous greens that can be used as a salad leaf, rocket contains anti-cancer compounds known as glucosinolates, which also stimulate detox enzymes. Rocket is rich in chlorophyll, which can stimulate haemoglobin and red blood cell production, helping to guard against anaemia. Walnuts are one of the best nuts for omega-3 fatty acids.

SERVES 2

75g (2½oz) rocket
½ head radicchio, shredded
1 small pear, peeled and thinly sliced
60g (2oz) goat's cheese, crumbled
2 tbsp walnuts, coarsely chopped
1 tbsp extra-virgin olive oil
1 tbsp balsamic vinegar
freshly ground pepper, to taste

1. Thoroughly wash and dry rocket and radicchio (pat with kitchen towel or use salad spinner) and place in medium salad bowl.
2. Add pear, goat's cheese and walnuts and gently toss.
3. Add oil, vinegar and pepper. Toss gently again.

Black Bean Salad

Black beans are particularly high in the energy-building mineral magnesium; and the cholesterol-lowering fibre in beans also prevents blood sugar levels from rising too rapidly after a meal. The folic acid and vitamin B6 in beans makes them protective against the development of artery plaque; and the oleic and linoleic acids in avocados can help lower cholesterol levels.

SERVES 2

1 tin (425g/15oz) black beans, drained and rinsed
100g (3½oz) cherry tomatoes, halved
½ avocado, diced
1 small red onion, diced
4 tbsp coriander, stems and leaves coarsely chopped
1 tbsp extra-virgin olive oil
1 lime, juiced
¼ tsp salt

Combine all the ingredients in a medium salad bowl and mix well.

Cucumber Wakame Salad

Cucumber contains a trace mineral called silica, necessary for the health of connective tissue (joints, muscles and ligaments, hair and nails). The sea vegetable wakame offers a broad range of minerals; cancer-protective lignans; and unique substances known as fucans (natural sulphated polysaccharides), which can lower the body's inflammatory response.

SERVES 2

1 large cucumber, peeled, seeded and thinly sliced
1 tbsp brown rice vinegar
½ lemon, juiced
2 tsp gomasio
8 tbsp dried wakame seaweed, cut into 1cm (½ inch) strips with scissors, soaked in 120ml (4 fl oz) cold water until soft (about 5 minutes) and drained

1. In medium bowl, combine cucumber slices, vinegar, lemon juice and gomasio.
2. Add drained wakame to bowl and toss.

Leafy Greens and Chickpea Salad

Chickpeas deliver heart-healthy fibre, and also contain a micronutrient trace mineral called molybdenum, crucial for the body's mechanism to detoxify sulphites – a common preservative found in wine and cold processed meats. Swiss chard packs in beneficial vitamins and minerals; including vitamin K (388.9 per cent of the daily value in one serving of cooked Swiss chard), essential for the maintenance of healthy bones.

SERVES 2

40g (11/4oz) Swiss chard
45g (11/2oz) baby spinach
15g (1/2oz) flat-leaf parsley leaves
200g (7oz) chickpeas, drained and rinsed
2 tbsp unsalted almonds, chopped
about 15 red grapes, halved

DRESSING
1 tbsp extra-virgin olive oil
½ tbsp mirin
2 tbsp brown rice vinegar
⅛ tsp salt

1. Thoroughly wash and dry chard, spinach and parsley (pat with paper towel or use salad spinner).
2. In a large bowl, combine all salad ingredients and toss well.
3. In a small bowl, whisk together dressing ingredients.
4. Dress the salad and toss.

Mediterranean Tuna Salad

Light tuna, tinned in water, is an excellent source of protein. It contains more of the heart-muscle healthy mineral selenium than any almost any other fish; and niacin, the B vitamin essential for replenishing energy, growth hormone production and nerve function. Dill is a 'chemoprotective' food that can help neutralize certain carcinogens, including cigarette and charcoal grill smoke.

SERVES 2

1 tin low-salt tuna chunks in spring water
1 tbsp fresh dill, chopped
2 tbsp spring onions, thinly sliced
1 tbsp extra-virgin olive oil
1 tbsp red wine vinegar
1 tbsp lime juice
pinch of salt
freshly ground pepper, to taste

CRISPY SALAD
145g (5oz) mixed salad leaves
1 tbsp lime juice

1. Drain tuna and place in medium bowl. Add remaining ingredients and mix well.
2. Thoroughly wash and dry the salad leaves (pat with kitchen towel or use salad spinner). In another bowl, toss with lime juice.
3. Serve tuna over crispy salad.

Mixed Salad Leaves with Balsamic Vinaigrette

Mixed leaves and parsley are good sources of chlorophyll, which promotes red blood cell production. Olive oil has a high level of monounsaturated fat, which helps lower LDL (bad) cholesterol, and is high in the essential fatty acid oleic acid, making it strongly anti-inflammatory.

SERVES 2

145g (5oz) mixed salad leaves
30g (1oz) flat leaf parsley, leaves and
  stems, coarsely chopped
1 tbsp extra-virgin olive oil
2 tsp balsamic vinegar (or more to taste)
½ lemon, juiced
freshly ground pepper, to taste

1. Thoroughly wash and dry the salad leaves and parsley (pat with kitchen towel or use salad spinner). Place in salad bowl.
2. Add remaining ingredients and toss.

Power Protein Mixed Green Salad

Small white beans tend to have the highest nutrient content of all beans, with more fibre, calcium, phosphorus and isoflavones (compounds with beneficial effects on hormone sensitive tissues such as breast and prostate) than their red and black bean cousins. Red peppers not only have more immune-boosting carotenes than their green counterparts, they also contain substances such as capsaicin and flavonoids, shown to prevent blood clot formation.

SERVES 2

1 tin (425g/15oz) white (cannellini) beans, drained and rinsed
½ red pepper, diced
¼ small red onion, diced (about 2 tbsp)
1 heaped tbsp fresh dill, chopped

DRESSING
1 tbsp extra-virgin olive oil
1½ tbsp brown rice vinegar
1½ tbsp red wine vinegar
pinch of salt
freshly ground pepper, to taste

BED OF SALAD LEAVES
145g (5oz) mixed salad leaves

1. In a medium bowl, combine beans, pepper, onion and dill.
2. In a small bowl, whisk together dressing ingredients and add to bean mixture, tossing well.
3. Thoroughly wash and dry the salad leaves (pat with kitchen towel or use salad spinner).
4. Serve bean mixture over bed of salad leaves.

Herby Chicken Salad

Organic, free-range chicken is a quality source of lean protein and all of the minerals that animal proteins contain, including niacin, selenium and the B vitamins. Thyme, oregano and basil are all rich in beneficial volatile oils that possess significant antioxidant and antibacterial properties.

SERVES 2

340g (12oz) Herb-Marinated Chicken, chopped (page 333)
1 tsp rapeseed oil mayonnaise
1 tsp Dijon mustard
1 tbsp capers
1 tsp caper juice
1 tbsp red onion, diced
2 thin slices avocado
2 wheat-free tortilla wraps, 18–20 cm (7–8 inches) in diameter

1. Chop chicken into bite-sized pieces.
2. In a small bowl, combine all ingredients (except for avocado and wraps) and mix well.
3. Serve in a wheat-free wrap with avocado slices.

Sweet Spinach Salad

Raw spinach has the highest concentration of the powerful antioxidant lutein of all vegetables. This confers it with cancer protective effects as well as promoting eye health and helping to prevent macular degeneration. Pine nuts are unusual among nuts for their arginine, magnesium and potassium content, all of which provide powerful protection against heart disease.

SERVES 2

200g (7oz) baby spinach
½ small red onion, thinly sliced
½ avocado, cubed
2 tbsp pine nuts, toasted

DRESSING
1 tbsp extra-virgin olive oil
1 lemon, juiced
½ tsp maple syrup
pinch of salt
freshly ground pepper, to taste

1. Thoroughly wash and dry spinach (pat with kitchen towel or use salad spinner). Place in large salad bowl with onion and avocado.
2. To toast pine nuts, toss constantly in small frying pan over low flame until golden (about 3 minutes). Add to salad.
3. In a small bowl, whisk together olive oil, lemon juice and maple syrup.
4. Dress salad and toss. Season with salt and pepper.

Vegetarian Cobb Salad

Watercress is a member of the cabbage family, and thus one more way to ingest this vegetable family's cancer protective phytochemicals. The health-giving oleic acid in olives and alpha-linolenic acid (ALA) in flaxmeal are important for lowering systemic inflammation, linked with many chronic diseases including heart disease, strokes and cancer.

SERVES 2

2 eggs
1 head romaine lettuce, coarsely chopped
1 bunch watercress, ends trimmed and coarsely chopped
½ avocado, cubed
100g (3½ oz) cherry tomatoes, halved
2 tbsp stoned Kalamata olives, chopped
60g (2oz) goat's cheese, crumbled
1 tbsp ground flax (linseed) meal

DRESSING
1 tbsp extra-virgin olive oil
1½ tbsp white balsamic vinegar (or regular balsamic)
1 tsp Dijon mustard
½ tbsp fresh thyme

1. Place two eggs in small pan with cold water. Simmer for 10 minutes. Remove and cool. Discard yolks; chop whites.
2. In a small bowl, combine dressing ingredients and mix well.

3. Thoroughly wash and dry the salad leaves (pat with kitchen towel or use salad spinner). Place in large salad bowl and toss with half the dressing. Add remaining ingredients (including chopped egg whites) and drizzle with remaining dressing.

Warm Hijiki Salad

Hijiki is an excellent source of calcium and it is rich in iodine, which plays a crucial role in supporting the thyroid gland. It also contains anti-inflammatory lignans. Tamari is a type of soy sauce that contains the B vitamin niacin, and iron and manganese among other minerals – all of which are needed for energy creation.

SERVES 2

8 tbsp dried hijiki seaweed
2 tsp sesame oil
½ small onion, thinly sliced
1 small carrot, cut into half moons
½ tbsp mirin
1 tsp low-salt tamari soy sauce
1 tbsp sesame seeds

1. Soak seaweed according to instructions on package.
2. In a large pan, heat oil on medium. Fry onion and carrot until lightly browned (about 5 minutes). Drain hijiki and add to pan with mirin, tamari and sesame seeds; mix well.

Watercress Rocket Salad

Two of the most nutrient-dense lettuces, watercress and rocket have cancer-protective properties. Red onions support the body's detox system. Oregano delivers multiple antioxidants and antibacterial phytochemicals. Feta cheese is a relatively low-fat alternative to cow's milk cheese and it is beneficial to both the skeletal and immune systems.

SERVES 2

40g (1¼oz) rocket, coarsely chopped
40g (1¼oz) watercress, coarsely chopped
115g (4oz) romaine lettuce, coarsely chopped
100g (3½oz) cherry tomatoes, halved
½ small red onion, thinly sliced
2 tbsp stoned Kalamata olives, chopped
60g (2oz) goat's milk feta cheese, crumbled

DRESSING
1 tbsp extra-virgin olive oil
1 tbsp red wine vinegar
1 tsp dried oregano
freshly ground pepper, to taste

1. Thoroughly wash and dry salad leaves (pat with paper towel or use salad spinner). Place in medium bowl.
2. Add remaining vegetables, olives and goat's cheese. Gently toss.
3. In a small bowl, combine dressing ingredients and whisk with fork. Add to salad and toss.

Side Recipes

Braised Chard

One of the most powerful anti-cancer foods, Swiss chard packs a powerful combination of immune supporting vitamin A and bone-building vitamin K. It also delivers lots of fibre and other phytochemicals. Studies are underway into its noted ability to protect against colon cancer.

SERVES 2

1 small bunch Swiss chard, leaves coarsely chopped
1 tsp extra-virgin olive oil
2 tsp water or low-salt vegetable stock
2 tsp gomasio

1. Thoroughly wash and dry chard (pat with kitchen towel or use salad spinner).
2. In a large frying pan, heat oil on medium.
3. Fry chard for 3 to 5 minutes, tossing while cooking.
4. Finish with gomasio.

Cinnamon Roasted Acorn Squash

Rich in potassium, it's also high in carotenes, which makes this squash supportive of immune and reproductive health. Like other carotene-rich vegetables, winter squash has been shown to have a protective effect against lung cancer and type 2 diabetes.

SERVES 2

1 acorn squash, halved and seeded
2 tsp extra-virgin olive oil
1 tsp cinnamon

1. Preheat oven to 180°C/350°F/gas 4.
2. Cut squash in half (cut off ends, place vertically on chopping board, guide knife down middle of squash and split open). Scoop out seeds and pulp.
3. Brush entire squash with olive oil and sprinkle with cinnamon.
4. Place squash flesh side down onto baking dish.
5. Bake for 30 minutes or until you can easily poke fork through the skin.

Crunchy Pak Choi with Tangy Chilli Vinaigrette

Pak choi (also known as Chinese broccoli) is good for bones; one serving has almost a full day's supply of bone-healthy vitamin K, and nearly 10 per cent of calcium. It's also full of water, so good for dieters. Chilli powder is a combination of cayenne, cumin, turmeric, ginger and oregano, making it a powerhouse of cancer and infection-fighting phytochemicals.

SERVES 2

1 small head pak choi, trimmed and shredded
1 small carrot, shredded or julienned
½ small red onion, thinly sliced

DRESSING
1 tbsp extra-virgin olive oil
1 tbsp brown rice vinegar
1 tsp Dijon mustard
1 lime, juiced
⅛ tsp chilli powder
pinch of salt
freshly ground pepper, to taste

1. Trim top and bottom of pak choi. Holding bunch together, thinly slice. Place in large bowl. Add carrot and onion and toss.
2. In a small bowl, combine dressing ingredients.
3. Toss dressing with vegetables. Season with salt and pepper.

Garlic Roasted Asparagus

Asparagus contains more of the B vitamin folate than any other vegetable besides spinach, making it healthy for the heart and for pregnant women.

SERVES 2

1 bunch asparagus, trimmed
½ tbsp extravirgin olive oil
1 lemon, juiced
2 cloves garlic, coarsely chopped

1. Preheat oven to 180°C/350°F/gas 4.
2. Cut bottom ends off asparagus (about 2.5 cm/1 inch). Place asparagus in small baking dish.
3. Add olive oil, lemon juice and garlic to baking dish and toss, gently coating asparagus.
4. Bake, uncovered, for 15 to 20 minutes.

Harvest Wild Rice

Of all the rice products available, wild rice is the best choice for energy creation. It offers a significant amount of all of the B vitamins, a host of minerals required for energy creation, a balance of anti-inflammatory omega-3 and omega-6 fatty acids, and slightly more protein and less fat than its closest cousin, brown rice.

SERVES 2

    100g (3½oz) wild rice (100% wild rice)
    350ml (1½ cups) water
    1 vegetable stock cube, low-salt
    ½ tbsp extra-virgin olive oil
    2 tbsp flat leaf parsley; coarsely chopped
    3 tbsp currants, optional
    2 tbsp pecans, coarsely chopped
    pinch of salt
    freshly ground pepper, to taste

1. In a small pan, combine rice, water and stock cube. Cover pan and bring to the boil on medium to high. Turn to low and simmer for 40 to 50 minutes (or until all water is absorbed).
2. Chop parsley and pecans.
3. When rice is cooked, add olive oil, parsley, currants and pecans and mix well. Season with salt and pepper.

Juicy Sweet Roasted Broccoli (no kidding!)

One of the most nutrient-dense foods, cooked broccoli delivers more vitamin C than any other green vegetable; anti-inflammatory omega-3 and -6 fatty acids, lutein, a powerful form of immune-boosting carotenes; and some of nature's best anti-cancer compounds, which enhance the liver's ability to flush out the form of oestrogen linked to breast cancer.

SERVES 2

    ½ head broccoli, cut into small pieces
    1 tbsp extra-virgin olive oil
    pinch of salt or 1 tbsp gomasio

1. Preheat oven to 180°C/350°F/gas 4.
2. Trim 2.5cm (1 inch) from bottom of broccoli stem. Cut half into small pieces using the stem and florets. Place in small baking dish and drizzle with olive oil and salt or gomasio. Toss to coat.
3. Cover dish with foil. Bake in oven, tossing occasionally, for about 15 minutes until brown (or less for crunchier broccoli).

Quinoa with Spring Onions and Toasted Sesame Oil

Wheat and gluten-free, quinoa is probably the least allergenic of all grains. It's a higher protein grain than any type of rice. Quinoa provides 15 per cent of your daily requirement for iron in one serving, and significant amounts of B vitamins necessary for energy creation. Spring onions, like all members of the onion family, activate the body's detox systems.

SERVES 2

100g (3½oz) quinoa
180ml (6 fl oz) water
½ tbsp sesame oil
1 tsp toasted sesame oil
2 tbsp spring onions, thinly sliced
1 tbsp gomasio or ⅛ tsp salt

1. Place quinoa in fine mesh sieve and rinse with water. In a small pan, combine water and quinoa. Place covered pan on medium/high and bring to the boil. Then simmer, covered, until grain is light and fluffy (about 10 minutes).
2. Clean and slice spring onions.
3. When quinoa is finished cooking, add sesame oils and gomasio or salt and mix well.

Quinoa with Sliced Avocado

By adding omega fatty acid-rich avocado to nutrient-dense quinoa, you increase the dish's anti-inflammatory abilities. Avocado also delivers bone-building vitamin K, and is an excellent source of the antioxidant vitamin E family.

SERVES 2

100g (3½oz) quinoa
180ml (6 fl oz) water
½ avocado, thinly sliced
2 tsp extra-virgin olive oil
pinch of salt

1. Place quinoa in fine mesh sieve and rinse with water. In a small pan combine water and quinoa. Place covered pan on medium/high and bring to the boil. Then simmer, covered, until grain is light and fluffy (about 10 minutes).
2. Slice avocado.
3. When quinoa is finished, add olive oil and season with salt.
4. Serve topped with avocado slices.

Quinoa Tabbouleh

The vitamin C in orange juice and powerful antioxidants in mint boost this nutrient-rich tabbouleh so that it supports the immune system and provides complex carbohydrates for slow-burning energy.

SERVES 2

100g (3½oz) quinoa
180ml (6 fl oz) water
½ small cucumber, peeled, seeded and
  diced
2 tbsp spring onions, thinly sliced
2 tbsp mint leaves, coarsely chopped
½ orange, juiced
½ lime, juiced
1 tbsp extra-virgin olive oil
pinch of salt
freshly ground pepper, to taste

1. Place quinoa in fine mesh sieve and rinse with water. In a small pan, combine water and quinoa. Place covered pan on medium/high and bring to the boil. Then simmer, covered, until grain is light and fluffy (about 10 minutes).
2. Prepare vegetables and mint and place in small bowl with olive oil and citrus juices.
3. When quinoa is finished, add to bowl and gently toss. Season with salt and pepper.

Sautéed Kale with Garlic

A descendent of wild cabbage, kale is a nutrition powerhouse. It is an excellent source of carotenes and vitamin C, making it a wonderful staple during cold and flu season; adding garlic to the dish makes it even more immune-boosting. Kale has the same anti-cancer properties as broccoli, and is packed with chlorophyll, which enriches red blood cells.

SERVES 2

1 tbsp extra-virgin olive oil
1 clove garlic, finely chopped
1 bunch leafy green kale*, pulled from
  stems and coarsely chopped
½ lemon, juiced
1 tbsp water
pinch of salt

1. Heat oil on medium to low in a large frying pan. Add garlic and sauté until lightly browned.
2. Thoroughly wash and dry kale (pat with kitchen towel or use salad spinner).
3. Chop kale and add to pan with lemon juice and water and sauté for 3 to 5 minutes, tossing regularly to cook evenly without burning.
4. Finish with a pinch of salt.

* You can also use lacinato kale (sometimes called dinosaur kale); it's the sweetest variety.

Scrumptious Brussels Sprouts

Brussels are part of the cancer-fighting brassica (or cruceriferous) family. They are rich in the breast protective compound Indole-3-carbinol; and are a good source of vitamin C and the powerful antioxidant lutein, which is thought to help prevent macular · degeneration, which causes loss of eyesight in old age.

SERVES 2

   1 small container Brussels sprouts, quartered
   ½ tbsp extra-virgin olive oil
   pinch of salt
   freshly ground pepper, to taste

1. Preheat oven to 180°C/350°F/gas 4.
2. Slice off bottom of sprouts and peel off outer leaves. Slice into quarters (or shave thin) and place in roasting tin with olive oil, salt and pepper. Toss and spread sprouts evenly across tin.
3. Bake for 20 to 30 minutes, turning occasionally, until soft and crispy.

Spiced Coconut Cauliflower

Cauliflower is another cancer-fighting cruciferous vegetable. Cumin enhances the liver's detoxification systems. Some 50 per cent of the fat in light coconut milk is beneficial lauric acid; which is an antiviral, antibacterial and antiprotozoal substance thought to destroy a wide variety of disease-causing organisms.

SERVES 2

   ½ head cauliflower, cut into bite-sized pieces
   ½ tbsp rapeseed oil
   1½ tsp brown mustard seeds
   1½ tsp cumin seeds
   ½ cinnamon stick
   3 whole cloves
   2 cardamom pods
   ⅛ tsp crushed chillies
   240ml (8 fl oz) light coconut milk
   ⅛ tsp salt

1. In a large frying pan, heat oil on medium to low and add all spices. Cook for about 3 minutes, stirring frequently to avoid burning.
2. Add cauliflower to pan with coconut milk and mix thoroughly.
3. Cover pan and simmer for 15 minutes.
4. Season with salt.

Steamed Artichokes with Lemon Aioli

Members of the thistle family, artichokes contain carbohydrates in the beneficial form of inulin, which helps regulate blood sugar. They contain active compounds (called caffeoylquinic acids) that strengthen many of the liver's functions.

SERVES 2

2 medium artichokes

AIOLI
115g (4oz) plain low-fat Greek yogurt
1 lemon, juiced
1 small clove garlic, finely chopped
½ tbsp extra-virgin olive oil
¼ tsp salt
freshly ground pepper, to taste

1. Slice off 1cm (½ inch) at bottom of artichoke stem and discard. Pull off and discard smaller leaves at the base.
2. In large pan, place 8cm (3 inches) of water. Add artichokes so that they stand (preferably in a steaming basket). Cover and bring to the boil, then reduce heat and simmer for 30 minutes.
3. In a small bowl, combine aioli ingredients. Place in refrigerator.
4. When artichokes are ready (you should be able to pull out the leaves easily) serve with aioli dip.

Sweet and Spicy Kale

Kale has more calcium than nearly any other vegetable (about one-third that of a glass of milk.) The uniquely high ratio of calcium to phosphorous (4:1) promotes the body's retention of calcium for bone-building. Kale is also an excellent source of carotenes, and are second only to spinach in terms of the concentration of the powerful antioxidants lutein and zeaxanthin in the cooked leaves.

SERVES 2

1 bunch kale, finely shredded
4 cloves garlic, finely chopped
¼ tsp crushed chillies
1 tbsp extra-virgin olive oil
2 tbsp apple juice
pinch of salt

1. In a large frying pan, heat oil on medium. Add garlic and chillies and fry until garlic is lightly browned.
2. Rinse kale and pat dry with kitchen towel.
3. Slice kale leaves off stems. Place leaves on top of one another, fold in half lengthwise and roll tightly, going from top of leaf to bottom. Firmly holding rolled kale, thinly slice (will look like spaghetti strands).
4. Add kale to pan with apple juice and simmer, covered, on low for 15 minutes, tossing occasionally.
5. Season with salt.

Warm Puy Lentils

Lentils have slightly more protein per calorie than classic beans such as white beans, and they are an excellent source of a wide range of minerals. Like beans, lentils contain lignans, fibre compounds that can increase the production of a protein (called sex hormone-binding globulin) that regulates oestrogen levels by removing excess oestrogen from the body.

SERVES 2

115g (4oz) Puy lentils
350ml (12 fl oz) water
10–15 cherry tomatoes, quartered
30g (1oz) spring onions, thinly sliced
1 tbsp red onion, finely chopped
1 small clove garlic, finely chopped
15g (½oz) flat leaf parsley, coarsely chopped
1 large lemon, juiced
1 tbsp extra-virgin olive oil
pinch of salt
freshly ground pepper, to taste

1. Place lentils and water in a small pan. Cover and bring to the boil on medium heat. Reduce to a simmer and cook, covered, for about 15 minutes.
2. In a small bowl, combine remaining ingredients and mix well.
3. When lentils are ready (chewy but not hard), drain using a fine mesh sieve, rinse with warm water and add to bowl. Mix well and season with salt and pepper.

MAIN MEALS

FISH RECIPES

Halibut Puttanesca

The risk of heart attack can be cut by almost half by increasing consumption of fish rich in omega-3 fatty acids. Halibut has lower levels of mercury than fattier fish (mercury tends to concentrate in the fat). Garlic and onions activate the body's detox systems; and lycopene in the tomoatoes is a powerful anti-oxidant.

SERVES 2

340g (12oz) halibut fillet (also works well with cod or other white fish)
½ lemon, juiced
1 tsp salt
1 tbsp extra-virgin olive oil
1 clove garlic, finely chopped
1 smallonion, thinly sliced
400g (14oz) cherry tomatoes
2 tbsp stoned Kalamata olives, chopped
2 tbsp capers
1 tbsp caper liquid
2 tbsp flat leaf parsley, coarsely chopped

1. Preheat oven to 180°C/350°F/gas 4.
2. In a small frying pan, heat olive oil on medium. Fry garlic and onion until golden brown.
3. Add tomatoes, olives, capers and caper liquid and simmer, covered, stirring occasionally for 15 minutes or until tomatoes have softened.

4. While puttanesca simmers, wash fish with salt and lemon juice, rinse under cold water and pat dry with a paper towel. Place in baking dish.
5. Add parsley to finished puttanesca sauce. Pour over fish and bake in oven for 20 minutes.

Miso-Baked Cod

Cod is similar to halibut in that it has moderate amounts of beneficial fats and relatively low mercury levels. Miso is a fermented soya-bean paste that is a good source of iron, zinc and copper and the B vitamins, all of which are important for manufacturing energy. As a soya-food, miso is thought to protect oestrogen-sensitive tissues like the breast and prostate.

SERVES 2

340g (12oz) cod (also works well with salmon)
½ lemon, juiced
1 tsp salt
1 tbsp white miso (not sweet variety)
1 tbsp honey
1 tsp low-salt tamari soy sauce
2 tsp fresh ginger root, peeled and finely chopped

1. Preheat oven to 190°C/375°F/gas 5.
2. Wash fish with salt and lemon juice, rinse under cold water and pat dry with kitchen towel. Place in baking dish.
3. In a small bowl, mix miso, honey tamari and ginger so that it becomes a paste. Spread evenly over fish.
4. Bake uncovered for 15 to 20 minutes, then finish under grill for 5 to 7 minutes.

Trout with Lemon and Herbs

Freshwater trout has a significant amount of beneficial omega-3 fats and lower mercury levels than larger fish. Thyme and oregano add anti-viral and anti-bacterial properties to this dish.

SERVES 2

340g (12oz) rainbow trout (also works well with flounder or sole)
½ lemon, juiced
1 tsp salt
2 tsp extra-virgin olive oil
1 lemon, juiced
2 sprigs fresh thyme
2 sprigs fresh oregano
¼ tsp salt
freshly ground pepper to taste

1. Preheat oven to 180°C/350°F/gas 4.
2. Cut two rectangles of greaseproof paper, approximately 33 by 38cm (13 by 15 inches).
3. Wash fish with salt and lemon juice, rinse under cold water and pat dry with a kitchen towel. Split fish into two equal servings.
4. Place fish on greaseproof paper.

Drizzle each piece with olive oil, lemon juice and place a sprig each of thyme and oregano on top of fish. Season with salt and pepper.

5. Seal greaseproof paper by bringing together the two lengthwise ends and folding them down like you'd fold a brown paper bag to close; then twist the ends of the packet like a sweet wrapper. Place on baking dish and bake for 20 minutes.

6. Remove fish from paper to serve.

Walnut-Pesto Wild Salmon

Salmon is one of the best sources of heart-healthy omega-3 fatty acids. Wild salmon is devoid of the PCBs, antibiotics, pesticides and artificial colourants present in most farm-raised salmon. Walnuts are particularly high in omega-3 fatty acids, adding to the strong anti-inflammatory properties of this dish.

SERVES 2

340g (12oz) wild Alaskan salmon fillet (also works well with any other fish)
1 lemon, juiced
1 tsp salt

PESTO*
90g (3oz) basil leaves, rinsed
4 cloves garlic, whole, peeled
60g (2oz) walnuts, shelled
6 tbsp extra-virgin olive oil

1. Preheat oven to 180°C/350°F/gas 4.
2. Combine all pesto ingredients in food processor and purée.
3. Wash fish with salt and lemon juice, rinse under cold water and pat dry with a kitchen towel. Place fish in baking dish.
4. Use half of the pesto to generously coat the top of each fillet.
5. Cover baking dish with tightly fitting top or aluminium foil and bake for 20 to 25 minutes (15 minutes for rare).

* Save half walnut pesto for a snack another day. Can be stored in airtight container in fridge for up to 1 week or immediately freeze for up to 3 months.

POULTRY RECIPES

Curry Roasted Chicken

There are numerous powerful antioxidant spices in curry powder, including turmeric, which has significant anti-inflammatory activity, and is helpful for preventing conditions like cancer and heart disease. Turmeric has also been shown to reduce the accumulation of beta-amyloid plaque – one of the main pathological processes leading to Alzheimer's disease.

SERVES 4

Small whole chicken (about 1.4kg/3 lb)
1 lemon, juiced
2 tsp salt
1 large onion, quartered

CURRY RUB
120ml (4 fl oz) extra-virgin olive oil
2 tsp salt
3 tbsp curry powder
1 bunch coriander, coarsely chopped

1. Preheat oven to 190°C/375°F/gas 4; place rack in the centre of the oven.
2. Discard any spare parts inside of chicken. Wash chicken with salt and lemon juice, rinse under cold water and pat dry with kitchen towel. Place chicken in large baking dish, breast-side up.
3. Quarter unpeeled onion and place inside cavity.
4. In a small bowl, combine rub ingredients; mix well.
5. Rub the curry mixture all over the chicken, placing some under the breast skin by creating a pocket between skin and flesh with your fingers.
6. Bake for 1 hour and 30 minutes. Baste regularly during baking (about every 20 to 30 minutes). When done, remove chicken from oven, cover with foil, and let it sit for 15 minutes.

Herb-Marinated Chicken

Chicken is a good source of lean animal protein that is lower in inflammatory arachadonic acid than beef (especially when you remove the skin). The powerful trio from the mint family – thyme, oregano, basil – add antioxidant and antibacterial properties to this dish.

SERVES 4 (includes leftovers)

685g (½ lb) skinless, boneless chicken
  breast, cubed
1 tsp salt
½ lemon, juiced

MARINADE
2 tbsp extra-virgin olive oil
1 clove garlic, finely chopped
1 lemon, juiced
1 tbsp fresh thyme, remove from stem
1 tbsp fresh oregano, chopped
1 tbsp fresh basil, chopped
¼ tsp salt
1 tbsp extra-virgin olive oil, for cooking

1. Wash chicken with salt and lemon juice; rinse under cold water and pat dry with kitchen towel.
2. Combine marinade ingredients in a large bowl; mix well.
3. Place chicken into the marinade and coat completely. (Can refrigerate at this point for up to a day.)
4. To cook, heat the olive oil in a large frying pan on medium. Fry herb-marinated chicken until browned on all sides and cooked through (about 10 to 12 minutes).

Turkey Bolognese over Spaghetti Squash

Turkey breast meat is an excellent source of low-fat protein. Turkey contains the amino acid tryptophan, a building block of the calming brain compound serotonin, which can leave you feeling sleepy. Spaghetti squash is low in carbohydrates, making it a wheat-and-gluten-free, low-calorie alternative to spaghetti.

SERVES 2

230g (8oz) minced turkey
1 tsp extra-virgin olive oil
1 clove garlic, finely chopped
1 small onion, thinly sliced
1 tsp dried or fresh thyme
1 tsp dried or fresh oregano
1 tsp dried or finely chopped fresh rosemary
450g (16oz) tin chopped tomatoes
2 tbsp tomato paste
Pinch of salt
2 tsp Parmesan cheese, grated (optional)
1 small spaghetti squash, halved and
  seeded
1 tsp extra-virgin olive oil

1. Preheat oven to 180°C/350°F/gas 4 for spaghetti squash.
2. Split spaghetti squash in half (cut off ends, place vertically on chopping board, guide knife down middle of squash and split open). Remove seeds, rub with olive oil and place face down on a baking tray. Bake for 30 minutes until fork easily pierces skin. (For microwave, pierce skin

with fork and cook on high for 15 minutes, turning once; allow to cool before opening.)

3. While spaghetti squash is cooking, heat olive oil in a large frying pan on medium. Fry garlic and onions until lightly browned. Add dried herbs and fry for another 2 minutes (if using fresh herbs, add with crushed tomatoes). Add minced turkey, breaking apart with fork as you continue to fry for 5 minutes, until lightly browned. Add crushed tomatoes, tomato paste, salt (and fresh herbs if using) and simmer, uncovered, for 20 minutes.

4. Scoop 'spaghetti' out of squash; top with bolognese and a sprinkle of Parmesan if desired.

VEGETARIAN RECIPES

Lemon Parsley Hummus Wrap

The combination of chickpeas, avocado, tomatoes and sprouts packs this dish with powerful phytochemicals, healthy fats and protein. Chickpeas support the body's detox system. Bean sprouts contain some of the most potent known cancer-fighting compounds and alfalfa sprouts, packed with beneficial phyto-oestrogens, are a close second.

SERVES 2

8 tbsp Lemon Parsley Hummus (page 340)*
½ avocado, stoned, removed from skin, thinly sliced
1 small vine-ripened tomato, thinly sliced
30g (1oz) beansprouts, rinsed and patted dry with kitchen towel**
2 wheat-free tortilla wraps, 18–20 cm (7–8 inches) diameter

1. Spread 4 tbsp hummus on one side of tortilla.
2. Top with half the avocado, tomato and sprouts. Roll or fold. Repeat.

* Store-bought hummus with all-natural ingredients is fine. Watch out for those brands with preservatives such as potassium sorbate or potassium benzoate. ** Make sure sprouts are fresh, meaning that there are no browned or spoiled areas; they can carry harmful bacteria.

Red Curry Tofu with Basil

Ginger contains potent anti-inflammatory compounds called gingerols. Gingerols inhibit the formation of inflammatory chemical messengers of the immune system that in particular are responsible for the pain of rheumatoid or osteo-arthritis; regular ginger consumption has been shown to reduce pain in those conditions. SERVES 2

½ block extra firm tofu, cut into slabs*
½ tbsp sesame oil
1 clove garlic, finely chopped
½ tbsp fresh ginger root, finely chopped
30g (1oz) spring onions, thinly sliced
240ml (8 fl oz) light coconut milk
1 tsp red curry paste
½ lime, juiced
⅛ tsp salt
30g (1oz) basil leaves, coarsely chopped

1. In a small pan. Fry garlic and ginger in sesame oil on medium heat until golden.
2. Add remaining ingredients (except basil and tofu) and mix well until curry paste dissolves. Add basil and simmer, uncovered, for 10 minutes.
3. Drain tofu well. Cut into 5mm (¼ inch) slabs and cut each slab in half.
4. Place tofu in pan, making sure to cover with sauce. Continue simmering, covered, for 10 more minutes, gently stirring.

* Leftover tofu can be stored in an airtight container with fresh water; change water every 2 days.

Tofu Vegetable Stir-Fry

Eat tofu to help regulate oestrogen metabolism, onions to activate the detox system, carrots and courgettes to provide fibre and carotenes, broccoli to contribute numerous cancer-fighting phytochemicals. Gomasio is a seaweed-based alternative to salt, which means it is packed with beneficial minerals unique to sea vegetables, and it contains only a fraction of the sodium of table salt.

SERVES 2

½ block extra firm tofu*, cubed
1 tbsp sesame oil
1 small onion, thinly sliced
1 small carrot, cut into half moons, about 3mm (⅛ inch) thick
1 small courgette, cut into ½ moons, about 3mm (⅛ inch) thick
60g (2oz) broccoli florets, cut into small pieces
2 tsp low-salt tamari, wheat-free
2 tsp mirin
2 tbsp water
½ tsp toasted sesame oil
½ tbsp gomasio

1. In a large frying pan or wok, heat sesame oil on medium and fry onions until translucent.
2. Add remaining vegetables, tamari, mirin and water, mix well and cook for another 3 minutes.
3. Drain tofu well and cut into 1 cm (½ inch) cubes. Add tofu and water

to pan. Gently mix, cover pan, and simmer for 5 more minutes.

4. Turn off heat and season with toasted sesame oil and gomasio.

* Leftover tofu can be stored in an airtight container with fresh water; change water every 2 days.

Vegetable Biryani

In addition to a rainbow of nutrient-packed vegetables, this dish includes basmati rice, a complex carbohydrate that has about half the glycaemic load of white rice. The lower glycaemic load makes basmati an excellent choice for reducing inflammation and increasing stamina.

SERVES 2

100g (3½oz) brown basmati rice
240ml (8 fl oz) water
½ tin (about 200g/7oz) chickpeas, drained and rinsed
1 tbsp sesame oil
1 clove garlic, finely chopped
1 small onion, thinly sliced

SPICES
1½ tsp brown or yellow mustard seeds
1½ tsp whole cumin seeds
3 whole cardamom pods
3 whole cloves
½ cinnamon stick
1½ tsp curry powder

VEGETABLES (OR USE MIXED FROZEN VEGETABLES)
1 small carrot, sliced lengthwise and cut into half moons
60g (2oz) cauliflower, cut into small pieces
50g (1¾oz) mangetout, trimmed
90g (3oz) yellow squash, sliced lengthwise and cut into half moons
60ml (2 fl oz) vegetable stock or water
60ml (2 fl oz) light coconut milk
pinch of salt

1. In a small pan, combine water and rice, cover and bring to the boil; reduce to a simmer and cook, covered, for 40 to 50 minutes.

2. In a large frying pan, heat oil on medium to low; add garlic, onion and spices and fry for 3 to 5 minutes, stirring regularly to avoid burning. Turn off heat.

3. Prepare all other vegetables and add to pan with chickpeas, stock (or water) and coconut milk; mix well. Turn heat back on and simmer, uncovered, for 20 minutes.

4. Discard cinnamon stick, cardamom pods and cloves. Add rice to the pan. Cook, gently stirring, for another 2 minutes.

Vegetarian Chilli

The powerful anti-oxidant, lycopene, is increased when cooked in this dish. The garlic, onion, cumin, chilli powder and cinnamon all add powerful phytochemicals that support the immune system and reduce inflammation.

SERVES 4 (includes leftovers)*

- 1 tin (425g/15oz) red kidney beans, drained and rinsed
- 1 tin (425g/15oz) black beans, drained and rinsed
- 1 tbsp extra-virgin olive oil
- 2 cloves garlic, chopped
- 1 small onion, thinly sliced
- 1 tsp ground cumin
- 1 tsp chilli powder
- ¼ tsp ground cinnamon
- 75g (2½oz) red pepper, diced
- 1 small courgette, sliced lengthwise and cut into half moons
- 1 small yellow squash, sliced lengthwise and cut into half moons
- 1 tin (425g/15oz) diced tomatoes
- 1 tin (145g/5oz) tomato paste
- 8 tbsp coriander, chopped
- pinch of salt
- 225g (8oz) plain low-fat Greek yogurt (optional)

1. In a large pan, heat oil on medium. Add garlic and onion and fry until soft and slightly golden. Add spices, pepper, courgette and squash and continue to fry for 3 to 5 minutes.
2. Add beans to pan with diced tomatoes and tomato paste and stir well. Cover and simmer for 10 minutes. Remove cover and simmer for another 10 minutes.
3. Stir in coriander to finish. Season with salt.
4. Serve with dollop of plain Greek yogurt.

* Store leftovers in airtight container in fridge for up to 3 days or immediately freeze for up to 3 months.

Vegetarian Chilli Burritos

Yogurt contains probiotics (edible bacteria that is beneficial to immune health and digestion); and it is a good low-allergenic source of calcium. Avocado adds anti-inflammatory essential fatty acids, and additional vitamins and minerals.

SERVES 2

2 servings of Vegetarian Chilli (page 337)
4 tbsp Guacamole* (page 339)
4 tbsp plain low-fat Greek yogurt (optional)
2 wheat-free or corn tortillas

1. In small pan, heat chilli on medium.
2. Warm tortillas in oven.
3. Place a serving of chilli, half the guacamole and half the yogurt in centre of each tortilla. Tightly wrap and enjoy.

* Can use store-bought guacamole.

SNACK RECIPES

Burst of Energy Trail Mix

Due to their beneficial essential fatty acid content walnuts and almonds are anti-inflammatory. All seeds and nuts contain antioxidant flavonoids which means they guard against cell damage that causes cancer. Pumpkin seeds in particular are very prostate-healthy, with high zinc and healthy and protective fats. Cranberry protects bladder health, including reducing the ability of bacteria to cause infections.

SERVES 8 (includes leftovers)*

60g (2oz) walnuts
65g (2¼oz) raw almonds
70g (2½ oz) raw pumpkin seeds (also known as pepitas)
40g (1¼oz) unsalted sunflower seeds, shelled
40g (1¼oz) dried cranberries
40g (1¼oz) dried papaya, coarsely chopped

1. Place all ingredients in a bowl and toss.
2. Measure individual servings into small plastic bags and store in cool, dry place. Great for on-the-go eating.

* Make once for entire 21-Day Plan.

Guacamole

Avocado is dense in vitamins, minerals and anti-inflammatory fats. Coriander has been shown to be helpful in capturing and eliminating heavy metals from the gut.

SERVES 2

2 ripe avocados
1 lime, juiced (about 2 tbsp)
½ small red onion, diced
4 tbsp coriander, with stems, coarsely chopped
pinch of salt
freshly ground pepper, to taste

1. Peel and halve avocados. Remove pit and use spoon to scoop out flesh.
2. In large bowl, mash avocado with fork. Add all other ingredients and mix well. Season with salt and pepper.
3. Serve with vegetables, rice crackers or in vegetarian chilli burritos.

Lemon Parsley Hummus

Chickpeas confer many of the benefits of all beans, including delivering heart-healthy fibre, and they also contain a micronutrient trace mineral called molybdenum, which is crucial for the body's mechanism to detoxify sulphites, a common preservative found in wine, cold processed meats and dried fruits.

SERVES 4 (includes leftovers)*

1 tin (425g/15oz) chickpeas, drained and rinsed
2 lemons, juiced, about 4 tbsp
80ml (3 fl oz) extra-virgin olive oil
1 small clove garlic
2 tbsp parsley leaves
½ tsp salt

Place drained and rinsed beans in food processor with remaining ingredients and purée until smooth and creamy.

* Store leftovers in airtight container in fridge for up to three days.

DESSERT RECIPES

Berry Parfait

Greek yogurt has more protein and less lactose than regular yogurt. Honey is one of nature's best germicidal agents: now even used medicinally for wound healing. Berries and the nuts in granola provide numerous plant compounds that reduce inflammation and protect cells from free radical damage.
SERVES 2

1 cup plain low-fat Greek yogurt
2 tbsp honey
150g (5½oz) raspberries
150g (5½oz) blackberries
4 tbsp Power Up! Granola (page 310)

1. Using a stemmed champagne or parfait glass, layer first yogurt, then honey and finally berries.
2. Top with Power Up! Granola.

Citrus Mint Mixed Berries

Blackberries contain essential fatty acid, and are considered mildly anti-inflammatory, plus they are a good source of the antioxidant selenium, essential for heart muscle maintenance.
SERVES 2

75g (2½ fl oz) blackberries
60g (2oz) blueberries
75g (2½oz) strawberries, quartered
75g (2½oz) raspberries
60ml (2 fl oz) orange juice, freshly squeezed
2 tsp fresh mint leaves, coarsely chopped

In a medium bowl, gently combine berries with orange juice and mint.

Coco-nutty Banana

Bananas are high in potassium, which helps lower blood pressure and replenish electrolytes lost during sweating. Blueberries contain one of nature's most powerful antioxidants, and the medium-chain fats in coconut increase the body's metabolic rate, which helps burn calories.

SERVES 2

1 large banana, sliced into rounds and quartered
2 tbsp shredded unsweetened coconut
125g (4½oz) blueberries
½ lemon, juiced

1. Slice banana and place in medium bowl with lemon juice. Mix gently. Add coconut and mix again to coat bananas.
2. Divide between two small bowls and top with blueberries.

Dark Chocolate Chunk Almond Biscuits

Spelt flour is an 'Old World' wheat, containing a different, more easily digested type of gluten than commercial wheat, making it less allergenic than conventional wheat. It provides double the protein and fibre of conventional wheat, and a special type of carbohydrate, mucoplysaccharides, that stimulate the immune system.

ONE DOZEN*

250g (9oz) smooth almond butter
80ml (3 fl oz) canola oil
120ml (4 fl oz) maple syrup
1 tsp vanilla extract
200g (7oz) spelt flour
60g (2oz) dark chocolate, coarsely chopped

1. Cover baking tray with greaseproof paper (or brush lightly with rapeseed oil).
2. Preheat oven to 180°C/350°F/gas 4.
3. In a large bowl, mix almond butter, oil, maple syrup and vanilla extract. Add spelt flour to form dough. Stir in dark chocolate pieces.
4. Drop small balls of dough (about 2.5cm/1 inch diameter) onto baking tray. Press with spoon to form 5mm (¼ inch) thick biscuits.
5. Bake for 15 to 20 minutes until biscuits are lightly browned on edges.
6. Cool before removing from tray.

* Store in airtight container in cool dry place for up to 1 week or freeze for up to 3 months.

Dark Chocolate Dairy-Free Mousse

Cocoa powder is one of the highest antioxidant foods and is rich in plant compounds that promote heart health. It's been shown to lower blood pressure, prevent blood clots and reduce inflammation. Cocoa also improves mood, especially in women.

SERVES 2

1 box (340g/12oz) silken tofu
5 tbsp cocoa powder
1½ tsp pure vanilla extract
120ml (4 fl oz) plus 2 tbsp maple syrup
⅛ tsp cinnamon, optional

1. Place all ingredients into a food processor or blender and purée until smooth and creamy.
2. Chill for 1 hour or overnight.

Spiced Apples with Pecan Crumble

Apples are rich in pectin, a soluble fibre, which can lower cholesterol and has been shown to be beneficial for prostate health. Apples are rich in antioxidant flavonoids, such as quercetin, which inhibits the formation of histamines, the immune compound released when allergies occurs. Ginger and pecans are anti-inflammatory, and cinnamon helps the body metabolize sugar.

SERVES 2

2 small Gala apples (or Fuji), cored
480ml (16 fl oz) apple juice
4 whole cloves
3mm (⅛ inch) slice fresh ginger root, unpeeled

PECAN CRUMBLE
30g (1oz) pecans, coarsely chopped
¼ tsp ground cinnamon
1½ tsp dark brown sugar

1. Rinse and core apples do not peel. Place apples in a medium pan with apple juice, cloves and ginger. Bring to the boil, then simmer, covered, for 10 minutes (apples should be fork tender).
2. In a small bowl, combine pecans, cinnamon and brown sugar.
3. Remove apples from pan and serve warm, topped with crumble.

Drinks and Cocktail Recipes

Cool Mint Lemonade

SERVES 2

2½ lemons, juiced
600ml (1 pint) cold water
120ml (4 fl oz) warm water
2 tbsp honey
2 sprigs fresh mint

1. In a jug, dissolve honey in warm water by stirring vigorously.
2. Add remaining water and lemon juice and mix well.
3. Add mint. Refrigerate for at least an hour for mint to impart full flavour.
4. Serve on the rocks.

Cranberry Tea Infusion

SERVES 2

4 cranberry tea bags
600ml (1 pint) water
120ml (4 fl oz) apple juice
2 sprigs fresh mint
½ orange, sliced into wedges (optional)

1. Heat water to warm.
2. In a jug, add tea bags, warm water, apple juice and mint.
3. Refrigerate until cool.
4. Serve in stemmed glass on the rocks with an orange wedge.

Dr Merrell's Fruit Juice

SERVES 2

250g (9oz) fresh pineapple, peeled, cored and cut into large cubes (or fresh papaya)
125g (4½oz) mixed frozen berries
120ml (4 fl oz) pineapple juice (or pomegranate or cherry juice)
120ml (4 fl oz) water (optional)

Combine all ingredients in a blender and purée until smooth. Add water (small amounts at a time) if required to reach desired consistency.

Dr Merrell's Veggie Juice

SERVES 2

2 medium cucumbers, peeled
2 stalks celery
2 large carrots (or 2 small apples)
30g (1oz) flat leaf parsley
fresh ginger root, penny-sized piece
230g (8oz) kale
1 lemon, juiced

1. Juice all vegetables in a vegetable juicer.
2. Finish with lemon juice.

Mango-Peach Freeze

SERVES 2

2 large handfuls frozen peaches (or fresh
   chunks frozen in peach juice)
480ml (16 fl oz) mango nectar or juice
½ lime, cut in half

1. Combine peaches and mango in
   blender and purée until smooth.
2. Serve in stemmed glass with a squeeze
   of lime.

Papaya Fizz

SERVES 2

350ml (12 fl oz) papaya juice
350ml (12 fl oz) soda
1 lime, quartered

1. In a jug, combine juice and soda.
2. Serve on the rocks with a squeeze of
   lime (half a lime per serving).

Peach Spritzer with Cranberry Ice

SERVES 2

480ml (16 fl oz) peach nectar
240ml (8 fl oz) soda

CRANBERRY ICE CUBES
60ml (2 fl oz) cranberry concentrate
60ml (2 fl oz) water

1. To make ice cubes, mix cranberry
   concentrate with water in a measuring
   jug, then pour into ice cube tray and
   freeze overnight (makes four cubes).
2. In a jug, combine nectar and soda.
3. Serve over cranberry ice cubes.

Tangerine Spritzer with Papaya Ice

SERVES 2

350ml (12 fl oz) tangerine juice, freshly
   squeezed (or use orange juice)
350ml (12 fl oz) soda
½ lime, cut in half

PAPAYA ICE CUBES
120ml (4 fl oz) papaya juice

1. To make ice cubes, pour papaya juice
   into ice cube tray and freeze overnight
   (makes 4 ice cubes).
2. In a jug, combine tangerine juice (or
   orange juice) and soda.
3. Cut lime and squeeze juice into jug.
4. Serve over papaya ice cubes.

Recipe Index

Breakfast
Dr Merrell's morning shake 309
French toast 309
Power up granola 310
Scrambled tofu with vegetables 312
Vegetable goat's cheese egg-white
   omelette 311

Soups
Immune-boost soup 311
Quick Italian vegetable soup 312
Red lentil soup 313
Rosemary butternut squash soup 313
Shiitake-miso soup 314
White bean kale soup 315

Salads
Antioxidant fruit salad 315
Rocket salad with crushed walnuts and
   goat's cheese 316
Black bean salad 316
Cucumber wakame salad 317
Leafy greens and chickpea salad 317
Mediterranean tuna salad 318
Mixed salad leaves with balsamic
   vinaigrette 318
Power protein mixed green salad 318
Herby chicken salad 319
Sweet spinach salad 320
Vegetarian cobb salad 320
Warm hijiki salad 321
Watercress rocket salad 321

Sides
Braised chard 322
Cinnamon roasted acorn squash 322
Crunchy pak choi with tangy chilli
   vinaigrette 323
Garlic roasted asparagus 323
Harvest wild rice 324
Juicy sweet roasted broccoli 324
Quinoa with spring onions and toasted
   sesame oil 325
Quinoa with sliced avocado 325
Quinoa tabbouleh 326
Sautéed kale with garlic 326
Scrumptious Brussels sprouts 327
Spiced coconut cauliflower 327
Steamed artichokes with
   lemon aioli 328
Sweet and spicy kale 328
Warm Puy lentils 329

Main meals
Fish
Halibut puttanesca 329
Miso-baked cod 330
Trout with lemon and herbs 330
Walnut-pesto wild salmon 331

Poultry
Curry roasted chicken 332
Herb-marinated chicken 333
Turkey bolognese over spaghetti
   squash 333

Vegetarian

Lemon parsley hummus wrap 334
Red curry tofu with basil 335
Tofu vegetable stir-fry 335
Vegetable biryani 336
Vegetarian chilli 337
Vegetarian chilli burritos 338

Snacks

Burst of energy trail mix 338
Guacamole 339
Lemon parsley hummus 339

Desserts

Berry parfait 340
Citrus mint mixed berries 340
Coco-nutty banana 341
Dark chocolate chunk almond biscuits 341
Dark chocolate dairy-free mousse 342
Spiced apples with pecan crumble 342

Drinks

Cool mint lemonade 343
Cranberry tea infusion 343
Dr Merrell's fruit juice 343
Dr Merrell's veggie juice 343
Mango-peach freeze 344
Papaya fizz 344
Peach spritzer with cranberry ice 344
Tangerine spritzer with papaya ice 344

Acknowledgments

The energetic costs of writing a book are astronomical, and this one was no different. A multitude of thanks goes out to the community that gathered around to make *The Source* a reality. First, to my soul mate and writing partner, Kathy, you were the cornerstone of this project, and without you it would never have happened. I am grateful for this literary partnership, and thankful that we made it out intact! I am deeply indebted to Kim Witherspoon and Richard Pine for their persistence, patience, and guidance in honing the concept for this book and for knowing that Kathy and I could do this together. Monumental thanks go to Leslie Meredith for being our editorial champion and offering such thoughtful guidance, and to Dominick Anfuso for his unwavering support. I offer much gratitude to Donna Loffredo for her tireless effort and attention to detail throughout the process, and to Carol de Onís for her incredible labors and detailed reading.

Deep gratitude goes out to the many masters who have taught me the value of using lifestyle changes and energetic management as healing modalities. In particular I want to thank Jeff Bland, Larry Dossey, and Dan Goleman for their friendship and visionary leadership in the healing arts. For years, Mehmet Oz and Christiane Northrup have shared ideas and collaborated in bringing integrative medicine to a greater audience. Specifically for this book I received invaluable input from Marion Nestle, Alan Hipkiss, and Harold Koenig, all of whom took time to speak with me about their pioneering work.

I am eternally grateful to my parents, June and Charles Merrell, for their unconditional love and for giving me my earliest lessons in healing energy. Deep thanks go to Kathy's parents, Donald and Colleen Healy, for their thoughtful input on the book, constant cheerleading and loving support throughout. Christian Wright gave her characteristically insightful commentary as well as inspiration for the title and for this we are deeply grateful. Many thanks go to Stefanie Bryn Sacks for offering her culinary magic and precious time.

Last but not least, I am forever grateful to all of my patients, for teaching me in countless ways how to create energy.

Index

A

acupuncture 21, 25, 36, 49–51, 189, 190, 199
adaptogens 92–4
aeroplanes 125–6
alcohol 78, 85, 97, 131, 173, 187, 190–1, 253–4
allergies 76, 82–3, 84, 95–6, 188–9, 194, 243, 244, 270
ANS (autonomic nervous system) 28–9, 31–2, 50, 52, 93
antibiotics 83, 84, 115, 116, 118, 192
antidepressants 30, 56, 146–7, 192, 193
antioxidants 69, 77, 78, 86, 90, 91, 92, 93, 94, 102, 107, 130, 131, 133, 200, 249, 265, 281, 289
see also detox
ATP (adenosine triphosphate) 13–14, 63–5, 91, 100, 144, 167, 168, 176

B

Benson, Dr Herbert 27, 32, 39, 234
biofeedback 46–7
blood sugar 30, 79, 80, 81, 130, 168, 235, 263, 292
breathing techniques 21, 23, 38, 39, 40–2, 162, 169
  see also t'ai chi; yoga
Buddhism 45, 207–8

C

caffeine 58–9, 70, 85, 105–6, 191, 250
cancer 44, 56, 78–9, 89, 101, 112, 114, 121, 207–8, 215, 224
carbohydrates 75–6, 79, 81, 84, 87, 167, 257–8
  complex 67, 68, 70–1, 80–1, 84, 166
carpets 121–2, 244
cars 125, 126
chamomile 56–7
chemicals and toxins 98–102, 108–9, 111–13, 117–19, 120–8, 237, 243, 244, 258, 291
  see also detox; diet
chicken and poultry 115–16, 281
chocolate 86, 265–6
chronic fatigue syndrome 10
cleaning products 122–3, 243, 244
coffee 85, 105–6, 254 *see also* caffeine
colonics 138
community and health 217–19, 264
cortisol 29–30, 54, 93, 150, 183–4
cosmetics 126–7, 243, 244

D

depression and anxiety 27, 54, 56, 146–7, 209
  see also antidepressants; relaxation techniques; stress
detox 15, 56, 85, 93, 94, 128–9, 132, 134–7
  see also chemicals and toxins; diet; gut health; juice cleanse; liver; supplements; 21-day plan
diet 15, 58–60, 166
calories 66–7, 68
chicken and poultry 115–16, 281
detox foods 110, 111–12, 113, 129–31, 241, 274

energy boosting food 61–3, 85–8
energy production 63–6
fish 69–70, 87, 117–19, 258–9
juice cleanse 134–7, 271, 273
meat 61, 68, 83, 114–15, 262–3, 280–1
organic food 87, 109, 110, 111–12, 113,
    114, 115, 126, 138
processed food 112–14
    see also carbohydrates, EFAs, fats, fibre;
    herbs; milk; protein; sugar; supplements;
    21-day plan; vitamins and minerals
digestion 29, 31, 32, 54, 63, 105, 133, 242,
    268–9, 289
DNA 13, 14, 25, 28, 31, 64, 77, 141
chemical damage 98, 99, 100, 134
diet 60, 61, 62, 69–70, 71, 75, 76, 83, 135
    see also mitochondria
Dossey, Dr Larry 213–14, 227
dreams 192, 255–6

E

EFAs (essential fatty acids) 68, 73, 77, 86,
    91, 117, 118, 130, 169, 275–6, 281,
    284
enemas 138, 139
environment see chemicals and toxins
exercise 15, 51–5, 70, 140–5, 146–50,
    163–5, 169–71
core training 152–3, 154, 155, 171
equipment 157–8
food supplements 166–9
martial arts 158–62
overtraining 151
strength training 153–4, 156–8
target heart rate 259
    see also relaxation techniques; stress;
    21-day plan; walking; yoga

F

family 220–1
fasting 134–7
fats 67, 68, 69, 70, 71, 73, 75, 79–80, 83,
    84, 85, 86, 87, 115
    see also diet, EFAs, meat
feng shui 282
fibre 71, 81, 85, 86, 87, 103, 130, 131, 137
fish 69–70, 87, 117–19, 258–9
food see diet
free-radicals 65, 66, 77, 78, 83, 84, 89, 91,
    100
    detox 104, 107–8, 130, 131, 169, 175
    exercise 144, 145, 151
fruit see diet (detox, energy and organic
    foods)

G

genetically modified crops (GMOs) 113, 116
GI (glycaemic index) 75–6, 79
ginseng 90, 93–4
GL (glycaemic load) 79, 80
glycation 66, 71, 79–81, 84
Goleman, Daniel 38, 218
'green' drinks 90
green tea 55–6, 77, 78, 85, 130, 249–50
guided imagery 47–9
gut health 102–3, 130, 137–9, 268–9

H

healing therapy 223–5, 286
heart disorders 16, 35, 63, 105, 135, 149,
    180, 185, 186, 209, 217, 272
heart rate 33, 54, 141–2, 148, 149, 150,
    165, 225, 259, 272

heavy metals 74, 90, 117, 118, 119, 128, 130, 133, 244
herbs 15, 56–7, 89–91, 92–5, 200, 201
    see also diet; supplements; vitamins and minerals
Hipkiss, Alan R 135, 145
holidays 283
homeopathy 57
HPA (hypothalamic-pituitary-adrenal) 28, 29–30, 31, 32, 50, 206

I

immune system 10, 23, 30, 35, 56, 82, 103, 140, 181, 190, 268
    inflammation 30, 61, 72, 74
    spirituality 206, 216, 217
    see also allergies; supplements
inflammation 29–30, 61, 66, 71, 72–7, 82, 83, 84, 93, 217, 263, 275, 292
insomnia see sleep
internet 219
Iyengar, B.K.S. 162, 170

J

jetlag 182–3
juice cleanse 16, 134–7, 271, 273

K

Koenig, Dr Harold 206, 210, 215, 216
Kreb's cycle 65–6, 92

L

light and dark therapy 44, 196–8
liver 104–8, 129, 130, 133, 139
    see also detox

M

martial arts 158–62, 224, 287
    see also yoga
massage 51, 256–7, 268
ME (myalgic encephalomyelitis) 10
meat 61, 68, 83, 114–15, 262–3, 280–1
meditation 15, 23, 27, 42–6, 161, 185, 198, 210, 234–5, 290–1
melatonin 196, 200, 272
milk and dairy 75, 82, 84, 114–15, 201
mind-body connection 22–7, 29, 30–4
    exercise 145
    martial arts 158–60, 162
    yoga 51–4, 162
    see also relaxation techniques; spirituality; stress
mitochondria 13, 14, 64–5, 66, 69, 79, 91, 92, 135, 141, 145, 154, 166, 181
music and art 164–5, 171, 222, 274–5

N

nature and health 222–3, 266
neuropeptides 26, 28, 30–1, 32, 33, 36, 50, 226
nightmares 192
Noetic Science 226–8
nutrients. see diet; supplements; 21-day plan; vitamins and minerals

O

organic food 87, 109, 110, 111–12, 113,
   114, 115, 126, 138
   see also diet; 21-day plan
Ornish, Dean 47, 217
oxidation 66, 70, 71, 77–9, 82, 83, 85, 292

P

paint 120–1, 244
PCBs (polychlorinated biphenyls) 117, 134
pesticides 110, 111, 112, 113, 117, 241,
   291
   see also chemicals
pharmaceuticals 10, 12, 24, 91, 92, 95, 103,
   109, 191–3
   see also antidepressants
plant foods see diet (detox, energy and
   organic foods)
plastics 123–5, 244
posture 155
poultry 115–16, 281
prayer and healing 211–14
prebiotics 132
pregnancy 16, 101, 118, 132, 257
probiotics 90, 133, 137, 268–9
processed food 112–14
protein 64, 67–8, 69, 79, 84, 85, 86, 87,
   145, 181
purge, digestive 138–9

Q

Qi 25, 49, 54
Qi gong 158–62, 171, 224
quiz (energy level) 17–18

R

Reiki 224–5, 286
relationships, intimate 220–1
relaxation techniques 32, 33, 37, 38, 39,
   40–49, 78, 234
   see also sleep; stress; 21-day plan
religion and healing 214–16

S

saunas 16, 129, 132, 134
serotonin 26, 30, 54, 56, 93, 176
sinus congestion 188–9
sleep 9–10, 70, 172–84
   acupuncture 199
   alcohol and caffeine 190–1
   chronic pain 190
   gastro-esophageal reflux disease 189
   inflammatory conditions 190
   pharmaceuticals 191–3
   pillows and mattress 194–6, 244, 270
   sleep apnoea 185–7, 279
   snoring 187, 188, 279
   stress 183–5, 260
   supplements 199–201
   therapies 196–8
   see also breathing techniques; diet;
   relaxation techniques; 21-day plan
smoking 27, 74, 78, 106–7
spices 263
spirituality and health 15, 202–10
   community 217–19, 252
   healers 223–5
   intimate relationships 220–1
   music and art 222
   prayer 211–14
   religion 214–16
stress 20–4, 26, 27, 33–4, 93, 94
   log keeping 238, 252, 262
   management 15, 35–9

mechanisms 28–31, 32, 50
  see also 21-day plan; exercise;
  relaxation techniques; sleeping problems;
  supplements
sugars 61, 63, 64, 66, 67, 69, 70–1,
  79–81, 84, 85, 93, 145, 159, 167
supplements 32, 64, 65, 88–94
  detox 131–2, 133
  exercise 166–9
  nervous system 55–7
  sleep 199–201
  see also diet; herbs; 21-day plan; vitamins
  and minerals

T

tai chi 54–5, 153, 158–62
teflon 243, 244
television 277
Thich Nhat Hanh 45, 290–1
toxins see chemicals
transfats 75, 83
21-day plan 230–3, 245–6
  diet 235, 241, 242, 247, 249–50, 258–9,
    262–3, 265–6, 275–6, 280–1, 284
  eating habits 235, 242, 257–8, 264, 278,
    292
  emotional health 252, 260, 274–5, 276–7,
    282, 283, 288
  energy drains 243, 244, 254
  exercise 237, 243, 245, 247, 248, 250–2,
    259, 269–70, 272, 273, 274, 276, 279,
    287–8, 293
    juice cleanse 271, 273
    logs 238, 252, 262, 268, 278, 284
  morning routine 234–5, 239–40, 247,
    261–2
  relaxation and meditation 234–5, 240–1,
    245–6, 256–7, 260, 268, 277, 284,
    290–1

sleep 238–9, 245–6, 252–3, 255–6,
  260–1, 264, 266–7, 270, 272, 273, 284,
  286
supplements 268–9, 278–9, 284, 285,
  287, 289
water 236–7, 273

V

vegetables see diet (detox, energy and organic
  foods)
visualization 163–4, 171, 235
vitamins and minerals 64, 66, 71, 77, 88–9,
  92, 130, 133, 166–7, 285
  see also diet; herbs; supplements
volatile organic compounds (VOCs) 120–2,
  244

W

walking 169, 237, 245, 274
water 16, 78, 109, 129, 131, 236–7
wheat 84, 247, 249

Y

yoga 15, 51–4, 153, 158–62, 169–70, 247,
  248, 269–70
yogurt 138, 269